W9-BME-945

Medical Terminology
Express

A SHORT-COURSE APPROACH BY BODY SYSTEM

Second Edition

Barbara A. Gylys (GĬL-ĭs), BS, MEd, CMA-A (AAMA)
Professor Emerita
College of Health and Human Services
University of Toledo
Toledo, Ohio

Regina M. Masters, BSN, RN, MEd, CMA (AAMA)
Adjunct Nursing Faculty
Lourdes University
Sylvania, Ohio

F.A. Davis Company • Philadelphia

F. A. Davis Company
1915 Arch Street
Philadelphia, PA 19103
www.fadavis.com

Printed in the United States of America

Last digit indicates print number: 10 9 8 7 6 5

Publisher: Quincy McDonald
Manager of Content Development: George W. Lang
Developmental Editor: Robin Levin Richman
Design and Illustration Manager: Carolyn O'Brien

As new scientific information becomes available through basic and clinical research, recommended treatments and drug therapies undergo changes. The author(s) and publisher have done everything possible to make this book accurate, up to date, and in accord with accepted standards at the time of publication. The author(s), editors, and publisher are not responsible for errors or omissions or for consequences from application of the book, and make no warranty, expressed or implied, in regard to the contents of the book. Any practice described in this book should be applied by the reader in accordance with professional standards of care used in regard to the unique circumstances that may apply in each situation. The reader is advised always to check product information (package inserts) for changes and new information regarding dose and contraindications before administering any drug. Caution is especially urged when using new or infrequently ordered drugs.

Library of Congress Control Number: 2014945712

This Book Is Dedicated With Love

to my best friend, colleague, and husband, Dr. Julius A. Gylys

and

to my children, Regina Maria and Dr. Julius A. Gylys, II

and

to Andrew Masters, Dr. Julia Halm, Caitlin Masters, Anthony Bishop-Gylys, Matthew Bishop-Gylys, Liam Halm, Harrison Robert Halm, and the little one, Emmett Thomas Halm

— BARBARA GYLYS

to my mother, best friend, mentor, and co-author, Barbara A. Gylys

and

to my father, Dr. Julius A. Gylys

and

to my husband, Bruce Masters, and my children Andrew, Dr. Julia, and Caitlin, all of whom have given me continuous encouragement and support, and to my grandsons Liam, Harrison, and Emmett who bring me endless joy.

— REGINA MASTERS

Medical Terminology Express has evolved due to the growing demand for a straightforward, easy-to-understand short-course textbook. The book is written in an engaging, nontechnical language that relates to students of all backgrounds and levels of education. It is designed as an uncomplicated passageway to learning the language of medicine. No natural science background is needed to absorb the information in the textbook. Keeping in mind that the needs of students from various educational environments differ, this text and its associated electronic resources are constructed for use in colleges, universities, career schools, online courses, and other educational environments that offer a medical terminology course. The design and flexibility of Medical Terminology Express, second edition, enable its use as a self-instructional book, as an eBook, or as a text in traditional lecture and classroom environments.

Although Medical Terminology Express has a unique approach that differs from any other medical terminology books we have authored, it still includes the same fundamental concepts of learning medical terminology, primarily by applying the principles of medical word building. The textbook and its associated electronic resources are organized as competency-based instruments. The various learning tools enable students to evaluate their understanding of medical terminology based on guidelines required by the major allied health accrediting agencies. The word-building and competency-based approaches are always evident in the educational materials we have published. Because this system of learning medical terminology has been so effective in numerous teaching environments and widely well received by educators and students, we continue to use the word-building and competency-based approaches in the textbooks and electronic resources we author. We have personally witnessed the success of these educational configurations during our many years of teaching medical terminology.

Various types of learning reinforcements are found throughout the Medical Terminology Express textbook and the supplemental teaching aids available to students and instructors. The Activity Pack, Instructor's Resources, DavisPlus, and Medical Language Lab website contain activities to supplement material covered in the textbook. All of the teaching aids include testing tools to reinforce anatomy and physiology content. For readers who require anatomy and physiology coverage, two anatomy and physiology activities, Anatomy Focus and Tag the Elements, are included for the 12 body-system chapters in the TermPlus software, which can be purchased separately from FA Davis Company. Nevertheless, the textbook emphasizes the meaning of basic medical terms and demonstrates how the terms are used in the health care environment. The ability to communicate in the language of medicine provides students with additional confidence to become effective members of the health care team.

TEXTBOOK OVERVIEW

We have enhanced the popular, effective features found in the previous edition, so the learner can easily apply and process the language of medicine correctly in the health care setting. Each chapter begins with a set of objectives that outline the goals the student should be able to achieve upon completion of that chapter. By completing the reinforcing activities throughout the chapter, the student should be able to achieve the objectives in a structured fashion.

Chapters 1 and 2

Chapter 1 is an **introduction to medical word building,** followed by Chapter 2, which presents an **orientation to the body as a whole.** Knowledge of the descriptive terms introduced in Chapter 2 is an essential part of medical terminology and provides a basic foundation for a better understanding of the body-system chapters that follow. Most importantly, the descriptive terms are included in the language of medicine used by health care providers in the clinical environment.

Chapters 3 to 13

Chapters 3 to 13 **introduce medical terminology related to a specific body system.** Each body-system chapter is arranged in the following sequence:

- The **Vocabulary Preview** includes terms, pronunciations, and meanings of medical words especially relevant to that chapter's body system so the student can easily understand the material presented in the chapter.
- The preview is followed by a description of the **Medical Specialty** or specialties related to the body system or systems covered in the chapter.
- The body system **Quick Study** presents a summary of the organs and functions of the specific body system covered in the chapter.
- The **Medical Word Building** tables introduce combining forms, suffixes, and prefixes related to the body system covered in the chapter. Key word elements and their meanings are labeled on an anatomical illustration to reinforce visually the word elements introduced. Review activities are also included in each of these sections.
- The **Medical Vocabulary** section contains terms related to diseases and conditions. This is followed by a section of diagnostic, medical, and surgical procedures and pharmacology. Dynamic illustrations are included that visually illustrate the disease; the diagnostic procedures used to identify the disease; and the medical, surgical, and pharmacological treatments used to treat various diseases and disorders.
- The section called **A Closer Look** presents extra information and reinforces key pathologies, procedures, and treatments related to the terminology covered in the given chapter.
- The **Abbreviations** table summarizes common abbreviations associated with the body system covered in the chapter.
- The **Chart Notes** section includes authentic medical reports related to a medical specialty associated with the relevant body system to reinforce terminology covered in the chapter. The chart notes are followed by an analysis exercise with an answer key to verify competency.
- Lastly, to improve your retention level of the chapter, various icons guide you to the **DavisPlus** and **Medical Language Lab** websites, which have additional reinforcement activities for each chapter. These resources are discussed in greater detail in the "Teaching and Learning Package" section that follows.

Appendices

Several appendices supplement the material in the chapters with additional information that aids in the learning process or provides information essential to meeting course requirements. Appendices are as follows:

- **Appendix A: Glossary of Medical Word Elements** is a summary of word elements presented in the textbook as well as additional word elements that may be encountered in medical reports or discussions in the field of medicine.
- **Appendix B: Answer Key** contains all of the answers for the activities in the textbook.
- **Appendix C: Abbreviations and Symbols** is a summary of all the abbreviations with meanings presented in the textbook and additional abbreviations and symbols used in health care environments.
- **Appendix D: Drug Classifications** provides a quick reference of common drug categories, including prescription and over-the-counter drugs used to treat signs, symptoms, and diseases of each body system.
- **Appendix E: Medical Specialties** is a summary of medical specialties along with brief descriptions.
- **Appendix F: Index of Diagnostic, Medical, and Surgical Procedures** provides a list of the diagnostic, medical, and surgical procedures covered in the textbook along with page numbers.
- **Appendix G: Oncological Terms** provides a summary of oncology terms covered in the textbook along with page numbers.

TEACHING AND LEARNING PACKAGE

Numerous teaching aids are available free of charge to instructors who adopt Medical Terminology Express: A Short-Course Approach by Body System, second edition. These teaching aids contain an abundance of information and activities to help students retain what they have learned in a given chapter. Various types of electronic resources are designed to enhance course content and ensure a program of excellence in a medical terminology curriculum. These innovative activities also provide various types of presentations to reinforce the learning process. The teaching aids include the Web-based Medical Language Lab (MLL) and the DavisPlus Online Resource Center for both students and instructors.

Medical Language Lab

Included in every new copy of Medical Terminology Express: A Short-Course Approach by Body System, second edition, is access to the ultimate online medical terminology resource for students. The Medical Language Lab is a rich learning environment using proven language development methods to help students become effective users of the language of medicine. To access the Medical Language Lab, students go to http://www.medicallanguagelab.com and register using the access code provided in their new copies of Medical Terminology Express: A Short-Course Approach by Body System.

Each lesson on the Medical Language Lab enables students to develop skills to listen critically for important terms, respond to others using medical terminology, and generate their own terminology-rich writing style and speech. By following the activities in each lesson, students graduate from simple memorization to becoming stronger users of the medical language.

Designed to work seamlessly with Medical Terminology Express: A Short-Course Approach by Body System, second edition, each activity on the Medical Language Lab has been crafted with content specific to the textbook. Every chapter in the textbook has a corresponding lesson on the Medical Language Lab. A designated icon found within the chapters tells students when it is most advantageous to integrate the activities on the Medical Language Lab into their studies. Students can be confident that every activity on the Medical Language Lab is relevant to the language of medicine and helps facilitate the learning process.

DavisPlus Online Resource Center

The DavisPlus website is accessed at http://davisplus.fadavis.com. The website provides a variety of activities to accelerate learning and reinforce information presented in each chapter. A designated icon found within the chapters tells students when it is most advantageous to integrate the activities on the DavisPlus website into their studies. All online exercises provide instructions for completing the various activities.

The multimedia activities available at the DavisPlus Online Resource Center include student and instructor resources as enumerated below:

- **Audio exercises** of pronunciations and meanings of newly introduced medical terms from the word elements tables (Chapters 1 through 13), designed to strengthen spelling, pronunciation, and knowledge of meanings of selected medical terms and develop medical transcription skills. These exercises include spelling, pronunciation, and meaning of key terms and are downloadable to an iPod or MP3 player.
- **Medical record exercises** (Chapters 3 through 13) that allow students to click highlighted terms in the medical record and hear their correct pronunciations and meanings. The audio exercises are designed to strengthen the student's understanding of medical terms.
- **Animations,** such as exploration of the pathology of gastroesophageal reflux disease (GERD) or the various stages of pregnancy and delivery, to help students better understand complex processes and procedures in a stimulating format.
- **Study questions** for Chapters 1 through 13, which students can answer after completing a chapter to determine their competency level for the chapter. The various testing devices also help students prepare for their accreditation examinations.
- Medical secretarial and medical transcription students can also use the audio exercises to learn beginning transcription skills by typing each word as it is pronounced. After typing the words, they can correct spelling by referring to the textbook or a medical dictionary.
- Finally, to evaluate student competency, a **Pronunciation, Spelling, and Transcription Activity Template** is provided in the Activity Pack.

Instructor Online Resource Center

The Instructors' Resources include a robust collection of supplemental teaching aids for instructors to plan course work and enhance their presentations. It is also designed to help students learn the language of medicine commonly used in clinical environments. Instructors can easily implement the teaching tools in various educational settings, including the traditional classroom, distance learning, or independent studies. When instructors integrate the ancillary products into course content, they will help provide a sound foundation for students to develop an extensive medical vocabulary. In addition, its use guarantees a full program of excellence for students of all aptitudes, no matter their educational background. The Instructor's Online Resource Center consists of an Activity Pack, Image Resource, PowerPoint Lecture Notes, Electronic Test Bank, and a Resource Kit—all of which are described next.

Activity Pack

The printable Activity Pack is a resource full of instructional support for using the textbook and ancillary products. It has been broadened and enhanced to meet the challenges of today's instructional needs. The Activity Pack is available in PDF format on the Instructor's Online Resource Center. The second edition of the Activity Pack includes the following materials:

- **Course Outlines.** Suggested course outlines help the instructor determine a comfortable pace and plan the best method of covering the material presented in the textbook. There are course outlines for a 10-week and a 15-week course. Also included are course outlines for individuals who choose to purchase the separate TermPlus software to use along with the textbook.
- **Student- and Instructor-Directed Activities.** These activities offer a variety of activities for each body-system chapter. Activities can serve as course requirements or supplemental material. In addition, the instructor can assign them as individual or collaborative projects. For group projects, Peer Evaluation Forms are provided.
- **Anatomy Questions.** Anatomical structures from each body-system chapter are provided to review or use as test questions. An answer key is also included.
- **Able to Label.** This testing device labels and reinforces the combining forms associated with the structures in each body-system chapter.
- **Supplemental Chart Notes and Analysis.** These exercises are provided for each body-system chapter. The notes are related to the medical specialty that reinforces terminology covered in the chapter.
- **Clinical Connection Activities.** These activities integrate clinical scenarios in each chapter as a solid reinforcement of content. Instructors can feel free to select activities they deem suitable for their course and decide whether the students should complete the activity independently, with peers, or as a group project.
- **Oral and Written Research Projects.** The research projects provide an opportunity for students to hone their research skills. The Community and Internet Resources section offers an updated list of technical journals, community organizations, and Internet sources that students can use to complete the oral and written projects. This section also contains a peer evaluation template for the oral and written research projects. These projects add variety and interest to the course while reinforcing the learning process.
- **Pronunciation, Spelling, and Transcription Activity Template.** This template is designed to help evaluate student competency in pronunciation, spelling, and meaning of medical terms. It can also serve as an introduction to transcription skills.
- **Crossword Puzzles.** These fun, educational activities reinforce material covered in each body-system chapter. Instructors can use them for an individual or group activity, an extra credit opportunity, or just for fun. An answer key is included for each puzzle.
- **Anatomy Coloring Activities.** These activities are included for each body-system chapter to reinforce the positions of the main organs that compose a particular body system.
- **Chart Note Terminology Answer Keys.** This section contains the answers to the Terminology tables in the Chart Notes sections of the textbook. It provides instructional support in using the textbook and assists instructors in correcting the terminology assignments.

Image Resource

We have enhanced and expanded the **image bank,** a popular feature of the first edition, to meet the current demands of numerous instructors. The **image resource** is an electronic image bank that contains all illustrations from the textbook. It is fully searchable and allows users to zoom in and out and display a jpeg image of an illustration that can be copied into a word processing document or PowerPoint presentation.

PowerPoint Lecture Notes

Medical Terminology Express: A Short-Course Approach by Body System, second edition, contains a completely updated and expanded **PowerPoint Lecture Notes** presentation for each chapter in the textbook that instructors can easily integrate, modify, or enhance to meet their classroom needs. We have developed over 1,332 slides for this edition with 982 new slides. This includes numerous, full-color illustrations with captions from the textbook and other sources. The Lecture Notes include a variety of interactive exercises with color illustrations from the textbook, followed by questions and answers relevant to the topic being discussed. This method helps reinforce the functions of each body system, the clinical application of medical terms, and the medical word-building system. Instructors can zoom in to enlarge images and test students' knowledge as they lead discussion of the content. In addition, links to other resources such as the Image Bank and Animations are summarized in notes so instructors are able to swap or add an illustration as well as present a reinforcing animation or assign it for students to view on the Student Resource section of the DavisPlus website. With the exception of Chapters 1 and 2, all Lecture Notes presentations related to a given chapter share a uniform style as follows:

- Structure and function of the body system with an interactive exercise.
- Primary signs, symptoms, and diseases of the body system with an interactive clinically related exercise, including common treatments for the disease.
- Common diagnostic procedures used to diagnose and evaluate pathological conditions of the various structures of the body system with an interactive word-building exercise.
- Common medical and surgical procedures used to treat pathological conditions of the various structures of the given body system with an interactive clinically related exercise.
- Common medications prescribed for treatment of disorders of the body system discussed with an interactive clinically related exercise.

Electronic Test Bank

The electronic test bank uses ExamView Pro, a powerful, user-friendly test-generation program. It enables instructors to create custom-made or randomly generated tests in a printable format from a test bank of more than 1,170 test items, with 545 new test items for this edition. The test bank includes multiple-choice, matching, true-false, and medical word building questions. Because of the flexibility of the ExamView Pro test-generating program, instructors can edit questions in the test bank to meet their specific educational needs. If instructors wish to restate, embellish, or streamline questions or change distractors, they can do so with little effort. They can also add questions to the test bank. The ExamView Pro program is available for PC and Macintosh users.

Resource Kits

Resource Kits are available for various Learning Management Systems, such as Blackboard, Angel, Moodle, and SCORM-compliant systems.

Teaching Guide

The Teaching Guide is an extensive instructional aid matched to every lecture in a common single-term Medical Terminology course. It is filled with sample homework assignments, in-class activities, and extensive lecture notes with suggested topic durations. When viewed electronically, the Teaching Guide also provides live hyperlinks to the instructor resources on DavisPlus.

Davis Digital Version

Adopters have access to the complete content of the text online in a searchable format that can be book-marked and accessed wherever you have a browser with an Internet connection.

TermPlus

TermPlus 3.0 is a powerful, interactive CD-ROM program that is available for this edition as a separate product from F.A.Davis Company. TermPlus is a popular competency-based, self-paced, multimedia program that includes graphics, audio, and a dictionary culled from Taber's Cyclopedic Medical Dictionary, 22nd edition. Help menus provide navigational support. The software comes with numerous interactive learning activities, including the following:

- Anatomy Focus
- Tag the Elements
- Spotlight the Elements
- Concentration
- Build Medical Words
- Programmed Learning
- Medical Vocabulary
- Chart Notes
- Spelling
- Crossword Puzzles
- Word Scramble
- Terminology Teaser

All activities can be graded and the results printed or e-mailed to an instructor. This feature makes TermPlus especially valuable as a distance-learning tool because it provides evidence of student drill and practice in various learning activities.

Acknowledgments

The second edition of Medical Terminology Express: A Short-Course Approach by Body Systems was updated based on comments and suggestions the authors received from the users of the first edition—both educators and students. We also are grateful and acknowledge the valuable contributions of F. A. Davis's editorial and production team who were responsible for this project:

- Quincy McDonald, Publisher, provided the overall design and layout for the second edition. He was instrumental in assisting the authors in designing a wide variety of state-of-the-art pedagogical products within the text to aid students in their learning activities and to help instructors plan course work and presentations. These teaching aids are described in the Teaching and Learning Package section of the Preface.
- Elizabeth Schaeffer, Developmental Editor of Electronic Products, patiently and enthusiastically addressed our numerous questions and background queries to ensure the textbook and its ancillary products were appropriately updated and accurately revised.
- George W. Lang, Manager of Content Development, expertly guided the manuscript and Activity Pack through the developmental and production phases of the projects.
- Margaret Biblis, Editor-in-Chief, once again provided her support and efforts for the quality of the finished product.

We also acknowledge and thank our exceptionally dedicated publishing partners who helped guide and shape this versatile project into a product of excellence:

Nichole Liccio, Editorial Assistant
Sharon Lee, Production Manager
Kate Margeson, Illustrations Coordinator
Carolyn O'Brien, Design and Illustration Manager
Cynthia Breuninger, Managing Editor
Kirk Pedrick, Director of Digital Solutions
Elizabeth Y. Stepchin, Developmental Associate

We also extend our sincerest gratitude to Neil Kelly, Director of Sales, and his staff of sales representatives, whose continued efforts have undoubtedly contributed to the success of this textbook.

Acknowledgments

The authors extend a special thanks to the clinical and chapter reviewers and students who read and edited the manuscript and provided suggestions for improving the textbook. Their feedback undoubtedly helped improve the excellence of the final text and ancillary products.

Lastly, we extend our deepest gratitude to the students and to the following field testers who worked through the entire final copy of the textbook and field-tested the reviews and test banks for improving the second edition.

- Caitlin Masters, BA in Business Administration, Indiana University; MPH in Public Health, Boston University. Employed at Beacon Health Strategies as Account Operations Manager, Boston, Massachusetts.
- Andrew Masters, BS, Miami University, Oxford, Ohio, and a graduate student completing an MSW degree in social work.

We are confident that students will enjoy Medical Terminology Express and that they will find learning the language of medicine to be an exciting, rewarding process that will help them succeed in the field of medicine. We welcome instructors and students to send comments and suggestions to F. A. Davis Company, 1915 Arch Street, Philadelphia, PA 19103. This feedback will help us better meet your educational needs in the third edition.

BARBARA GYLYS
REGINA MASTERS

Contents at a Glance

Contents

APPENDICES

Introduction to Medical Terminology

Objectives

Upon completion of this chapter, you will be able to:

- Identify and define the four elements used to build medical words.
- Apply the basic rules to define and build medical terms.
- Define and provide examples of surgical, diagnostic, pathological, and related suffixes.
- Apply rules learned in this chapter to write singular and plural forms of medical words.
- Practice pronouncing the medical terms presented in this chapter.
- Demonstrate your knowledge by successfully completing the activities in this chapter.

The language of medicine is a specialized vocabulary used by health care providers. Many current medical word elements originated as early as the 4th century B.C., when Hippocrates practiced medicine. With technological and scientific advancements in medicine, new terms have evolved to reflect these innovations. For example, radiographic terms, such as magnetic resonance imaging (MRI) and ultrasound (US), are now used to describe current diagnostic procedures.

MEDICAL WORD ELEMENTS

A medical word consists of some or all of the following elements:

- word root
- combining form
- suffix
- prefix

How these elements are combined and whether all or some of them are present in a medical term determines the meaning of a word. To understand the meaning of medical words, it is important to learn how to divide them into their basic elements. This chapter covers the basic principles of medical word building and how to pronounce the terms correctly. Pronunciations are provided with all terms. In addition, pronunciation guidelines are located on the inside back cover of this book so you can refer to them throughout the chapters to help pronounce terms correctly.

Word Roots

A **word root** (WR) is the foundation of a medical term and contains its primary meaning. All medical terms have at least one word root. Examine the terms **tonsillitis, tonsillectomy, colitis,** and **colectomy** listed below to determine their basic elements (roots and suffixes) and meanings. You will note that the meaning of the word changes whenever you change one of the word elements. (In the examples that follow, word roots are in **boldface** and suffixes are in blue.)

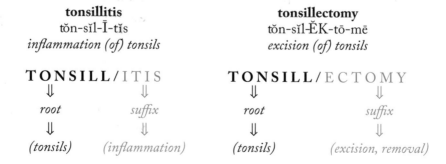

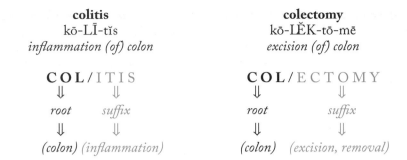

| Word Analysis | The roots *tonsill* and *col* indicate body parts, the tonsils and colon, respectively. The suffix *-itis* means *inflammation*; the suffix *-ectomy* means *excision, removal*. By adding a different suffix to the root, the meaning of the word changes, as shown in the above examples. |

Combining Forms

A **combining form (CF)** is created when a word root is combined with a vowel. The vowel, known as a combining vowel, is usually an *o*, but sometimes it is an *i* or *e*. The combining vowel has no meaning of its own but enables two word elements to be connected. Like the word root, the combining form is the basic foundation to which other word elements are added to build a complete medical word. In this text, a combining form will be listed as *word root/vowel* (such as *arthr/o, gastr/o, nephr/o, neur/o,* and *oste/o*), as illustrated in the following examples. The difficulty of pronouncing certain combinations of word roots requires insertion of a vowel. Like the word root, the combining form usually indicates a body part.

Examples of Combining Forms

Word Root	+	Combining Vowel	=	Combining Form	Meaning
arthr	+	o	=	**arthr/o**	*joint*
gastr	+	o	=	**gastr/o**	*stomach*
nephr	+	o	=	**nephr/o**	*kidney*
neur	+	o	=	**neur/o**	*nerve*
oste	+	o	=	**oste/o**	*bone*

Linking Suffixes

A CF links with a suffix that begins with a consonant. Examples of suffixes that begin with a consonant are *-centesis* and *-pathy*. This linking is illustrated below in the terms *arthr/o/centesis* and *gastr/o/pathy*.

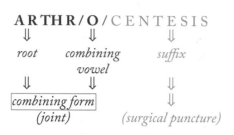

arthrocentesis
ăr-thrō-sĕn-TĒ-sĭs
surgical puncture of a joint

A R T H R / O / C E N T E S I S
⇓   ⇓   ⇓
root   *combining*   *suffix*
        vowel
          ⇓   ⇓   ⇓
    combining form   ⇓
        (joint)   *(surgical puncture)*

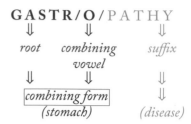

gastropathy
găs-TRŎP-ă-thē
disease of the stomach

G A S T R / O / P A T H Y
⇓   ⇓   ⇓
root   *combining*   *suffix*
        vowel
          ⇓   ⇓   ⇓
    combining form   ⇓
        (stomach)   *(disease)*

A WR links with a suffix that begins with a vowel. Examples of suffixes that begin with a vowel are *-itis* and *-ectomy*. This linking is illustrated below in the terms *arthr/itis* and *gastr/ectomy*.

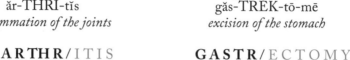

arthritis
ăr-THRĪ-tĭs
inflammation of the joints

A R T H R / I T I S
⇓   ⇓
root   *suffix*
(joint)   *(inflammation)*

gastrectomy
găs-TRĔK-tō-mē
excision of the stomach

G A S T R / E C T O M Y
⇓   ⇓
root   *suffix*
(stomach)   *(excision, removal)*

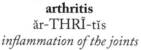
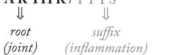
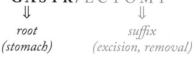

| **Word Analysis** | The roots *gastr* and *arthr* indicate body parts. The suffix *-itis* means *inflammation*; *-centesis* means *puncture*; *-pathy* means *disease*; and *-ectomy* means *excision, removal*. |

Suffixes

A **suffix** is a word element placed at the end of a word that changes the meaning of the word. In the terms mast/ectomy and mast/itis, the suffixes are *-ectomy* (excision, removal) and *-itis* (inflammation). Changing the suffix changes the meaning of the word. In medical terminology, a suffix usually describes a pathology (disease or abnormality), symptom, surgical or diagnostic procedure, or part of speech.

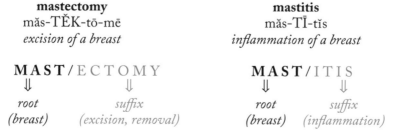

mastectomy
măs-TĔK-tō-mē
excision of a breast

M A S T / E C T O M Y
⇓   ⇓
root   *suffix*
(breast)   *(excision, removal)*

mastitis
măs-TĪ-tĭs
inflammation of a breast

M A S T / I T I S
⇓   ⇓
root   *suffix*
(breast)   *(inflammation)*

When studying medical terminology, try to learn the combining form rather than the root because the combining form makes most words easier to pronounce. In the example of arthrocentesis, the root without a connecting vowel would be written *arthrcentesis* (ăr-thr-sĕn-TĒ-sĭs). Spelled this way, the term is difficult to pronounce. By adding the vowel after the root, the word arthrocentesis (ăr-thrō-sĕn-TĒ-sĭs) is much easier to pronounce.

Word Analysis	The root *mast* indicates the body part, the breast. The suffix *-ectomy* means *excision, removal*; the suffix *-itis* means *inflammation*. Adding different suffixes to the root *mast* changes the meaning of the word.

Prefixes

A **prefix** is a word element attached to the beginning of a word or word root. However, not all medical terms have a prefix. Adding or changing a prefix changes the meaning of the word. The prefix usually indicates a number, time, position, direction, or negation. Prefixes do not require adding a connecting vowel. Many prefixes in medical terms are the same as the prefixes used in the English language. Consider the following terms. (In the examples that follow, word roots are in **boldface**, suffixes are in blue, and prefixes are in pink.)

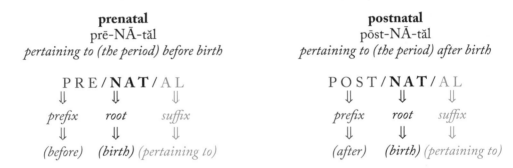

prenatal
prē-NĀ-tăl
pertaining to (the period) before birth

PRE / **NAT** / AL
⇓   ⇓   ⇓
prefix   *root*   *suffix*
⇓   ⇓   ⇓
(before) *(birth)* *(pertaining to)*

postnatal
pōst-NĀ-tăl
pertaining to (the period) after birth

POST / **NAT** / AL
⇓   ⇓   ⇓
prefix   *root*   *suffix*
⇓   ⇓   ⇓
(after) *(birth)* *(pertaining to)*

The prefixes *pre-* and *post-* indicate a state of time. Both prefixes are attached directly to the word root that follows. In the above examples, *pre-* and *post-* are attached to the root *nat*. In this text, whenever a prefix stands alone, it will be followed by a hyphen, as in *pre-* and *post-*. Whenever a suffix stands alone, it will be preceded by a hyphen, as in *-al*.

Word Analysis	The root *nat* means *birth*; the suffix *-al* means *pertaining to*.

Review Activity 1-1
Matching Word Elements

Match the numbered list items with their definitions in the right-hand column.

1. __*gj*__ pre- means   *a.* foundation of a word, such as *cardi* and *arthr*

2. __*d*__ basic components of words   *b.* end of a word

3. __*g*__ combining form   *c.* beginning of a word

4. __*h*__ combining vowel(s)   *d.* word root, suffix, combining form, and prefix

5. __*i*__ post- means   *e.* stomach

6. __*f*__ suffix -itis   *f.* inflammation

7. __*e*__ gastr means   *g.* arthr/o

8. __*c*__ location of prefixes   *h.* "o" and "i"

9. __*b*__ location of suffixes   *i.* after

10. __*a*__ word root   *j.* before

✓ **Competency Verification:** Check your answers in Appendix B, Answer Key, page 357. If you are not satisfied with your level of comprehension, review the terms in the table and retake the review.

Correct Answers: _____ × 10 = _____ **% Score**

Review Activity 1-2
Understanding Medical Word Elements

Fill in the following blanks to complete the sentences correctly.

1. The four elements used to form medical words are _word root, prefix, suffix, combining vowel_

2. A root is the main part or foundation of a word. In the words arthritis, arthroma, and arthroscope, the root is _arthr_

Identify the following statements as true or false by circling *True* or *False* for each statement. If false, rewrite the statement correctly on the line provided.

3. A combining vowel is usually an _i._   **True** (**False**)
    _o_

4. A ~~word root~~ links a suffix that begins with a consonant.   **True** (**False**)
    Combining form

5. A combining vowel enables two word elements to be connected.   (**True**) **False**

6. A combining form links a suffix that begins with a consonant.   (**True**) **False**

7. Whenever a prefix stands alone, it will be ~~preceded~~ by a hyphen.   **True** ~~**False**~~
    followed

8. In the term intramuscular, *intra-* is the prefix.   (**True**) **False**

Underline the word root in each of following combining forms.

9. splen/o (spleen)

10. hyster/o (uterus)

11. enter/o (intestine)

12. neur/o (nerve)

13. ot/o (ear)

14. dermat/o (skin)

15. hydr/o (water)

> **Competency Verification:** Check your answers in Appendix B, Answer Key, page 357. If you are not satisfied with your level of comprehension, review the terms in the table and retake the review.
>
> **Correct Answers:** _____ × **6.67** = _____ **% Score**

Review Activity 1-3
Identifying Word Roots and Combining Forms

Underline the word roots in the following terms.

Medical Word	**Meaning**
1. nephritis	*inflammation of the kidneys*
2. arthrodesis	*fixation of a joint*
3. dermatitis	*inflammation of the skin*
4. arthrocentesis	*surgical puncture of a joint*
5. gastrectomy	*excision of the stomach*

Underline the following elements that are combining forms.

6. nephr	kidney
7. hepat/o	liver
8. arthr	joint
9. oste/o/arthr	bone, joint
10. cholangi/o	bile vessel

> **Competency Verification:** Check your answers in Appendix B, Answer Key, page 357. If you are not satisfied with your level of comprehension, review the terms in the table and retake the review.
>
> **Correct Answers:** _____ × **10** = _____ **% Score**

DEFINING AND BUILDING MEDICAL WORDS

Defining and building medical words are crucial skills in mastering medical terminology. Following the basic guidelines will help develop these skills.

Defining Medical Words

Here are three steps for defining medical words using the term oste/o/arthr/itis (ŏs-tē-ō-ăr-**THRĪ**-tĭs) as an example.

1. Define the **suffix**, or last part of the word. In this case, the suffix *-itis* means *inflammation*.
2. Define the first part of the word (**word root** or **combining form**, or **prefix**). In this case, the combining form *oste/o* means *bone*.
3. Define the middle parts of the word (**word root** or **combining form**). In this case, *arthr* means *joint*. Table 1-1 further illustrates this process.

TABLE I-I **Defining Osteoarthritis**		
This table illustrates the three steps of defining a medical word using the example osteoarthritis.		
Combining Form	**Middle**	**Suffix**
oste/o	arthr	-itis
bone	*joint*	*inflammation*
(rule 2)	(rule 3)	(rule I)

Therefore, oste/o/arthr/itis is an *inflammation of bone(s) and joint(s).*

Building Medical Words

There are three rules for building medical words.

Rule #I

A word root links a suffix that begins with a vowel.

Word Root	+	Suffix	=	Medical Word	Meaning
append *appendix*	+	**-ectomy** *excision, removal*	=	**append/ectomy** ăp-ĕn-DĔK-tō-mē	*excision of the appendix*
gastr *stomach*	+	**-itis** *inflammation*	=	**gastr/itis** găs-TRĪ-tĭs	*inflammation of the stomach*

Rule #2

A combining form (root + *o*) links a suffix that begins with a consonant.

Combining Form	+	Suffix	=	Medical Word	Meaning
colon/o *colon*	+	-scope *instrument for examining*	=	colon/o/scope kō-LŎN-ō-skōp	*instrument for examining the colon*

Rule #3

A combining form (root + *o*) links a root to another root to form a compound word. This rule holds true even if the next root begins with a vowel, as in gastroenteritis. Keep in mind that the rules for linking multiple roots to each other are slightly different from the rules for linking roots and combining forms to suffixes. Following are several examples.

Combining Form	+	Word Root	+	Suffix	=	Medical Word	Meaning
gastr/o *stomach*	+	enter *intestine (usually small intestine)*	+	-itis *inflammation*	=	gastr/o/enter/itis găs-trō-ĕn-tĕr-Ī-tĭs	*inflammation of stomach and intestine (usually small intestine)*
gastr/o *stomach*	+	col colon	+	-itis inflammation	=	gastr/o/col/itis găs-trō-kō-LĪ-tĭs	*inflammation of stomach and colon*
oste/o *(bone)*	+	chondr *cartilage*	+	-itis *inflammation*	=	osteochondritis ŏs-tē-ō-kŏn-DRĪ-tĭs	*inflammation of bone and cartilage*
oste/o *(bone)*	+	arthr *joint*	+	-itis *inflammation*	=	osteoarthritis ŏs-tē-ō-ăr-THRĪ-tĭs	*inflammation of bone and joint*

Review Activity 1-4
Defining Medical Words

Use the following table to complete the statements below. The first one is completed for you.

Combining Forms	Suffixes and Prefixes	Meaning
append/o		appendix
arthr/o		joint
col/o, colon/o		colon
enter/o		intestine (usually small)
gastr/o		stomach
mast/o		breast
oste/o		bone
	-centesis	surgical puncture
	-itis	inflammation
	-pathy	disease
	-scope	instrument to view or examine
	pre-	before
	post-	after

1. Mast/ectomy is an excision of a _breast_____.
2. Tonsill/itis is an __inflammation_____ of the tonsils.
3. A colon/o/scope is an instrument to examine the __colon_____.
4. Oste/o/malacia is a softening of a __bone_____ (singular).
5. Post/nat/al means pertaining to (the period) __after_____ birth.
6. Arthr/o/centesis is a surgical puncture of a __joint_____.
7. Arthr/o/pathy is a __disease_____ of the joints.
8. A prefix that means *before* is __pre_____.
9. The combining form for *stomach* is __gastr/o_____.
10. The suffix for *disease* is __-pathy_____.
11. The combining form for *breast* is __mast/o_____.
12. The suffix that means *instrument to examine* is __-scope_____.
13. The combining form *append/o* refers to the __appendix_____.

14. Gastro/enter/itis is an inflammation of the stomach and the_intestine_____.

15. The suffix for *surgical puncture* is_centesis_____.

Competency Verification: Check your answers in Appendix B, Answer Key, page 357. If you are not satisfied with your level of comprehension, review the terms in the table and retake the review.

Correct Answers: _____ × **6.67** = _____ **% Score**

Review Activity 1-5
Defining and Building Medical Words

The three steps for defining medical words are:

1. Define the last part of the word, or **suffix**.

2. Define the first part of the word, or **prefix, word root,** or **combining form.**

3. Define the middle of the word.

First pronounce the term aloud. Then apply the above three steps to define the terms in the following table. If you are uncertain of a definition, refer to Appendix A of this textbook, which provides an alphabetical list of word elements and their definitions. The first one is completed for you.

Term	Definition
1. col/itis kō-LĪ-tĭs	*inflammation (of) colon*
2. gastr/o/scope GĂS-trō-skōp	instrument to examine the stomach
3. hepat/itis hĕp-ă-TĪ-tĭs	inflammation of the liver
4. pre/nat/al prē-NĀ-tăl	before birth
5. tonsill/ectomy tŏn-sĭl-ĔK-tō-mē	removal of the tonsils
6. tonsill/itis tŏn-sĭl-Ī-tĭs	inflammation of the tonsils

Refer to the section "Building Medical Words" on page 8 to complete this activity. Write the number for the rule that applies to each listed term and a short summary of the rule. Use the abbreviations *WR* to designate a word root and *CF* to designate *combining form*. The first one is completed for you.

Term	Rule	Summary of Rule
7. append/ectomy ăp-ĕn-DĔK-tō-mē	*1*	*A WR links a suffix that begins with a vowel.*
8. arthr/o/centesis ăr-thrō-sĕn-TĒ-sĭs		
9. col/ectomy kō-LĔK-tō-mē		
10. colon/o/scope kō-LŎN-ō-skōp		
11. gastr/itis găs-TRĪ-tĭs		
12. gastr/o/enter/o/col/itis găs-trō-ĕn-tĕr-ō-kŏl-Ī-tĭs		
13. arthr/o/pathy ăr-THRŎP-ă-thē		
14. oste/o/arthr/itis ŏs-tē-ō-ăr-THRĪ-tĭs		
15. oste/o/chondr/itis ŏs-tē-ō-kŏn-DRĪ-tĭs		

 Competency Verification: Check your answers in Appendix B, Answer Key, page 358. If you are not satisfied with your level of comprehension, review the terms in the table and retake the review.

Correct Answers: _____ × **6.67** = _____ **% Score**

PRONUNCIATION GUIDELINES

Although pronunciation of medical words usually follows the same rules that govern pronunciation of English words, some medical words may be difficult to pronounce when first encountered. Therefore, selected terms in this book include a phonetic pronunciation. Diacritical marks and capitalization are used to aid pronunciation of terms throughout the text and to help you understand pronunciation marks used in most dictionaries.

Pronunciation guidelines are located on the inside back cover of this book and at the end of selected tables. Use them whenever help is needed with pronunciation of medical words.

Review Activity 1-6
Understanding Pronunciations

Review the pronunciation guidelines (located inside the front cover of this book) and underline the correct answer in each of the following statements.

1. The diacritical mark ‾ is called a (breve, macron).

2. The diacritical mark ˘ is called a (breve, macron).

3. The ‾ indicates the (short, long) sound of vowels.

4. The ˘ indicates the (short, long) sound of vowels.

5. The combination *ch* is sometimes pronounced like *(k, chiy)*. Examples are *ch*olesterol, *ch*olemia.

6. When *pn* is at the beginning of a word, it is pronounced only with the sound of *(p, n)*. Examples are *pn*eumonia, *pn*eumotoxin.

7. When *pn* is in middle of a word, the *p (is, is not)* pronounced. Examples are ortho*pn*ea, hyper*pn*ea.

8. When *i* is at the end of a word, it is pronounced like *(eye, ee)*. Examples are bronch*i*, fung*i*, nucle*i*.

9. For *ae* and *oe*, only the (first, second) vowel is pronounced. Examples are burs*ae*, pleur*ae*.

10. When *e* and *es* form the final letter or letters of a word, they are commonly pronounced as (combined, separate) syllables. Examples are syncop*e*, systol*e*, nar*es*.

 Competency Verification: Check your answers in Appendix B, Answer Key, page 359. If you are not satisfied with your level of comprehension, review the terms in the table and retake the review.

Correct Answers: _____ × 10 = _____ % Score

Review Activity 1-7
Plural Suffixes

When a word changes from a singular to a plural form, the suffix of the word is the part that changes. For example, the medical report may list one diagno*sis* or several diagno*ses*. The rules for forming plurals starting from the singular forms of the words are listed on the inside back cover of this book. When in doubt about singular and plural word formations, refer to these rules or use a medical dictionary. Review the rules and use them to complete this activity. The first word is completed for you.

Singular	Plural	Rule
1. sarcoma săr-KŌ-mă	*sarcomata*	*Retain the* ma *and add* ta.
2. thrombus THRŎM-bŭs	thrombi	
3. appendix ă-PĔN-dĭks	appendices	
4. diverticulum dī-vĕr-TĬK-ū-lŭm	diverticula	
5. ovary Ō-vă-rē	ovaries	
6. diagnosis dī-ăg-NŌ-sĭs	diagnoses	
7. lumen LŪ-mĕn	lumina	
8. vertebra VĔR-tĕ-bră	vertebre	
9. thorax THŌ-răks	~~thora~~ thorces	
10. spermatozoon spĕr-măt-ō-ZŌ-ŏn	Spermatazoa	

Competency Verification: Check your answers in Appendix B, Answer Key, page 359. If you are not satisfied with your level of comprehension, review the terms in the table and retake the review.

Correct Answers: _____ × 10 = _____ **% Score**

Review Activity 1-8
Common Suffixes

In previous material, you were introduced to the principles of medical word building. You learned that a combining form is a word root + vowel and that the combining form is the main part or foundation of a medical term. Examples of combining forms are *gastr/o* (stomach), *dermat/o* (skin), and *nephr/o* (kidney). You also learned that a suffix is an element located at the end of a word and a prefix is an element located at the beginning of a word. This section presents common suffixes and prefixes used to construct medical terms. Some of these elements have already been introduced, but they are now reinforced in the appropriate categorized tables below. Similar tables are included for each chapter in the book. The common elements in this section of the chapter will be reinforced throughout the textbook in numerous medical terms.

Surgical Suffixes

Common suffixes associated with surgical procedures, their meanings, and an example of a related term are listed in the following table. First, study the suffix and its meaning and practice pronouncing the term aloud. Then use the information provided to complete the meaning of each term. You may also refer to *Appendix A: Glossary of Medical Word Elements* to complete this exercise. To build a working vocabulary of medical terms and understand how those terms are used in the health care industry, it is important that you complete all of these exercises. The first one is completed for you.

Suffix	Term	Meaning
-centesis surgical puncture	arthr/o/**centesis** ăr-thrō-sĕn-TĒ-sĭs *arthr/o:* joint	*Surgical puncture of a joint*
-clasis to break; surgical fracture	oste/o/**clasis** ŏs-tē-ŎK-lă-sĭs *oste/o:* bone	surgical fracture of a bone
-desis binding, fixation (of a bone or joint)	arth r/o/**desis** ăr-thrō-DĒ-sĭs *arthr/o:* joint	binding of a joint
-ectomy excision, removal	append/**ectomy** ăp-ĕn-DĔK-tō-mē *append:* appendix	removal of the appendix
-lysis separation; destruction; loosening	thromb/o/**lysis** thrŏm-BŎL-ĭ-sĭs *thromb/o:* blood clot	separation of a blood clot
-pexy fixation (of an organ)	mast/o/**pexy** MĂS-tō-pĕks-ē *mast/o:* breast	fixation of a breast
-plasty surgical repair	rhin/o/**plasty** RĪ-nō-plăs-tē *rhin/o:* nose	surgical repair of the nose
-rrhaphy suture	my/o/**rrhaphy** mī-OR-ă-fē *my/o:* muscle	suture of a muscle

(Continued)

Suffix	Term	Meaning
-stomy forming an opening (mouth)	trache/o/**stomy** trā-kē-ŎS-tō-mē *trache/o:* trachea (windpipe)	*forming an opening of the trachea*
-tome instrument to cut	oste/o/**tome** ŎS-tē-ō-tōm *oste/o:* bone	*instrument to cut a bone*
-tomy incision	trache/o/**tomy** trā-kē-ŎT-ō-mē *trache/o:* trachea (windpipe)	*incision in the trachea*
-tripsy crushing	lith/o/**tripsy** LĬTH-ō-trĭp-sē *lith/o:* stone, calculus	*crushing of the calculus*

Pronunciation Help	Long Sound Short Sound	ā in rāte ă in ălone	ē in rēbirth ĕ in ĕver	ī in īsle ĭ in ĭt	ō in ōver ŏ in nŏt	ū in ūnite ŭ in cŭt

 Competency Verification: Check your answers in Appendix B, Answer Key, page 359. If you are not satisfied with your level of comprehension, review the terms in the table and retake the review.

Diagnostic Suffixes

Common suffixes associated with diagnostic procedures, their meanings, and an example of a related term are listed in the following table. First, study the suffix and its meaning and practice pronouncing the term aloud. Then use the information provided to complete the meaning of each term. You may also refer to *Appendix A: Glossary of Medical Word Elements* to complete this exercise. To build a working vocabulary of medical terms and understand how those terms are used in the health care field, it is important that you complete all of these exercises. The first one is completed for you.

Suffix	Term	Meaning
-gram record, writing	electr/o/cardi/o/**gram** ē-lĕk-trō-KĂR-dē-ō-grăm *electr/o:* electricity *cardi/o:* heart	*Record of electrical activity of the heart*
-graph instrument for recording	cardi/o/**graph** KĂR-dē-ō-grăf *cardi/o:* heart	*instrument for recording activity of the heart*
-graphy process of recording	angi/o/**graphy** ăn-jē-ŎG-ră-fē *angi/o:* vessel (usually blood or lymph)	*recording activity of a vessel*

Suffix	Term	Meaning
-meter instrument for measuring	pelv/i/**meter*** pĕl-VĬM-ĕ-tĕr *pelv/i:* pelvis	instrument for measuring the pelvis
-metry act of measuring	pelv/i/**metry*** pĕl-VĬM-ĕ-trē *pelv/i:* pelvis	act of measuring the pelvis
-scope instrument for examining	endo/**scope** ĔN-dō-skōp *endo-:* in, within	instrument for examining inside the body
-scopy visual examination	endo/**scopy** ĕn-DŎS-kō-pē *endo-:* in, within	examining the inside of the body

Pronunciation Help	Long Sound	ā in rāte	ē in rēbirth	ī in īsle	ō in ōver	ū in ūnite
	Short Sound	ă in ălone	ĕ in ĕver	ĭ in ĭt	ŏ in nŏt	ŭ in cŭt

**The i in pelv/i/meter and pelv/i/metry are exceptions to the rule of using the connecting vowel o.*

 Competency Verification: Check your answers in Appendix B, Answer Key, page 360. If you are not satisfied with your level of comprehension, review the terms in the table and retake the review.

Pathological Suffixes

Common suffixes associated with pathological (disease) conditions, their meanings, and an example of a related term are listed in the following table. First, study the suffix and its meaning and practice pronouncing the term aloud. Then use the information provided to complete the meaning of each term. You may also refer to *Appendix A: Glossary of Medical Word Elements* to complete this exercise. To build a working vocabulary of medical terms and understand how those terms are used in the health care industry, it is important that you complete all of these exercises. The first one is completed for you.

Suffix	Term	Meaning
-algia, -dynia pain	neur/**algia** nū-RĂL-jē-ă *neur:* nerve	*Pain in a nerve*
	ot/o/**dynia** ō-tō-DĬN-ĕ-ă *ot/o:* ear	ear pain
-cele hernia, swelling	hepat/o/**cele** hĕ-PĂT-ō-sēl *hepat/o:* liver	liver swelling

(Continued)

Suffix	Term	Meaning
-ectasis dilation, expansion	**bronchi/ectasis** brŏng-kē-ĔK-tă-sĭs *bronchi:* bronchus (plural, bronchi)	dilation of the bronchi
-edema swelling	**lymph/edema** lĭmf-ĕ-DĒ-mă *lymph:* lymph	swelling of the lymph nodes
-emesis vomiting	**hyper/emesis** hī-pĕr-ĔM-ĕ-sĭs *hyper-:* excessive, above normal	excessive vomiting
-emia blood condition	**an/emia** ă-NĒ-mē-ă *an-:* without, not	abnormal blood condition
-iasis abnormal condition (produced by something specific)	**chol/e/lith/iasis*** kō-lē-lĭ-THĪ-ă-sĭs *chol/e:* bile, gall *lith:* stone, calculus	formation of gallstones
-itis inflammation	**gastr/itis** găs-TRĪ-tĭs *gastr:* stomach	inflammation of the stomach
-lith stone, calculus	**chol/e/lith*** KŌ-lē-lĭth *chol/e:* bile, gall	gallstones
-malacia softening	**chondr/o/malacia** kŏn-drō-mă-LĀ-shē-ă *chondr/o:* cartilage	softening of the cartilage
-megaly enlargement	**cardi/o/megaly** kăr-dē-ō-MĔG-ă-lē *cardi/o:* heart	enlargement of the heart
-oma tumor	**neur/oma** nū-RŌ-mă *neur:* nerve	nerve tumor
-osis abnormal condition; increase (used primarily with blood cells)	**cyan/osis** sī-ă-NŌ-sĭs *cyan:* blue	skin turns blue
-pathy disease	**my/o/pathy** mī-ŎP-ă-thē *my/o:* muscle	muscle disease

*The e in chol/e/lithiasis and chol/e/lith *are exceptions to the rule of using the connecting vowel o.*

Suffix	Term	Meaning
-penia decrease, deficiency	erythr/o/**penia** ĕ-rĭth-rō-PĒ-nē-ă *erythr/o:* red	decrease in red blood cells
-phobia fear	hem/o/**phobia** hē-mō-FŌ-bē-ă *hem/o:* blood	fear of blood
-plegia paralysis	hemi/**plegia** hĕm-ē-PLĒ-jē-ă *hemi-:* one half	half-body paralysis
-rrhage, -rrhagia bursting (of)	hem/o/**rrhage** HĔM-ĕ-rĭj *hem/o:* blood	excessive bleeding
	men/o/**rrhagia** mĕn-ō-RĀ-jē-ă *men/o:* menses, menstruation	excessive bleeding during menstruation
-rrhea discharge, flow	dia/**rrhea** dī-ă-RĒ-ă *dia-:* through, across	excessive defecation
-rrhexis rupture	arteri/o/**rrhexis** ăr-tē-rē-ō-RĔK-sĭs *arteri/o:* artery	rupture in an artery
-stenosis narrowing, stricture	arteri/o/**stenosis** ăr-tē-rē-ō-stĕ-NŌ-sĭs *arteri/o:* artery	narrowing of an artery
-toxic poison	hepat/o/**toxic** HĔP-ă-tō-tŏk-sĭk *hepat/o:* liver	toxic liver
-trophy nourishment, development	dys/**trophy** DĬS-trō-fē *dys-:* bad; painful; difficult	bad development

Pronunciation Help	Long Sound	ā in rāte	ē in rēbirth	ī in īsle	ō in ōver	ū in ūnite
	Short Sound	ă in ălone	ĕ in ĕver	ĭ in ĭt	ŏ in nŏt	ŭ in cŭt

 Competency Verification: Check your answers in Appendix B, Answer Key, pages 360–361. If you are not satisfied with your level of comprehension, review the terms in the table and retake the review.

Review Activity 1-9
Common Prefixes

Common prefixes, their meanings, and an example of a related term are listed in the following table. First, study the prefix and its meaning and practice pronouncing the term aloud. Then use the information in the following table to complete the meaning of the terms. You may also refer to *Appendix A: Glossary of Medical Word Elements* to complete this exercise. To understand the meaning of medical terms, it is important to engage actively in activities of this type. Complete all of the exercises, and you will master medical terminology. The first one is completed for you.

Prefix	Term	Meaning
a-*, an-† without, not	**a**/mast/ia ă-MĂS-tē-ă *mast:* breast *-ia:* condition	*Without a breast*
	an/esthesia ăn-ĕs-THĒ-zē-ă *-esthesia:* feeling	w/o feeting
circum-, peri- around	**circum**/duction sĕr-kŭm-DŬK-shŭn *-duction:* act of leading, bring- ing, conducting	act of bringing around
	peri/odont/al pĕr-ē-ō-DŎN-tăl *odont:* teeth *-al:* pertaining to	pertaining to around the teeth
dia-, trans- through, across	**dia**/therm/y DĪ-ă-thĕr-mē *therm:* heat *-y:* condition, process	Procerr of neating across
	trans/vagin/al trăns-VĂJ-ĭn-ăl *vagin:* vagina *-al:* pertaining to	pertaining to across the vagina

Prefix	Term	Meaning
dipl-, diplo- double	**dipl**/opia dĭp-LŌ-pē-ă *-opia:* vision	double vision *(handwritten)*
	diplo/bacteri/al dĭp-lō-băk-TĔR-ē-ăl *bacteri:* bacteria *-al:* pertaining to	Pertaining to double bacteria *(handwritten)*
dys- bad, painful, difficult	**dys**/phonia dĭs-FŌ-nē-ă *-phonia:* voice	bad/painful/difficult voice *(handwritten)*
endo-, intra- in, within	**endo**/crine ĔN-dō-krĭn *-crine:* secrete	Secrete within *(handwritten)*
	intra/muscul/ar ĭn-tră-MŬS-kū-lăr *muscul:* muscle *-ar:* pertaining to	Pertaining to within the muscle *(handwritten)*
homo-, homeo- same	**homo**/graft HŌ-mō-grăft *-graft:* transplantation	transplantation of the same *(handwritten)*
	homeo/plasia hō-mē-ō-PLĀ-zē-ă *-plasia:* formation, growth	formation of the same *(handwritten)*
hypo- under, below, deficient	**hypo**/derm/ic hī-pō-DĔR-mĭk *derm:* skin *-ic:* pertaining to	below the skin *(handwritten)*
macro- large	**macro**/cyte MĂK-rō-sīt *-cyte:* cell	large cell *(handwritten)*
micro- small	**micro**/scope MĪ-krō-skōp *-scope:* instrument for examining	instrument for examining small things *(handwritten)*
mono-, uni- one	**mono**/therapy MŎN-ō-thĕr-ă-pē *-therapy:* treatment	one therapy *(handwritten)*

(Continued)

Prefix	Term	Meaning
	uni/nucle/ar ū-nĭ-NŪ-klē-ăr *nucle:* nucleus -*ar:* pertaining to	one cell
post- after, behind	**post**/nat/al pōst-NĀ-tăl *nat:* birth -*al:* pertaining to	after birth
pre-, pro- before, in front of	**pre**/nat/al prē-NĀ-tăl *nat:* birth -*al:* pertaining to	before birth
	pro/gnosis prŏg-NŌ-sĭs -*gnosis:* knowing	knowing before
primi- first	**primi**/gravida prī-mĭ-GRĂV-ĭ-dă -*gravida:* pregnant woman	first-time pregnant women
retro- backward, behind	**retro**/version rĕt-rō-VĔR-zhŭn -*version:* turning	turning backward
super- upper, above	**super**/ior soo-PĒ-rē-or -*ior:* pertaining to	pertaining to above

Pronunciation Help	Long Sound	ā in rāte	ē in rēbirth	ī in īsle	ō in ōver	ū in ūnite
	Short Sound	ă in ălone	ĕ in ĕver	ĭ in ĭt	ŏ in nŏt	ŭ in cŭt

The prefix a- is usually used before a consonant. †The prefix an- is usually used before a vowel.

 Competency Verification: Check your answers in Appendix B, Answer Key, pages 361–362. If you are not satisfied with your level of comprehension, review the terms in the table and retake the review.

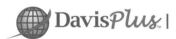 Visit the *Medical Terminology Express* online resource center at *DavisPlus* for an audio exercise of the terms in this table. Other activities are also available to reinforce content.

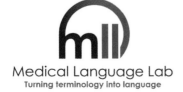
Medical Language Lab
Turning terminology into language

Visit the Medical Language Lab at *medicallanguagelab.com* to enhance your study and reinforce this chapter's word elements with the flash-card activity. We recommend you complete the flash-card activity before continuing with the next section.

Medical Vocabulary Recall

Match the medical term(s) below with the definitions in the numbered list.

appendectomy   gastritis   hyperemesis   neuroma   primigravida
chondromalacia   hepatocele   mastopexy   pelvimetry   rhinoplasty
dysphonia   hemophobia   myopathy   postnatal   tracheotomy

1. **rhinoplasty** is a surgical repair of the nose (to change shape or size).
2. **primigravida** refers to a woman pregnant for the first time.
3. **pelvimetry** is the act of measuring the pelvis.
4. **hepatocele** refers to a hernia or swelling of the liver.
5. **appendectomy** is an excision of the appendix.
6. **hyperemesis** means excessive or above abnormal vomiting.
7. **mastopexy** is a surgical fixation of the breast(s).
8. **gastritis** is an inflammation of the stomach.
9. **myopathy** refers to a disease of muscle(s).
10. **postnatal** pertains to (the period) after birth.
11. **dysphonia** means difficulty in speaking.
12. **tracheotomy** is an incision of the trachea.
13. **neuroma** is a tumor composed of nerve cells.
14. **chondromalacia** means a softening of cartilage.
15. **hemophobia** refers to a fear of blood.

Competency Verification: Check your answers in Appendix B, Answer Key, page 363. If you are not satisfied with your level of comprehension, review the terms in the table and retake the review.

Correct Answers: _____ × **6.67** = _____ **% Score**

kyphoplasty
primigravida
perimetry
nephrocele
appendectomy
hypertensis
mastopexy
gastritis
myopathy
postnatal
dysphonia
tracheotomy
neuroma
chondromalacia
hemophilia

Body Structure

Objectives

Upon completion of this chapter, you will be able to:

- List the levels of organization of the human body.
- Understand the meanings and usage of terms related to direction, planes, quadrants, and regions of the body.
- Describe the standard positions of body placement that are used to perform patient examinations, x-rays, and medical and surgical procedures.
- Identify combining forms, suffixes, and prefixes associated with body structure.
- Recognize, pronounce, build, and spell medical terms and abbreviations associated with body structure.
- Demonstrate your knowledge of this chapter by successfully completing the activities in this chapter.

VOCABULARY PREVIEW

Term	Meaning
anterior ăn-TĒR-ē-or *anter:* anterior, front *-ior:* pertaining to	Toward the front of the body, organ, or structure
anteroposterior ăn-tĕr-ō-pōs-TĒR-ē-or	Pertaining to the front and back of the body or passing from the front to the back of the body
inferior ĭn-FĒ-rē-or *infer:* lower, below *-ior:* pertaining to	Pertaining to below, lower, or toward the tail
scan skăn	Process of using a moving device or a sweeping beam of radiation to produce images of an internal area, organ, or tissue of the body

Pronunciation Help	Long Sound	ā in rāte	ē in rēbirth	ī in īsle	ō in ōver	ū in ūnite
	Short Sound	ă in ălone	ĕ in ĕver	ĭ in ĭt	ŏ in nŏt	ŭ in cŭt

OVERVIEW

This chapter provides an orientation to the body as a whole. Descriptive terms are used to describe the structural organization of the body. Terms that specify direction, position, and location of various organs in relationship to each other are included. Knowledge of these descriptive terms is an essential part of medical terminology and provides a basic foundation for a better understanding of the body system chapters that follow. Most importantly, these terms are included in the language of medicine used by health care providers in the clinical environment.

Levels of Organization

The human body consists of several structural and functional levels of organization. Each higher level increases in complexity because it incorporates the structures and functions of the previous levels. Eventually, all levels contribute to the structure and function of the entire organism. (See Figure 2-1.) The levels of organization from the least to the most complex are the:

- **cellular level**, molecules combine to form cells, the basic structural and functional units of the body
- **tissue level**, groups of cells that work together to perform a specialized function
- **organ level**, structures that are composed of two or more different types of tissue; they have specific functions and usually have recognizable shapes
- **system level**, related organs with a common function; also called *organ-system level*
- **organism level**, collection of body systems that makes up the most complex level: a living human being. All parts of the human body functioning together constitute the total organism.

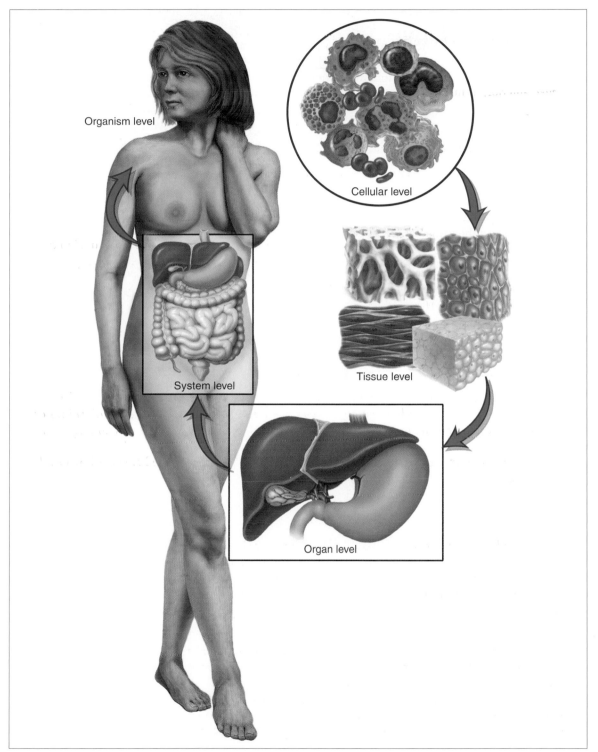

Organism level

Cellular level

Tissue level

System level

Organ level

Figure 2-1 Levels of organization of the human body. The body system illustrated is the digestive system.

Anatomical Position

Health care providers use directional terms to identify accurately the location of diseases in the body. These terms also indicate the position of the body when performing diagnostic, surgical, and therapeutic procedures. However, without a standard position, directional terms are meaningless. That's why health care providers must visualize the body in a standard position. In the field of medicine, the standard reference position of the body is known as the *anatomical position*. In anatomical position, the person stands erect, the eyes look straight ahead, the arms are at the sides of the body with the palms of the hand turned forward, and the feet are parallel to one another and flat on the floor. (See Figure 2-2.)

Directional Terms

Directional terms describe the relationship of one body part to another in reference to the anatomical position. For example, if a person is in anatomical position, the toes are **anterior** to the ankle, and the legs are **inferior** to the trunk. Locate the directional terms *anterior* and *inferior* in Figure 2-2. Physicians

Figure 2-2 Anatomical position, directional terms, and body planes.

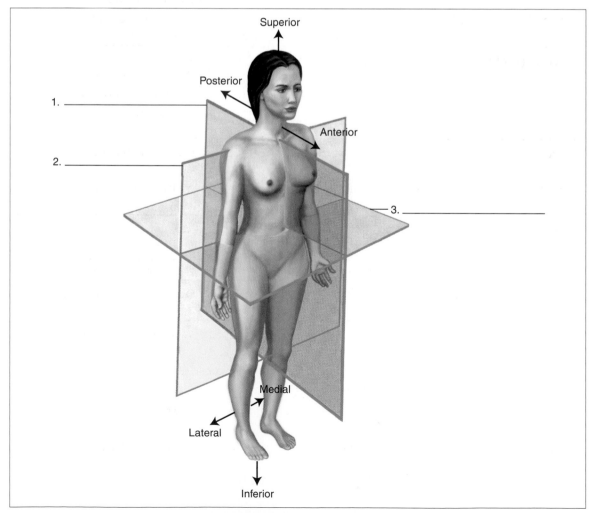

commonly use such terms in medical reports and to communicate with other health care providers and patients. For example, to explain the location, or position, of the liver to a patient who knows where the heart is, you can say that the heart is *superior* to, or *above*, the liver. You can also say the esophagus (throat) is *posterior* to, or *behind*, the trachea (windpipe).

Review Table 2-1 for a comprehensive summary of directional terms along with their definitions. These terms are used to describe the locations of organs in relationship to one another throughout the

TABLE 2-1 **Directional Terms**		
Term	**Definition**	**Example**
Adduction	Movement toward the midline of the body	The arm moves from shoulder height to the side of the body.
Abduction	Movement away from the midline of the body	The arm moves from the side of the body to shoulder height.
Superior (cephalic, cranial)	Above or higher; toward the head	The chest is superior to the abdomen. The heart is superior to the stomach.
Inferior (caudal)	Below or lower; toward the tail	The intestines are inferior to the stomach. The legs are inferior to the trunk.
Anterior (ventral)	Front of the body; toward the front	The navel is on the anterior side of the body. The toes are anterior to the ankle.
Posterior (dorsal)	Back of the body; toward the back	The spinal column is on the posterior side of the body. The heel is posterior to the toes.
Medial	Pertaining to the middle; toward the midline	The mouth is medial to the cheeks.
Lateral	Pertaining to the side; toward the side	The eyes are lateral to the nose.
External	Outside, exterior to	The ribs are external to the lungs.
Internal	Within, interior to	The brain is internal to the skull.
Superficial	Toward or on the surface	A scrape from a fall is a superficial wound.
Deep	Away from the surface	A bullet wound can penetrate deep into the abdomen.
Proximal	Near the point of attachment to the trunk or a structure	The ankle is proximal to the foot.
Distal	Farther from the point of attachment to the trunk or a structure	The toes are distal to the ankle.
Parietal	Pertaining to the outer wall of a cavity	The parietal pleura lines the chest cavity.
Visceral	Pertaining to the organs within a cavity	The visceral pleura covers the lungs.

body. In Table 2-1, opposing terms are presented consecutively to aid memorization. A graphic illustration of some of these terms is also depicted in Figure 2-2.

BODY PLANES

A **plane** is an imaginary flat surface that separates two portions of the body or an organ. Reference of body planes helps you understand the anatomical relationship of one body part to another. They are used to denote the clinical divisions of the abdomen as well as the location of organs contained within the divisions.

Body planes are also used to describe the location of x-ray images. For example, an **anteroposterior** chest x-ray is taken in the frontal (coronal) plane. Before the development of computed tomography (CT) scanning, which displays an image along a transverse plane, conventional x-ray images were on a vertical plane. The dimensions of body irregularities were difficult, if not impossible, to ascertain.

Label the three body planes in Figure 2-2 as you read the following material.

1. **Median plane** — vertical plane that passes through the midline of the body and divides the body or organ into equal right and left sides; also called *midsagittal plane.*
2. **Frontal plane** — plane that divides the body into **anterior** (front) and **posterior** (back) portions; also called *coronal plane.*
3. **Horizontal plane** — plane that separates the body into **superior** (upper) and **inferior** (lower) portions; also called *transverse plane.*

BODY CAVITIES

Body cavities are hollow spaces within the body that help protect, separate, and support internal organs. The body has two main cavities—the **dorsal (**back of the body) and the **ventral** (front of the body). Refer to the cavities in Figure 2-3 as you read the following information. The dorsal cavity is divided into the (1) **cranial** and (2) **spinal** cavities and contains the brain and the spinal cord. The (3) **diaphragm,** a dome-shaped muscle, separates the thoracic and abdominal cavities and plays an important role in breathing.

The **ventral** cavity is subdivided into the (4) **thoracic** cavity, which contains the heart and lungs, and the (5) **abdominopelvic** cavity. The abdominopelvic cavity is further subdivided into the (6) **abdominal** and (7) **pelvic** cavities and contains organs of the digestive and reproductive systems. Clinicians use the cavities to locate internal organs and to identify abnormalities within the cavities.

QUADRANTS AND REGIONS

To describe the location of the many abdominal and pelvic organs more easily, anatomists and clinicians use two methods of dividing the abdominopelvic cavity into smaller areas. These divisions are known as **quadrants** and **regions.** The nine-region division is more widely used for anatomical studies, and quadrants are more commonly used by clinicians to describe the site of abdominopelvic pain, tumor, or other abnormalities.

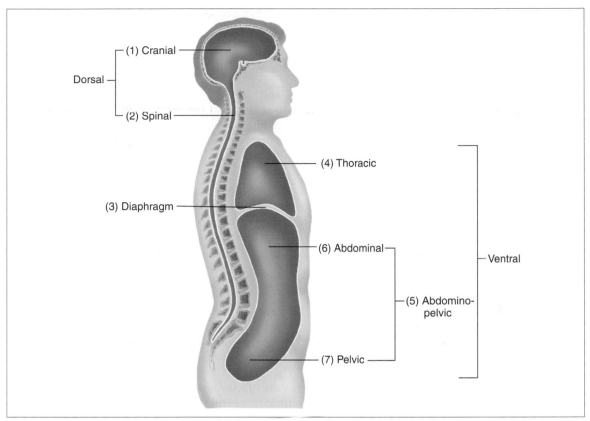

Figure 2-3 Body cavities, with the ventral (anterior) cavities located in the front of the body and the dorsal (posterior) cavities located in the back of the body.

Abdominopelvic Quadrants

Four quadrants identify the placement of internal organs in the abdominopelvic cavity. Generally, quadrants are used to report the findings of a clinical examination or an exploratory surgery. For example, a physician may describe a patient's abdominal pain in the left upper quadrant (LUQ). This quadrant indicates different clinical possibilities than if the pain were in the right lower quadrant (RLQ). Quadrants are also used to describe the location of surgical procedures, incision sites, or tumors.

Use the following abbreviations to label the quadrants in Figure 2-4A.

1. **Right upper quadrant (RUQ)** — contains the right lobe of the liver, the gallbladder, part of the pancreas, and part of the small and large intestine.
2. **Right lower quadrant (RLQ)** — contains part of the small and large intestine, the appendix, the right ovary, the right fallopian tube, and the right ureter.
3. **Left upper quadrant (LUQ)** — contains the left lobe of the liver, the stomach, the spleen, part of the pancreas, and part of the small and large intestine.
4. **Left lower quadrant (LLQ)** — contains part of the small and large intestine, the left ovary, the left fallopian tube, and the left ureter.

Abdominopelvic Regions

The abdominopelvic cavity can be divided into nine regions. Quadrants are normally used to describe and diagnose conditions, whereas region designations are used mainly to indicate the location of internal organs. For example, the liver is located in the epigastric and right hypochondriac regions.

Identify the nine regions in Figure 2-4B as you read the following information.

1. **Right hypochondriac** — upper right region located under the cartilage of the ribs.
2. **Left hypochondriac** — upper left region located under the cartilage of the ribs.
3. **Right lumbar** — middle right region located near the waist.
4. **Left lumbar** — middle left region located near the waist.
5. **Right iliac** — lower right region located near the groin (also called *right inguinal region*).
6. **Left iliac** — lower left region located near the groin (also called *left inguinal region*).
7. **Epigastric** — middle region located above the stomach.
8. **Umbilical** — middle region located in the area of the umbilicus, or navel.
9. **Hypogastric** — lower middle region located below the stomach and umbilical region.

POSITIONING FOR EXAMINATIONS AND TREATMENTS

To provide a comfortable environment for patients during an examination, surgery, or therapeutic treatment, it is customary to expose only the body part that is being examined or treated. Draping

Figure 2-4 Quadrants and regions. (A) Four quadrants are formed when an imaginary horizontal and vertical line cross at the umbilicus (belly button). (B) Nine regions are formed with two imaginary horizontal and vertical lines that form a square around the umbilicus.

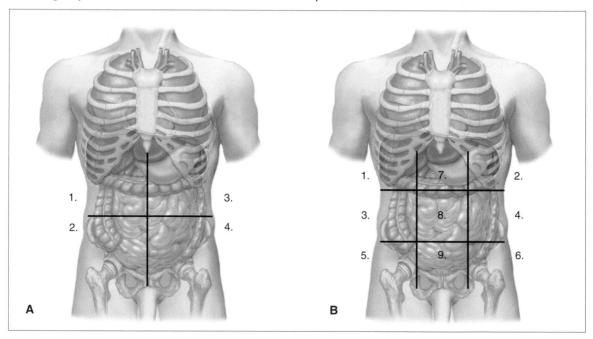

sheets are used to cover the body while the patient lies on the examining table as well as before surgery.

Various body positions are employed during medical examinations, x-rays, surgeries, and therapeutic treatments. The position used depends on the procedure or treatment and the sex of the patient. Seven basic patient positions used for medical examinations, therapeutic treatments, and surgeries are illustrated in Figure 2-5 and discussed below. These terms are found in different types of medical reports, including the physical examination, radiographic report, and operative report:

1. **Knee-chest position.** The patient is assisted into a kneeling position with the buttocks elevated. The head and chest are on the table, and the arms are extended above the head and flexed at the elbow. This position facilitates examination of the rectum.

2. **Lithotomy position.** The patient is assisted into a **supine** (lying on the back) position. The legs are sharply flexed at the knees, and the feet are placed in stirrups. This position is used for vaginal examination and the Papanicolaou (Pap) test.

3. **Dorsal recumbent position.** The patient is assisted into a supine position. The legs are sharply flexed at the knees, and the feet are placed on the table. This position is used to examine the vagina and rectum in a female patient and the rectum in a male patient.

4. **Sims position.** The patient is assisted into a side-lying position on the left side. The left arm is placed behind the body, and the right arm is moved forward and flexed at the elbow. Both legs are flexed at the knee, but the right leg is sharply flexed and positioned next to the left leg, which is slightly flexed. This position is used to examine the vagina and rectum in a female patient and the rectum in a male patient. Sims position is also used to administer an enema.

5. **Prone position.** The patient is assisted to lie flat on the abdomen with the head turned slightly to the side. The arms are extended above the head or alongside the body. Prone position is used to examine the back, spine, and lower extremities.

6. **Fowler position.** The patient is assisted into a semisitting position. The head of the examination table is tilted to produce a 45- to 60-degree angle with the patient's knees bent or not bent. An angle of 45 degrees or more is considered *high Fowler position*; an angle of approximately 30 degrees is considered *semi-Fowler position*. This position promotes lung expansion. It is used if the patient has difficulty breathing.

7. **Supine position.** The patient is assisted to lie flat on the back with arms at the sides. This position is used to examine the chest, heart, abdomen, and extremities. It is also used to examine the head and neck as well as in certain neurological reflex testing.

Two other commonly used positions are the erect standing position and Trendelenburg position. The **erect standing position,** also referred to as the *anatomical position*, is illustrated in Figure 2-2. In anatomical position, and depending on the type of examination, the patient may be instructed to bend over, walk, or move specific body parts in a particular manner. The physician observes these movements to determine the patient's level of coordination, strength, flexibility, balance, and range of motion. In the **Trendelenburg position**, the patient is lying flat on the back, and the entire examination table is tilted with the head of the table down. This position is used for therapeutic treatments, such as postural drainage in patients who have thick respiratory secretions.

 Competency Verification: Check your labeling of Figure 2-2, and Figure 2-4A in Appendix B, Answer Key, page 363.

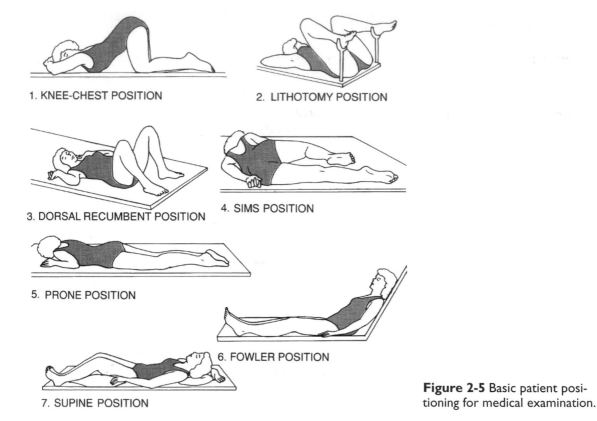

1. KNEE-CHEST POSITION

2. LITHOTOMY POSITION

3. DORSAL RECUMBENT POSITION

4. SIMS POSITION

5. PRONE POSITION

6. FOWLER POSITION

7. SUPINE POSITION

Figure 2-5 Basic patient positioning for medical examination.

ALERT: An extensive self-paced anatomy and physiology multimedia review is included in *TermPlus*, a powerful, interactive CD-ROM program that can be purchased separately from F.A. Davis Company.

MEDICAL WORD BUILDING

Constructing medical words using word elements (combining forms, suffixes, and prefixes) related to body structure will enhance your understanding of those terms and reinforce your ability to use terms correctly.

Combining Forms

Begin your study of body structure terminology by reviewing associated combining forms (CFs) as outlined in the following tables. This introductory study of CFs provides an understanding of the construction and meanings of medical terms related to body regions and body structures as well as the use of directional terms. You may also refer to *Appendix A: Glossary of Medical Word Elements* to complete this exercise. The first one is completed for you.

Combining Form	Meaning	Medical Word	Meaning
Body Regions			
abdomin/o	abdomen	**abdomin/al** (ăb-DŎM-ĭ-năl) *-al:* pertaining to	*pertaining to the abdomen*
caud/o	tail	**caud/ad** (KAW-dăd) *-ad:* toward	toward the tail
cephal/o	head	**cephal/ad** (SĔF-ă-lăd) *-ad:* toward	toward the head
cervic/o	neck; cervix uteri (neck of uterus)	**cervic/al** (SĔR-vĭ-kăl) *-al:* pertaining to	pertaining to the neck
crani/o	cranium (skull)	**crani/al** (KRĀ-nē-ăl) *-al:* pertaining to	pertaining to the head
gastr/o	stomach	**gastr/ic** (GĂS-trĭk) *-ic:* pertaining to	pertaining to the stomach
ili/o	ilium (lateral, flaring portion of the hip bone)	**ili/ac** (ĬL-ē-ăk) *-ac:* pertaining to	pertaining to the ilium
inguin/o	groin	**inguin/al** (ĬNG-gwĭ-năl) *-al:* pertaining to	pertaining to the groin
lumb/o	loins (lower back)	**lumb/ar** (LŬM-băr) *-ar:* pertaining to	pertaining to the lower back
pelv/i*	pelvis	**pelv/i/meter** (pĕl-VĬM-ĕ-tĕr) *-meter:* instrument for measuring	instrument for measuring pelvis
pelv/o		**pelv/ic** (PĔL-vĭc) *-ic:* pertaining to	pertaining to the pelvis
spin/o	spine	**spin/al** (SPĪ-năl) *-al:* pertaining to	pertaining to the spine

*The *i* in *pelv/i/meter* is an exception to the rule of using the connecting vowel o.

(Continued)

Combining Form	Meaning	Medical Word	Meaning
Body Regions			
thorac/o	chest	**thorac/ic** (thō-RĂS-ĭk) -*ic*: pertaining to	Pertaining to the chest
umbilic/o	umbilicus, navel	**umbilic/al** (ŭm-BĬL-ĭ-kăl) -*al*: pertaining to	pertaining to the naval
Directional Terms			
anter/o	anterior, front	**anter/ior** (ăn-TĔR-ē-or) -*ior*: pertaining to	pertaining to the front
dist/o	far, farthest	**dist/al** (DĬS-tăl) -*al*: pertaining to	pertaining to the farthest
dors/o	back (of the body)	**dors/al** (DOR-săl) -*al*: pertaining to	Pertaining to the back
infer/o	lower, below	**infer/ior** (ĭn-FĒ-rē-or) -*ior*: pertaining to	pertaing to below
later/o	side, to one side	**later/al** (LĂT-ĕr-ăl) -*al*: pertaining to	pertaining to the side
medi/o	middle	**medi/al** (MĒ-dē-ăl) -*al*: pertaining to	pertaining to the middle
poster/o	back (of the body), behind, posterior	**poster/ior** (pŏs-TĔR-ē-or) -*ior*: pertaining to	~~to~~ pertaining to the back
proxim/o	near, nearest	**proxim/al** (PRŎK-sĭm-ăl) -*al*: pertaining to	pertaining to the nearest
super/o**	upper, above	**super/ior** (soo-PĒ-rē-or) -*ior*: pertaining to	pertaining to above
ventr/o	belly, belly side	**ventr/al** (VĔN-trăl) -*al*: pertaining to	pertaing to the belly

**The CF *super/o* can also be used as prefix.

Combining Form	Meaning	Medical Word	Meaning
Other Combining Forms Related to Body Structure			
cyt/o	cell	**cyt**/o/**meter** (sī-TŎM-ĕ-tĕr) *-meter:* instrument for measuring	*instrument for measuring cells*
hist/o	tissue	**hist**/o/**lysis** (hĭs-TŎL-ĭ-sĭs) *-lysis:* separation; destruction; loosening	*destruction of tissue*
nucle/o	nucleus	**nucle**/**ar** (NŪ-klē-ăr) *-ar:* pertaining to	*pertaining to the nucleus*
radi/o	radiation, x-ray; radius (lower arm bone on the thumb side)	**radi**/o/**graphy** (rā-dē-ŎG-ră-fē) *-graphy:* process of recording	*Process of recording an x-ray*

Suffixes and Prefixes

In the following table, suffixes and prefixes are listed alphabetically, and other word parts are defined as needed. Review the medical word and study the elements that make up the term. Then complete the meaning of the medical words in the right-hand column. You may also refer to *Appendix A: Glossary of Medical Word Elements* to complete this exercise.

Word Element	Meaning	Medical Words	Meaning
Suffixes			
-ad	toward	medi/**ad** (MĒ-dē-ăd) *medi/o:* middle	*toward the middle*
-al	pertaining to	coron/**al** (kŏ-RŌN-ăl) *coron:* heart	*Pertaining to the heart*
-algia	pain	cost/**algia** (kŏs-TĂL-jē-ă) *cost:* ribs	*pain in ribs*
-dynia		thorac/o/**dynia** (thō-răk-ō-DĬN-ē-ă) *thorac/o:* chest	*Chest pain*

(Continued)

Word Element	Meaning	Medical Words	Meaning
Suffixes			
-gen	forming, producing, origin	path/o/**gen** (PĂTH-ō-jĕn) *path/o:* disease	*disease forming*
-genesis		carcin/o/**genesis** (kăr-sĭ-nō-JĔN-ĕ-sĭs) *carcin/o:* cancer	*cancer forming*
-logist	specialist in the study of	hist/o/**logist** (hĭs-TŎL-ō-jĭst) *hist/o:* tissue	*tissue specialist*
-logy	study of	eti/o/**logy** (ē-tē-ŎL-ō-jē) *eti/o:* cause	*study of cause*
-lysis	separation; destruction; loosening	cyt/o/**lysis** (sī-TŎL-ĭ-sĭs) *cyt/o:* cell	*destruction of a cell*
-meter	instrument used to measure	therm/o/**meter** (thĕr-MŎM-ĕ-tĕr) *therm/o:* heat	*instrument used to measure heat*
-plasia	formation, growth	hyper/**plasia** (hī-pĕr-PLĀ-zē-ă) *hyper-:* excessive, above normal	*excessive growth*
-toxic	poison	hepat/o/**toxic** (HĔP-ă-tō-tŏk-sĭk) *hepat/o:* liver	*poison to liver*
Prefixes			
bi-	two	**bi**/later/al (bī-LĂT-ĕr-ăl) *later:* side, to one side *-al:* pertaining to	*pertaining to two sides*
epi-	above, on	**epi**/gastr/ic (ĕp-ĭ-GĂS-trĭk) *gastr:* stomach *-ic:* pertaining to	*pertaining to above the stomach*
infra-	below, under	**infra**/cost/al (ĭn-fră-KŎS-tăl) *cost:* ribs *-al:* pertaining to	*pertaining to below the ribs*

Word Element	Meaning	Medical Words	Meaning
Prefixes			
trans-	across, through	**trans**/vagin/al (trăns-VĂJ-ĭn-ăl) *vagin:* vagina —*al:* pertaining to	*Pertaining to across the vagina*

 Competency Verification: Check your answers in Appendix B, Answer Key, pages 363–365. If you are not satisfied with your level of comprehension, review the terms in the table and retake the review.

DavisPlus | Visit the *Medical Terminology Express* online resource center at *DavisPlus* for an audio exercise of the terms in this table. Other activities are also available to reinforce content.

Medical Language Lab
Turning terminology into language

Visit the Medical Language Lab at *medicallanguagelab.com* to enhance your study and reinforce this chapter's word elements with the flash-card activity. We recommend you complete the flash-card activity before continuing with the next section.

Medical Terminology Word Building

In this section, combine the word parts you have learned to construct medical terms related to body structures. The first one is an example completed for you.

Use **caud/o (tail)** to build words that mean:

1. toward the tail *caudad*

2. pertaining to the tail _Caudal_

Use **thorac/o (chest)** to build words that mean:

3. surgical puncture of the chest _thoracocentesis_

4. pertaining to the chest _thoracic_

5. surgical repair of the chest _thoracopexy_

Use **gastr/o (stomach)** to build words that mean:

6. pertaining to the stomach _gastric_

7. surgical repair of the stomach _gastropexy_

Use **pelv/i (pelvis)** to build words that mean:

8. pertaining to the pelvis _pelvic_

9. instrument to measure the pelvis _pelvimeter_

Use *abdomin/o* (**abdomen**) to build words that mean:

10. pertaining to the abdomen _abdominal_

11. surgical repair of the abdomen _abdominopexy_

Use *crani/o* (**cranium [skull]**) to build words that mean:

12. pertaining to the cranium (skull) _cranial_

13. surgical repair of the cranium (skull) _craniopexy_

Use *medi/o* (**middle**) to build words that mean:

14. pertaining to the middle _medial_

15. toward the middle _mediad_

Use *cyt/o* (**cell**) to build words that mean:

16. study of cells _cytology_

17. specialist in the study of cells _cytologist_

18. destruction, dissolution, or separation of a cell _cytolysis_

Use *hist/o* (**tissue**) to build words that mean:

19. study of tissues _histology_

20. specialist in the study of tissues _histologist_

Competency Verification: Check your answers in Appendix B, Answer Key, on page 365. Review material that you did not answer correctly.

Correct Answers: _____ × 5 = _____ %

MEDICAL VOCABULARY

The following tables consist of selected terms related to the body as a whole. Recognizing and learning these terms will help you understand the connection between diseases and diagnostic procedures. Word analysis for selected terms is also provided.

Diseases and Conditions

adhesion ăd-HĒ-zhŭn	Band of scar tissue binding anatomical surfaces that are normally separate from each other (See Figure 2-6.)
inflammation ĭn-flă-MĀ-shun	Protective response of body tissues to irritation, infection, or allergy
sepsis SĔP-sĭs	Body's inflammatory response to infection in which there is fever, elevated heart and respiratory rates, and low blood pressure

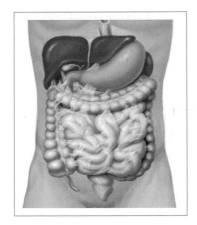

Figure 2-6 Abdominal adhesions. Adhesions most commonly form in the abdomen after abdominal surgery, inflammation, or injury.

Diagnostic Procedures

endoscopy
ĕn-DŎS-kō-pē
endo-: in, within
-scopy: visual examination

Visual examination of the interior of organs and cavities with a specialized lighted instrument called an *endoscope* (See Figure 2-7.)

fluoroscopy
floo-or-ŎS-kō-pē
fluor/o: luminous,
        fluorescence
-scopy: visual examination

Radiographic procedure that uses a fluorescent screen instead of a photographic plate to produce a visual image from x-rays that pass through the patient, resulting in continuous imaging of the motion of internal structures and immediate serial images

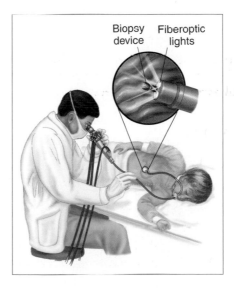

Biopsy device   Fiberoptic lights

Figure 2-7 Endoscopy.

magnetic resonance imaging (MRI) măg-NĔT-ĭc RĔZ-ĕn-ăns ĬM-ĭj-ĭng	Radiographic technique that uses electromagnetic energy to produce multiplanar cross-sectional images of the body (See Figure 2-8E.)
nuclear scan NŪ-klē-ăr	Diagnostic technique that produces an image of an organ or area by recording the concentration of a radiopharmaceutical substance called a *tracer*, usually introduced into the body by ingestion, inhalation, or injection (See Figure 2-8C.)

radiography
rā-dē-ŎG-ră-fē
  radi/o: radiation, x-ray; radius (lower arm bone on the thumb side)
  -graphy: process of recording
	Production of captured shadow images on photographic film through the action of ionizing radiation passing through the body from an external source (See Figure 2-8A.)

Figure 2-8 Medical imaging. (A) Chest radiography. (B) Ultrasonography of blood flow with color indicating direction. (C) Nuclear scan of liver and spleen. (D) CT scan of eye (lateral view). (E) MRI scan of head. (F) PET scan of brain.

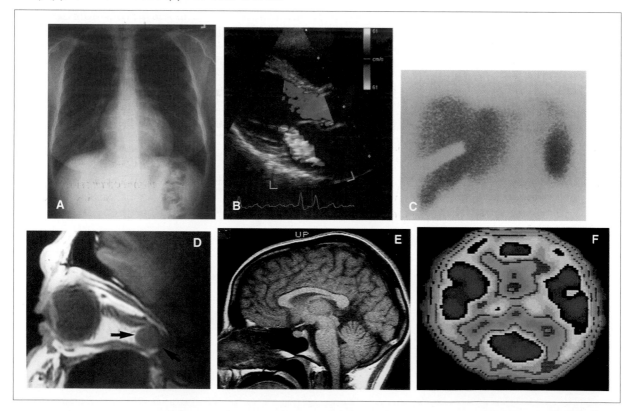

radiopharmaceutical
rā-dē-ō-fărm-ă-SŪ-tĭ-kăl
    radi/o: radiation,
          x-ray; radius
          (lower arm
          bone on
          thumb side)
pharmaceutic: drug,
          medicine
    -al: pertaining to
	Drug that contains a radioactive substance, which travels to an area or a specific organ that will be scanned

tomography
tō-MŎG-ră-fē
    tom/o: to cut
  -graphy: process of
         recording
	Radiographic technique that produces a film representing a detailed cross-section of tissue structure at a predetermined depth

computed tomography (CT) scan
kŏm-PŪ-tĕd tō-MŎG-ră-fē
    tom/o: to cut
  -graphy: process of
         recording
	Narrow beam of x-rays with a contrast medium (provides more detail) or without a contrast medium that targets a specific organ or body area to produce multiple cross-sectional images for detecting pathological conditions such as tumors or metastases (See Figure 2-8D.)

positron emission tomography (PET) scan
PŎZ-ĭ-trŏn ē-MĬSH-ŭn tō-MŎG-ră-fe
    tom/o: to cut
  -graphy: process of
         recording
	Nuclear imaging study that combines CT with radiopharmaceuticals to produce a cross-sectional image of radioactive dispersions in a section of the body to reveal the areas where the radiopharmaceutical is being metabolized and where there is a deficiency in metabolism; useful in evaluating Alzheimer disease and epilepsy (See Figure 2-8F.)

single-photon emission computed tomography (SPECT) scan
SĬNG-gŭl FŌ-tŏn ē-MĬ-shŭn cŏm-PŪ-tĕd tō-MŎG-ră-fē
    tom/o: to cut
  -graphy: process of
         recording
	Nuclear imaging study that scans organs after injection of a radioactive tracer and employs a specialized gamma camera that detects emitted radiation to produce a three-dimensional image from a composite of numerous views; used to show how blood flows to an organ and helps determine how well the organ is functioning

(Continued)

ultrasonography (US)
ŭl-tră-sŏn-ŎG-ră-fē
  -ultra: excess, beyond
   son/o: sound
 -graphy: process of
      recording
	Imaging technique that uses high-frequency sound waves (ultrasound) that bounce off body tissues and are recorded to produce an image of an internal organ or tissue (See Figure 2-8B.)

Pronunciation Help	Long Sound	ā in rāte	ē in rēbirth	ī in īsle	ō in ōver	ū in ūnite
	Short Sound	ă in ălone	ĕ in ĕver	ĭ in ĭt	ŏ in nŏt	ŭ in cŭt

Medical Vocabulary Recall

Match the medical terms below with the definitions in the numbered list.

adhesion   fluoroscopy   PET   SPECT

CT scan   inflammation   radiography   tomography

endoscopy   MRI   radiopharmaceutical   US

endoscope   nuclear scan   sepsis

1. **CT scan** _____ uses a narrow beam of x-rays to generate multiple views of a specific organ or body area in cross-sectional images.

2. **fluoroscopy** _____ directs x-rays through the body to a fluorescent screen to view organs in motion, such as the digestive tract and heart.

3. **US** _____ employs high-frequency sound waves to produce images of internal structures of the body.

4. **MRI** _____ employs magnetic energy to produce cross-sectional images.

5. **PET** _____ is a type of nuclear scan that uses radiopharmaceuticals to reveal areas where the radiopharmaceutical is metabolized.

6. **endoscope** _____ is a lighted instrument to view interior of organs and cavities.

7. **inflammation** _____ is the body's protective response to irritation, infection, or allergy.

8. **SPECT** _____ is similar to PET, but employs a specialized gamma camera that detects emitted radiation to produce a three-dimensional image.

9. **tomography** _____ produces a film representing a detailed cross-section of tissue structure at a predetermined depth; three types include CT, PET, and SPECT.

10. **radiopharmaceutical** _____ is a drug that contains a radioactive substance that travels to an area or a specific organ to be scanned.

11. **endoscopy** _____ is a procedure to enable visualization of the interior of organs and cavities with a lighted instrument.

12. <u>nuclear scan</u> employs a tracer to diagnose a disease.

13. <u>adhesion</u> is a band of scar tissue that binds anatomical surfaces that normally are separate from each other.

14. <u>radiography</u> is production of shadow images on photographic film.

15. <u>sepsis</u> is the body's inflammatory response to infection.

Competency Verification: Check your answers in Appendix B, Answer Key, on page 365. Review material that you did not answer correctly.

Correct Answers: _____ × **6.67** = _____ %

Pronunciation and Spelling

Use the following list to practice correct pronunciation and spelling of medical terms. First practice the pronunciation aloud. Then write the correct spelling of the term. The first word is completed for you.

Pronunciation	Spelling
1. bī-LĂT-ĕr-ăl	*bilateral*
2. ăd-HĒ-zhŭn	adhesion
3. SĔR-vĭ-kăl	cervical
4. KRĀ-nē-ăl	cranial
5. DĬS-tăl	distal
6. ĕn-DŎS-kō-pē	endoscopy
7. floo-or-ŎS-kō-pē	fluoroscopy
8. ĭn-flă-MĀ-shun	inflammation
9. LŬM-băr	lumbar
10. rā-dē-ō-fărm-ă-SŪ-tĭ-kăl	radiopharmaceutical
11. rā-dē-ŎG-ră-fē	radiography
12. SĔP-sĭs	sepsis
13. sĭg-MOY-dō-skōp	sigmoidoscope
14. SPĔK-ū-lŭm	speculum
15. tō-MŎG-ră-fē	tomography

Competency Verification: Check your answers in Appendix B, Answer Key, on page 365. Review material that you did not answer correctly.

Correct Answers: _____ × **6.67** = _____ %

ABBREVIATIONS

This section introduces abbreviations associated with body structure and radiology.

Abbreviation	Meaning	Abbreviation	Meaning
Body Structure and Related			
ant	anterior	LLQ	left lower quadrant
AP	anteroposterior	LUQ	left upper quadrant
Bx, bx	biopsy	PA	posteroanterior
CXR	chest x-ray; chest radiograph	RLQ	right lower quadrant
LAT, lat	lateral	RUQ	right upper quadrant
Radiology			
CT	computed tomography	PET	positron emission tomography
CXR	chest x-ray, chest radiograph	US	ultrasound; ultrasonography
MRI	magnetic resonance imaging	SPECT	single-photon emission computed tomography

Demonstrate What You Know!

To evaluate your understanding of body regions and directional terms, match each term in Column A with its meaning in Column B.

Column A

1. umbilical _i_
2. iliac _n_
3. cervical _j_
4. cephalad _h_
5. cranial _a_
6. epigastric _m_
7. thoracic _c_
8. inguinal _b_
9. anterior _d_
10. proximal _e_
11. lateral _f_
12. posterior _o_
13. caudad _l_
14. ventral _f_
15. distal _g_

Column B

a. pertaining to the skull
b. pertaining to the groin
c. pertaining to the chest
d. toward the front (of the body)
e. nearest the point of attachment
f. pertaining to the belly side or front of the body
g. farthest from the point of attachment
h. toward the head
i. middle region located near the navel
j. pertaining to the neck
k. pertaining to the side
l. toward the tail
m. middle region located above the stomach
n. pertaining to the ilium
o. pertaining to the back (of body), behind

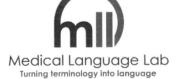

Medical Language Lab
Turning terminology into language

If you are not satisfied with your retention level of the body structure chapter, visit *DavisPlus* Student Online Resource Center and the Medical Language Lab at *medicallanguagelab.com* to complete the website activities linked to this chapter.

Integumentary System

Objectives

Upon completion of this chapter, you will be able to:

- Describe types of medical treatment provided by dermatologists.
- List three primary functions of the skin.
- Identify the two layers and the three accessory organs of the skin.
- Identify three underlying structures of the skin.
- Identify combining forms, suffixes, and prefixes associated with the integumentary system.
- Recognize, pronounce, build, and spell medical terms and abbreviations associated with the integumentary system.
- Demonstrate your knowledge by successfully completing the activities in this chapter.

VOCABULARY PREVIEW

Term	Meaning
cutaneous kū-TĀ-nē-ŭs *cutane:* skin *-ous:* pertaining to	Pertaining to the skin
lesion LĒ-zhŭn	Wound, injury, or pathological change in body tissue
systemic sĭs-TĔM-ĭk	Pertaining to a system or the whole body rather than a localized area
therapeutic thĕr-ă-PŪ-tĭk *therapeut:* treatment *-ic:* pertaining to	Pertaining to treating, remediating, or curing a disorder or disease

Pronunciation Help	Long Sound	ā in rāte	ē in rēbirth	ī in īsle	ō in ōver	ū in ūnite
	Short Sound	ă in ălone	ĕ in ĕver	ĭ in ĭt	ŏ in nŏt	ŭ in cŭt

MEDICAL SPECIALTY OF DERMATOLOGY

The integumentary system is associated with the medical specialty of **dermatology**. Physicians who specialize in treating integumentary disorders are called **dermatologists**. These specialists focus on diseases of the skin and the relationship of a **cutaneous lesion** to a **systemic** disease.

Various surgical and **therapeutic** procedures are used to treat integumentary disorders, including skin transplantations, ultraviolet light therapy, and various medications. The dermatologist's practice includes treatment of skin disorders caused by internal diseases of the body. Examples are pressure ulcers that result from poor circulation and skin lesions that result from diabetes or syphilis. The dermatologist's scope of practice also includes management of skin cancers, moles, and other skin tumors. The dermatologist employs various techniques to enhance and correct cosmetic skin defects and prescribes measures to maintain healthy skin.

INTEGUMENTARY SYSTEM QUICK STUDY

The term **integument**, also known as **skin**, is derived from the Latin word *integumentum*, which means a *covering*. The skin is the largest organ of the body, consisting of several kinds of tissues that are structurally arranged to function together. Its elaborate system of distinct tissues includes glands that produce several types of secretions, nerves that transmit impulses, and blood vessels that help regulate body temperature. The skin is essentially composed of two layers:

1. The **epidermis,** the outer layer of the skin, forms the protective covering of the body. It is thinnest on the eyelids and thickest on the palms of the hands. The epidermis is also the nonsensitive layer of the skin and has neither a blood supply nor a nerve supply (avascular). It is dependent on the dermis' network of capillaries for nourishment.

2. The **dermis,** the inner layer of the skin, is rich with blood vessels (vascular), nerve endings, sebaceous (oil) and sudoriferous (sweat) glands, and hair follicles. The subcutaneous tissue, which lies just beneath the dermis, binds the dermis to underlying structures. The main functions of the subcutaneous tissue are to protect the tissues and organs underneath it and to prevent heat loss.

Anatomical structures known as the accessory organs of the skin are also located within the dermis. They include nails, sweat glands, and sebaceous glands. (See *Integumentary System*, below.)

ALERT: An extensive self-paced anatomy and physiology multimedia review is included in *TermPlus,* a powerful, interactive CD-ROM program that can be purchased separately from F.A. Davis Company.

MEDICAL WORD BUILDING

Constructing medical words using word elements (combining forms, suffixes, and prefixes) related to the integumentary system will enhance your understanding of those terms and reinforce your ability to use terms correctly.

Combining Forms

Begin your study of integumentary terminology by reviewing the organs and their associated combining forms (CFs), which are illustrated in the figure *Integumentary System* that follows.

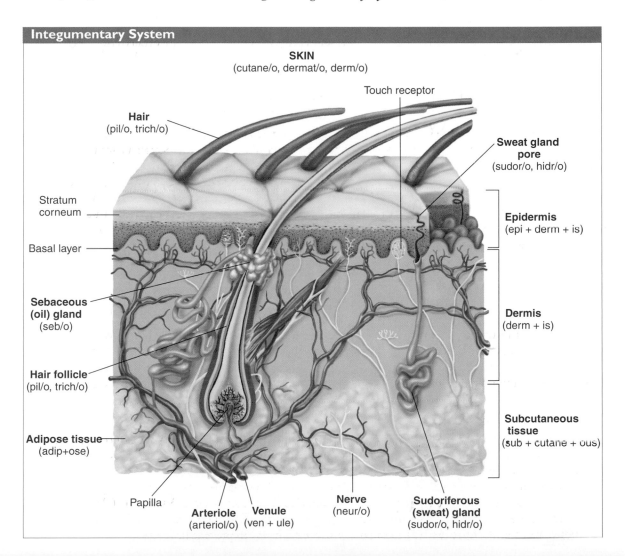

Integumentary System

SKIN
(cutane/o, dermat/o, derm/o)

Touch receptor

Hair
(pil/o, trich/o)

Sweat gland pore
(sudor/o, hidr/o)

Stratum corneum

Epidermis
(epi + derm + is)

Basal layer

Sebaceous (oil) gland
(seb/o)

Dermis
(derm + is)

Hair follicle
(pil/o, trich/o)

Subcutaneous tissue
(sub + cutane + ous)

Adipose tissue
(adip+ose)

Papilla

Arteriole
(arteriol/o)

Venule
(ven + ule)

Nerve
(neur/o)

Sudoriferous (sweat) gland
(sudor/o, hidr/o)

In the table that follows, CFs are listed alphabetically, and other word parts are defined as needed. Review the medical word and study the elements that make up the term. Then complete the meaning of the medical words in the right-hand column. The first one is completed for you. You may also refer to *Appendix A: Glossary of Medical Word Elements* to complete this exercise.

Combining Form	Meaning	Medical Word	Meaning
adip/o	fat	adip/o/cele (ĂD-ĭ-pō-sēl) *-cele:* hernia, swelling	*hernia containing fat or fatty tissue*
lip/o	fat	lip/o/cyte (LĬP-ō-sīt) *-cyte:* cell	fat cell
steat/o	fat	steat/oma (stē-ă-TŌ-mă) *-oma:* tumor	tumor of a fat cell
cutane/o	skin	sub/cutane/ous (sŭb-kū-TĀ-nē-ŭs) *sub-:* under, below *-ous:* pertaining to	Pertaining to below the Skin
dermat/o	Skin	dermat/o/logist (dĕr-mă-TŎL-ō-jĭst) *-logist:* specialist in the study of	Skin Specialist
derm/o	Skin	hypo/derm/ic (hī-pō-DĔR-mĭk) *hypo-:* under, below, deficient *-ic:* pertaining to	Pertaining to below the Skin
cyan/o	blue	cyan/osis (sī-ă-NŌ-sĭs) *-osis:* abnormal condition; increase (used primarily with blood cells)	blue Abnormal condition
erythem/o	red	erythem/a (ĕr-ĭ-THĒ-mă) *-a:* noun ending	reddening
erythemat/o	red	erythemat/ous (ĕr-ĭ-THĔM-ă-tŭs) *-ous:* pertaining to	Pertaining to red
erythr/o	red	erythr/o/cyte (ĕ-RĬTH-rō-sīt) *-cyte:* cell	red cell

Combining Form	Meaning	Medical Word	Meaning
hidr/o*	sweat	**hidr**/osis (hī-DRŌ-sĭs) -*osis:* abnormal condition; increase (used primarily with blood cells)	*increased sweating*
sudor/o	*sweat*	**sudor**/esis (sū-dō-RĒ-sĭs) -*esis:* condition	*sweat condition*
ichthy/o	dry, scaly	**ichthy**/osis (ĭk-thē-Ō-sĭs) -*osis:* abnormal condition; increase (used primarily with blood cells)	*dry abnormal condition*
kerat/o	horny tissue; hard; cornea	**kerat**/osis (kĕr-ă-TŌ-sĭs) -*osis:* abnormal condition; increase (used primarily with blood cells)	*abnormal condition of cornea*
melan/o	black	**melan**/oma (mĕl-ă-NŌ-mă) -*oma:* tumor	*black tumor*
myc/o	fungus (plural, *fungi*)	dermat/o/**myc**/osis (dĕr-mă-tō-mī-KŌ-sĭs) *dermat/o:* skin -*osis:* abnormal condition; increase (used primarily with blood cells)	*abnormal fungal condition of skin*
onych/o	nail	**onych**/o/malacia (ŏn-ĭ-kō-mă-LĀ-shē-ă) -*malacia:* softening	*nail softening*
pil/o	hair	**pil**/o/nid/al (pī-lō-NĪ-dăl) *nid:* nest -*al:* pertaining to	*pertaining to hair*
trich/o	*hair*	**trich**/o/pathy (trĭk-ŎP-ă-thē) -*pathy:* disease	*hair disease*

*Do not mistake hidr/o (sweat) for hydr/o (water).

(Continued)

Combining Form	Meaning	Medical Word	Meaning
scler/o	hardening; sclera (white of eye)	**scler/o**/derma (sklĕr-ō-DĔR-mă) *-derma:* skin	*hardening of skin*
seb/o	sebum, sebaceous	**seb/o**/rrhea (sĕb-or-Ē-ă) *-rrhea:* discharge, flow	*sebaceous discharge*
squam/o	scale	**squam**/ous (SKWĀ-mŭs) *-ous:* pertaining to	*pertaining to scale*
therm/o	heat	**therm**/al (THĔR-măl) *-al:* pertaining to	*pertaining to heat*
xer/o	dry	**xer/o**/derma (zē-rō-DĔR-mă) *-derma:* skin	*dry skin*

Suffixes and Prefixes

In the table that follows, suffixes and prefixes are listed alphabetically, and other word parts are defined as needed. Review the medical word and study the elements that make up the term. Then complete the meaning of the medical words in the right-hand column. You may also refer to *Appendix A: Glossary of Medical Word Elements* to complete this exercise.

Word Element	Meaning	Medical Word	Meaning
Suffixes			
-cyte	cell	leuk/o/**cyte** (LOO-kō-sīt) *leuk/o:* white	*white cell*
-derma	skin	py/o/**derma** (pī-ō-DĔR-mă) *py/o:* pus	*skin infection w/ pus*
-oma	tumor	carcin/**oma** (KĂR-sĭ-NŌ-mă) *carcin:* cancer Get a closer look at carcinomas on page 66 and page 67.	*cancerous tumor*

Word Element	Meaning	Medical Word	Meaning
Suffixes			
-phoresis	carrying, transmission	dia/**phoresis** (dī-ă-fō-RĒ-sĭs) *dia-:* through, across	carrying through
-plasty	surgical repair	dermat/o/**plasty** (DĔR-mă-tō-plăs-tē) *dermat/o:* skin	Surgical repair of skin
-therapy	treatment	cry/o/**therapy** (krī-ō-THĔR-ă-pē) *cry/o:* cold	cold treatment
Prefixes			
an-	without, not	**an**/hidr/osis (ăn-hī-DRŌ-sĭs) *hidr:* sweat *-osis:* abnormal condition; increase (used primarily with blood cells)	abnormal condition of not sweating
epi-	above, upon	**epi**/derm/oid (ĕp-ĭ-DĔR-moyd) *derm:* skin *-oid:* resembling	above the skin
homo-	same	**homo**/graft (HŌ-mō-grăft) *-graft:* transplantation	Same transplantation
hyper-	excessive, above normal	**hyper**/hidr/osis (hī-pĕr-hī-DRŌ-sĭs) *hidr:* sweat *-osis:* abnormal condition; increase (used primarily with blood cells)	excessive sweating condition

 Competency Verification: Check your answers in Appendix B, Answer Key, page 366. If you are not satisfied with your level of comprehension, review the terms in the table and retake the review.

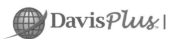 Visit the *Medical Terminology Express* online resource center at *DavisPlus* for an audio exercise of the terms in this table. Other activities are also available to reinforce content.

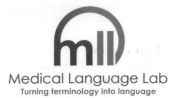

Medical Language Lab
Turning terminology into language

Visit the Medical Language Lab at *medicallanguagelab.com* to enhance your study and reinforce this chapter's word elements with the flash-card activity. We recommend you complete the flash-card activity before continuing with the next section.

Medical Terminology Word Building

In this section, combine the word parts you have learned to construct medical terms related to the integumentary system.

Use *adiplo* or *liplo* (fat) to build medical words that mean:

1. tumor consisting of fat _lipoma_

2. cell consisting of fat _lipocyte_

Use *ichthylo* (dry, scaly) to build a word that means:

3. abnormal condition of dry, scaly (skin) _ichthyosis_

Use *onychlo* (nail) to build medical words that mean:

4. tumor of the nail _onychoma_

5. disease of nails _onychopathy_

6. softening of nails _onychomalacia_

Use *trichlo* (hair) to build medical words that mean:

7. disease of the hair _trichopathy_

8. abnormal condition of the hair _trichosis_

Use *xerlo* (dry) to build medical words that mean:

9. skin that is dry _xeroderma_

10. abnormal condition of dryness _xerosis_

Use the suffix **-cyte** (cell) to build medical words that mean:

11. red cell _erythrocyte_

12. white cell _leukocyte_

13. black cell _melanocyte_

Use prefixes **an-** (without, not) or **hyper-** (excessive, above normal) to build medical words that mean:

14. abnormal condition without sweat _anhidrosis_

15. abnormal condition of excessive sweat _hyperhidrosis_

Competency Verification: Check your answers in Appendix B, Answer Key, on page 367. Review material that you did not answer correctly.

Correct Answers: _____ × 6.67 = _____ %

MEDICAL VOCABULARY

The following tables consist of selected terms that pertain to diseases and conditions of the integumentary system. Terms related to diagnostic, medical, and surgical procedures are included as well as pharmacological agents used to treat diseases. Recognizing and learning these terms will help you understand the connection between diseases and their treatments. Word analyses for selected terms are also provided.

Diseases and Conditions

abrasion ă-BRĀ-zhŭn	Scraping or rubbing away of a surface, such as skin, by friction
abscess ĂB-sĕs	Localized collection of pus at the site of an infection (characteristically a staphylococcal infection)
furuncle FŪ-rŭng-kl	Abscess that originates in a hair follicle; also called *boil*
carbuncle KĂR-bŭng-kl	Cluster of furuncles in the subcutaneous tissue (See Figure 3-1.)
acne ĂK-nē	Inflammatory disease of sebaceous follicles of the skin, marked by comedos (blackheads), papules, and pustules (small skin lesion filled with purulent material) (See Figure 3-2.)
alopecia ăl-ō-PĒ-shē-ă	Absence or loss of hair, especially of the head; also known as *baldness*

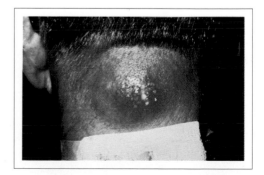

Figure 3-1 Dome-shaped abscess that has formed a furuncle in hair follicles of the neck. (From Goldsmith, LA, Lazarus, GS, and Tharp, MD: *Adult and Pediatric Dermatology: A Color Guide to Diagnosis and Treatment.* FA Davis, Philadelphia, 1997, p 364, with permission.)

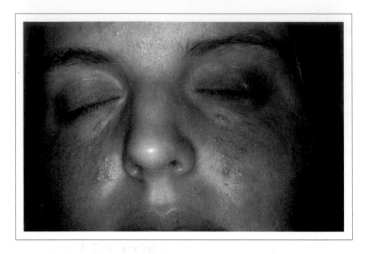

Figure 3-2 Acne vulgaris. (From Goldsmith, LA, Lazarus, GS, and Tharp, MD: *Adult and Pediatric Dermatology: A Color Guide to Diagnosis and Treatment.* FA Davis, Philadelphia, 1997, p 227, with permission.)

burn	Tissue injury caused by contact with a thermal, chemical, electrical, or radioactive agent
first-degree (superficial)	Mild burn affecting the epidermis and characterized by redness and pain with no blistering or scar formation
second-degree (partial thickness)	Burn affecting the epidermis and part of the dermis and characterized by redness, blistering or larger bullae, and pain with little or no scarring (See Figure 3-3.)
third-degree (full thickness)	Severe burn characterized by destruction of the epidermis and dermis with damage to the subcutaneous layer, leaving the skin charred black or dry white in appearance with insensitivity to touch

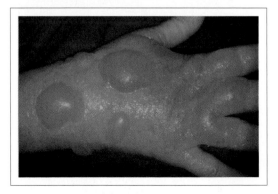

Figure 3-3 Second-degree (partial thickness burn). (From Goldsmith, LA, Lazarus, GS, and Tharp, MD: *Adult and Pediatric Dermatology: A Color Guide to Diagnosis and Treatment.* FA Davis, Philadelphia, 1997, p 318, with permission.)

carcinoma kăr-sĭ-NŌ-mă *carcin:* cancer *-oma:* tumor	Uncontrolled growth of abnormal cells in the body; also called *malignant cells*
melanoma měl-ă-NŌ-mă *melan:* black *-oma:* tumor	Malignant tumor that originates in melanocytes and is considered the most dangerous type of skin cancer, which, if not treated early, becomes difficult to cure and can be fatal Get a closer look at carcinomas, page 66 and page 67.
comedo KŎM-ē-dō	Discolored, dried sebum plugging an excretory duct of the skin; also called *blackhead*
cyst SĬST	Closed sac or pouch in or under the skin with a definite wall that contains fluid, semifluid, or solid material
pilonidal pī-lō-NĪ-dăl	Growth of hair in a dermoid cyst or in a sinus opening on the skin
sebaceous sē-BĀ-shŭs	Cyst filled with sebum (fatty material) from a sebaceous gland
eczema ĔK-zĕ-mă	Redness of skin caused by swelling of the capillaries (See Figure 3-4.)

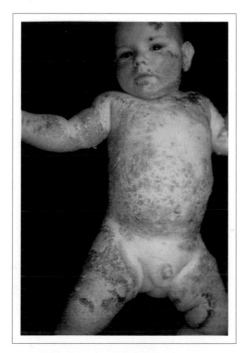

Figure 3-4 Scattered eczema of the trunk of an infant. (From Goldsmith, LA, Lazarus, GS, and Tharp, MD: *Adult and Pediatric Dermatology: A Color Guide to Diagnosis and Treatment.* FA Davis, Philadelphia, 1997, p 243, with permission.)

gangrene GĂNG-grēn	Death of tissue, usually resulting from loss of blood supply
hemorrhage HĔM-ĕ-rĭj *hem/o:* blood *-rrhage:* bursting forth (of)	External or internal loss of a large amount of blood in a short period
contusion kŏn-TOO-zhŭn	Hemorrhage of any size under the skin in which the skin is not broken; also known as a *bruise*
ecchymosis ĕk-ĭ-MŌ-sĭs	Skin discoloration consisting of a large, irregularly formed hemorrhagic area with colors changing from blue-black to greenish brown or yellow; commonly called a *bruise* (See Figure 3-5.)
petechia pē-TĒ-kē-ă	Minute, pinpoint hemorrhagic spot of the skin that is a smaller version of an ecchymosis
hematoma hēm-ă-TŌ-mă *hemat:* blood *-oma:* tumor	Elevated, localized collection of blood trapped under the skin that usually results from trauma
hirsutism HŬR-sūt-ĭzm	Excessive growth of hair in unusual places, especially in women; may be due to hypersecretion of testosterone

ichthyosis
ĭk-thē-Ō-sĭs
 ichthy/o: dry, scaly
  -osis: abnormal
    condition;
    increase (used
    primarily with
    blood
    cells)
	Genetic skin disorder in which the skin is dry and scaly, resembling fish skin because of a defect in keratinization (See Figure 3-6.)

impetigo ĭm-pĕ-TĪ-gō	Bacterial skin infection characterized by isolated pustules that become crusted and rupture

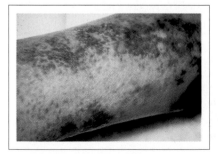

Figure 3-5 Ecchymosis. (From Harmening, DM: *Clinical Hematology and Fundamentals of Hemostasis,* ed 4. FA Davis, Philadelphia, 2001, p 489, with permission.)

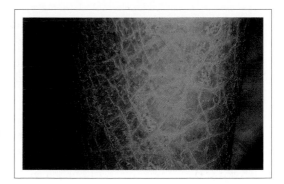

Figure 3-6 Ichthyosis. (From Goldsmith, LA, Lazarus, GS, and Tharp, MD: *Adult and Pediatric Dermatology: A Color Guide to Diagnosis and Treatment.* FA Davis, Philadelphia, 1997, p 129, with permission.)

keloid KĒ-lŏyd	Overgrowth of scar tissue at the site of a skin injury (especially a wound, surgical incision, or severe burn) caused by excessive collagen formation during the healing process
psoriasis sō-RĪ-ă-sĭs	Chronic skin disease characterized by itchy red patches covered with silvery scales (See Figure 3-7.)
scabies SKĀ-bēz	Contagious skin disease transmitted by the itch mite
skin lesions LĒ-zhŭnz	Areas of pathologically altered tissue caused by disease, injury, or a wound resulting from external factors or internal disease
tinea TĬN-ē-ă	Fungal infection whose name commonly indicates the body part affected, such as tinea pedis (athlcte's foot); also called *ringworm*

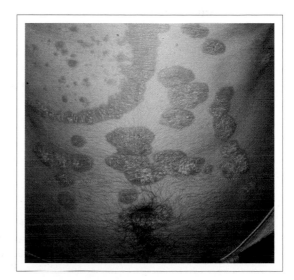

Figure 3-7 Psoriasis. (From Goldsmith, LA, Lazarus, GS, and Tharp, MD: *Adult and Pediatric Dermatology: A Color Guide to Diagnosis and Treatment.* FA Davis, Philadelphia, 1997, p 258, with permission.)

ulcer ŬL-sĕr	Lesion of the skin or mucous membranes marked by inflammation, necrosis, and sloughing of damaged tissues
pressure ulcer	Skin ulceration caused by prolonged pressure, usually in a patient who is bedridden; also known as *decubitus ulcer* or *bedsore*. (See Figure 3-8.)
urticaria ŭr-tĭ-KĂR-ē-ă	Allergic reaction of the skin characterized by eruption of pale red elevated patches that are intensely itchy; also called *wheals (hives)* (See Figure 3-9.)
verruca vĕr-ROO-kă	Rounded epidermal growth caused by a virus; also called *wart*

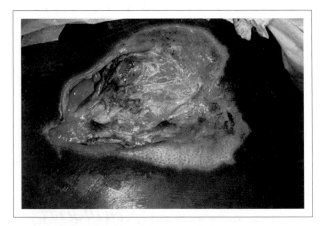

Figure 3-8 Pressure ulcer. Deep pressure ulcer over a bony prominence in a bedridden patient. (From Goldsmith, LA, Lazarus, GS, and Tharp, MD: *Adult and Pediatric Dermatology: A Color Guide to Diagnosis and Treatment.* FA Davis, Philadelphia, 1997, p 445, with permission.)

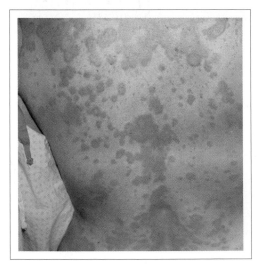

Figure 3-9 Urticaria. (From Goldsmith, LA, Lazarus, GS, and Tharp, MD: *Adult and Pediatric Dermatology: A Color Guide to Diagnosis and Treatment.* FA Davis, Philadelphia, 1997, p 209, with permission.)

vesicle VĔS-ĭ-kl	Small blister-like elevation on the skin containing a clear fluid; large vesicles arc called *bullae* (singular, bulla)
vitiligo vĭt-ĭl-Ī-gō	Localized loss of skin pigmentation characterized by milk-white patches; also called *leukoderma* (See Figure 3-10.)
wheal hwēl	Smooth, slightly elevated skin that is white in the center with a pale red periphery; also called *hives* if itchy

Diagnostic Procedures

biopsy (bx) BĪ-ŏp-sē *bi:* life *-opsy:* view of	Removal of a small piece of living tissue from an organ or other part of the body for microscopic examination to confirm or establish a diagnosis, estimate prognosis, or follow the course of a disease
skin test	Any test in which a suspected allergen or sensitizer is applied to or injected into the skin to determine the patient's sensitivity to it (See Figure 3-11.)

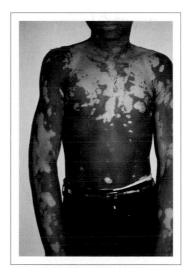

Figure 3-10 Vitiligo. (From Goldsmith, LA, Lazarus, GS, and Tharp, MD: *Adult and Pediatric Dermatology: A Color Guide to Diagnosis and Treatment.* FA Davis, Philadelphia, 1997, p 121, with permission.)

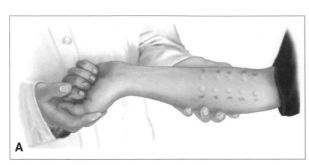
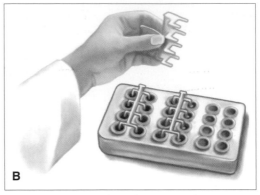

Figure 3-11 Skin tests. (A) Intradermal allergy test reactions. (B) Scratch (prick) skin test kit for allergy testing.

Medical and Surgical Procedures

cryosurgery krī-ō-SĚR-jĕr-ē *cry/o:* cold	Use of subfreezing temperature, commonly with liquid nitrogen, to destroy abnormal tissue cells, such as unwanted, cancerous, or infected tissue
débridement dĭ-BRĒD-mĕnt	Removal of foreign material, damaged tissue, or cellular debris from a wound or burn to prevent infection and promote healing
fulguration fŭl-gū-RĀ-shŭn	Tissue destruction by means of high-frequency electrical current; also called *electrodesiccation*
incision and drainage (I&D)	Incision of a lesion, such as an abscess, followed by the drainage of its contents
Mohs surgery MŌZ	Surgical procedure used primarily to treat skin neoplasms in which tumor tissue fixed in place is removed layer by layer for microscopic examination until the entire tumor is removed
skin graft	Surgical procedure to transplant healthy tissue by applying it to an injured site

allograft
    ĂL-ō-grăft
      allo-: other, differing
           from normal
      -graft: transplantation
	Transplantation of healthy tissue from one person to another person; also called *homograft*

autograft
    AW-tō-grăft
      auto-: self, own
      -graft: transplantation
	Transplantation of healthy tissue from one site to another site in the same individual

synthetic sĭn-THĔT-ĭk	Transplantation of artificial skin produced from collagen fibers arranged in a lattice pattern

xenograft
ZĔN-ō-grăft
  xen/o: foreign, strange
  -graft: transplantation
	Transplantation (dermis only) from a foreign donor (usually a pig) and transferred to a human; also called *heterograft*

skin resurfacing	Procedure that repairs damaged skin, acne scars, fine or deep wrinkles, or tattoos or improves skin tone irregularities through the use of topical chemicals, abrasion, or laser
chemical peel	Use of chemicals to remove outer layers of skin to treat acne scarring and general keratoses as well as for cosmetic purposes to remove fine wrinkles on the face; also called *chemabrasion*
cutaneous laser kū-TĀ-nē-ŭs *cutane:* skin *-ous:* pertaining to	Any of several laser treatments employed for cosmetic and plastic surgery
dermabrasion DĔRM-ă-brā-zhŭn	Removal of acne scars, nevi, tattoos, or fine wrinkles on the skin through the use of sandpaper, wire brushes, or other abrasive materials on the epidermal layer

Pharmacology

antibiotics ăn-tĭ-bī-ŎT-ĭks	Kill bacteria that cause skin infections
antifungals ăn-tĭ-FŬNG-găls	Kill fungi that infect the skin
antipruritics ăn-tĭ-proo-RĬT-ĭks	Reduce severe itching
corticosteroids kor-tĭ-kō-STĔR-oyds	Anti-inflammatory agents that treat skin inflammation

Pronunciation Help	Long Sound	ā in rāte	ē in rēbirth	ī in īsle	ō in ōver	ū in ūnite
	Short Sound	ă in ălone	ĕ in ĕver	ĭ in ĭt	ŏ in nŏt	ŭ in cŭt

A Closer Look

Take a closer look at these integumentary disorders to enhance your understanding of the medical terminology associated with them.

Basal Cell Carcinoma

Basal cell carcinoma (BCC) is the most common form of skin cancer, caused by overexposure to sunlight. The tumor develops on skin that is exposed to the sun, such as on the head, neck, and back of the hands and commonly on the face. Skin cancer falls into two major groups: nonmelanoma and melanoma. BCC is a type of **nonmelanoma skin cancer** that is a **malignancy** of the basal layer of the epidermis, or hair follicles. Although BCCs rarely spread to other parts of the body (**metastasize**), they tend to recur—especially lesions that are larger than 2 cm. Nevertheless, BCCs can grow wide and deep, destroying skin tissue and bone. BCC is most prevalent in blond, fair-skinned men and is the most common malignant tumor affecting white people. Although these tumors grow slowly, they commonly ulcerate as they increase in size and develop crusting that is firm to the touch. Depending on the location, size, and depth of the lesion, treatment includes surgical excision, **curettage and electrodesiccation, cryosurgery,** or **radiation therapy.** The following illustration shows a BCC above the eye.

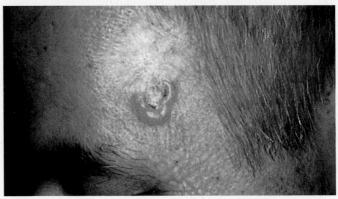

Basal cell carcinoma with pearly, flesh-colored papule with depressed center and rolled edge. (From Goldsmith, LA, Lazarus, GS, and Tharp, MD: *Adult and Pediatric Dermatology: A Color Guide to Diagnosis and Treatment.* FA Davis, Philadelphia, 1997, p 157, with permission.)

A Closer Look—cont'd

Squamous Cell Carcinoma

Squamous cell carcinoma (SCC) is the second most common form of nonmelanoma skin cancer after basal cell carcinoma. When detected and treated early, it rarely causes further problems. Untreated, SCC can grow large or metastasize, causing serious complications.

The incidence of skin cancers is increasing every year, likely as a result of increased sun exposure. Most SCCs result from prolonged exposure to **ultraviolet (UV) radiation,** either from sunlight or from tanning beds or lamps. Avoiding UV light as much as possible is the best protection. Sunscreen is an important part of a sun-safety program but by itself does not completely prevent SCC or other types of skin cancer. The following illustration shows SCC on the skin.

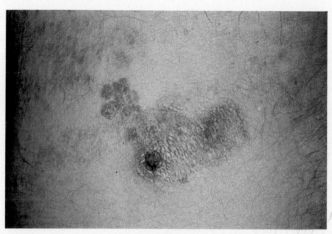

Squamous cell carcinoma on the skin. (From Goldsmith, LA, Lazarus, GS, and Tharp, MD: *Adult and Pediatric Dermatology: A Color Guide to Diagnosis and Treatment.* FA Davis, Philadelphia, 1997, p 237, with permission.)

Medical Vocabulary Recall

Match the medical terms below with the definitions in the numbered list.

alopecia   comedo   débridement   metastasize   tinea
autograft   cryosurgery   eczema   pressure ulcer   verruca
biopsy   dermabrasion   hirsutism   scabies   vitiligo

1. _verruca_ is a rounded epidermal growth caused by a virus.

2. _vitiligo_ is localized loss of skin pigmentation characterized by appearance of milk-white patches.

3. _tinea_ is a fungal skin disease, commonly called ringworm, whose name indicates the body part affected.

4. _pressure ulcer_ is ulceration caused by prolonged pressure; also called *decubitus ulcer*.

5. _eczema_ is a general term for an itchy red rash that may become crusted, thickened, or scaly.

6. _autograft_ is a type of skin graft taken from a different site of the same patient's body

7. _biopsy_ refers to excision of a small piece of living tissue from an organ or other part of the body for microscopic examination.

8. _dermabrasion_ refers to use of revolving wire brushes or sandpaper to remove superficial scars on the skin.

9. _hirsutism_ is excessive growth of hair, in unusual places, especially in women.

10. _cryosurgery_ refers to use of liquid nitrogen to destroy or eliminate abnormal tissue cells.

11. _débridement_ refers to removal of foreign material and dead or damaged tissue, especially in a wound.

12. _scabies_ is a contagious skin disease transmitted by the itch mite.

13. _alopecia_ is absence or loss of hair, especially of the head; baldness.

14. _comedo_ is a blackhead.

15. _metastasize_ means to spread or invade distant structures of the body.

Competency Verification: Check your answers in Appendix B, Answer Key, on page 367. Review material that you did not answer correctly.

Correct Answers: _____ × **6.67** = _____ %

Pronunciation and Spelling

Use the following list to practice correct pronunciation and spelling of medical terms. Practice the pronunciation aloud, and then write the correct spelling of the term. The first word is completed for you.

Pronunciation	Spelling
1. ă-BRĀ-zhŭn	*abrasion*
2. ĂB-sĕs	abscess
3. ĂK-nē	acne
4. ăl-ō-PĒ-shē-ă	alopecia
5. BĪ-ŏp-sē	biopsy
6. krī-ō-THĔR-ă-pē	cryotherapy
7. dī-ă-fō-RĒ-sĭs	diaphoresis
8. ĕp-ĭ-DĔR-moyd	epidermoid
9. ĕr-ĭ-THĔM-ă-tŭs	erythematous
10. FŪ-rŭng-kl	furuncle
11. KĒ-loyd	keloid
12. hēm-ă-TŌ-mă	hematoma
13. HŬR-sūt-ĭzm	hirsutism
14. LĒ-zhŭnz	lesion
15. ŏn-ĭ-kō-mă-LĀ-shē-ă	onychomalacia
16. pē-TĒ-kē-ă	petechia
17. SKĀ-bēz	scabies
18. sō-RĪ-ă-sĭs	psoriasis
19. sĕb-or-Ē-ă	seborrhea
20. vĭt-ĭl-Ī-gō	vitiligo

Competency Verification: Check your answers in Appendix B, Answer Key, on page 367. Review material that you did not answer correctly.

Correct Answers: _____ × 5 = _____ %

ABBREVIATIONS

The following table introduces abbreviations associated with the integumentary system.

Abbreviation	Meaning	Abbreviation	Meaning
BCC	basal cell carcinoma	I&D	incision and drainage; irrigation and débridement
Bx, bx	biopsy	PE	physical examination; pulmonary embolism; pressure-equalizing (tube)
DM	diabetes mellitus	SCC	squamous cell carcinoma
FH	family history	UV	ultraviolet

CHART NOTES

Chart notes comprise part of the medical record and are used in various types of health care facilities. The chart notes that follow were dictated by the patient's physician and reflect common clinical events using medical terminology to document the patient's care. Studying and completing the terminology and chart note analysis sections below will help you learn and understand terms associated with the medical specialty of dermatology.

Terminology

The following terms are linked to chart notes in the specialty of dermatology. First, practice pronouncing each term aloud. Then, use a medical dictionary such as *Taber's Cyclopedic Medical Dictionary; Appendix A: Glossary of Medical Word Elements*, or other resources to define each term.

Term	Meaning
Bartholin gland BĂR-tō-lĭn	two pea sized glands on posterior of vagina opening
colitis kō-LĪ-tĭs	inflammation of colon
diabetes mellitus dī-ă-BĒ-tēz MĔ-lĭ-tŭs	insufficient production of insulin
diaphoresis dī-ă-fō-RĒ-sĭs	sweating
enteritis ĕn-tĕr-Ī-tĭs	inflammation of intestine

Term	Meaning
erythematous ĕr-ĭ-THĔM-ă-tŭs	redness of skin
FH	family history
histiocytoma hĭs-tē-ō-sī-TŌ-mă	benign skin tumor of Langerhans cells
macules MĂK-ūlz	yellowish area around fovea
papules PĂP-ūlz	small, raised, solid pimple
pruritus proo-RĪ-tŭs	severe itching of skin
psoriasis sō-RĪ-ă-sĭs	skin condition that speeds up life cycle of cells
sclerosed sklĕ-RŌST	affected by sclerosis
syncope SĬN-kō-pē	fainting
vulgaris vŭl-GĂ-rĭs	common form of acne

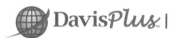 **DavisPlus** | Visit *Medical Terminology Express* at *DavisPlus* Online Resource Center. Use it to practice pronunciations and reinforce the meanings of the terms in this chart note.

Psoriasis

Read the following chart note aloud. Underline any term you have trouble pronouncing or cannot define. If needed, refer to the Terminology section above for correct pronunciations and meanings of terms.

This is a 32-year-old woman who experienced intermittent psoriasis since her early teens in various stages of severity. Her condition has become more troublesome over the past year because of an increase of symptoms after being exposed to the sun. Her past history indicates she had chronic sinusitis of 3 years' duration. Her Bartholin gland was excised in 20xx. She has had pruritus of the scalp and abdominal regions. There is no FH of psoriasis. An uncle has had diabetes mellitus since age 43. Patient has

(Continued)

occasional abdominal pains accompanied by diaphoresis and/or syncope. PE showed the patient has psoriatic involvement of the scalp, external ears, trunk, and, to a lesser degree, legs. There are many scattered erythematous (light ruby colored) thickened plaques covered by thick yellowish white scales. A few areas on the legs and arms show multiple, sclerosed, brown macules and papules.

Diagnoses:

1. Psoriasis vulgaris.
2. Multiple histiocytomas.
3. Abdominal pains, by history.
4. Rule out colitis, regional enteritis.

Chart Note Analysis

From the preceding chart note, select the medical word that means
1. discolored area on the skin that is not elevated: __macule__
2. condition that comes and goes: __intermittent__
3. fainting episode: __syncope__
4. common or ordinary: __vulgaris__
5. inflammation of the colon: __colitis__
6. of long duration: __chronic__
7. hardened: __sclerosed__
8. inflammation of small intestine: __enteritis__
9. severe itching: __pruritus__
10. mucous gland at the vaginal opening: __Bartholin glands__
11. skin disease characterized by itchy red patches covered with silvery scales: __psoriasis__
12. redness of the skin caused by capillary dilation: __erythematous__
13. inflammation of the sinus cavity: __sinusitis__
14. elevated lesion containing pus (as seen in acne and psoriasis): __papule__
15. synonymous with hyperhidrosis and sudoresis: __diaphoresis__

Competency Verification: Check your answers in Appendix B, Answer Key, on page 367. Review material that you did not answer correctly.

Correct Answers: _____ × 6.67 = _____ %

Demonstrate What You Know!

To evaluate your understanding of how medical terms you have studied in this and previous chapters are used in a clinical environment, complete the numbered sentences by selecting an appropriate term from the words below.

antibiotic	dermis	lipocyte	onychopathy	sebaceous
carcinoma	epidermis	mycosis	psoriasis	sudoriferous
dermatologist	ichthyosis	onychomalacia	pyoderma	xenograft

1. The _dermis_ is the layer of skin containing blood vessels, oil and sweat glands, and hair follicles.

2. When a person sweats, the _Sudoriferous_ glands are working.

3. If there is disease of the nail bed, the condition is charted _onychopathy_.

4. The Dx for a patient with a fungal infection of the skin is _mycosis_.

5. A skin transplantation from a foreign donor to a human is a(n) _xenograft_.

6. The layer of skin that does not have blood or nerve supplies is the _epidermis_.

7. A physician who specializes in treating skin disorders is known as a _dermatologist_.

8. _Sebaceous_ glands are oil-producing glands of the skin.

9. The Dx of a patient with a cancerous tumor is _carcinoma_.

10. A hereditary skin disorder characterized by fine, small flaky, white scales is called _ichthyosis_.

11. A patient who exhibits softening of the nails has the condition called _onychomalacia_.

12. A(n) _antibiotic_ kills bacteria that cause skin infections.

13. A fat-storing cell is called a(n) _lipocyte_.

14. A chronic skin disease characterized by itchy red patches covered with silvery scales is _psoriasis_.

15. The medical term for pus in the skin is _pyoderma_.

 Competency Verification: Check your answers in Appendix B, Answer Key, on page 368. Review material that you did not answer correctly.

Correct Answers: _____ × 6.67 = _____ %

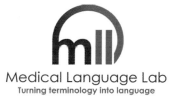

Medical Language Lab
Turning terminology into language

If you are not satisfied with your retention level of the integumentary system chapter, visit *DavisPlus* Student Online Resource Center and the Medical Language Lab to complete the website activities linked to this chapter.

Respiratory System

Objectives

Upon completion of this chapter, you will be able to:

- Identify four types of medical treatment provided by pulmonary specialists.
- List three primary functions of the respiratory system.
- Identify the primary structures of the respiratory system.
- Briefly describe the pathway of inhaled and exhaled air through the respiratory tract.
- Identify combining forms, suffixes, and prefixes associated with the respiratory system.
- Recognize, pronounce, build, and spell medical terms and abbreviations associated with the respiratory system.
- Demonstrate your knowledge by successfully completing the activities in this chapter.

VOCABULARY PREVIEW

Term	Meaning

diagnosis
dī-ăg-NŌ-sĭs
   dia-: through, across
   gnos: knowing
   -is: noun ending
	Identification of a disease or condition by a scientific evaluation of physical signs, symptoms, history, laboratory test results, and procedures

pulmonary
PŬL-mō-nĕ-rē
   pulmon: lung
   -ary: pertaining to
	Pertaining to the lungs or the respiratory system

respiration rĕs-pĭr-Ā-shŭn	Molecular exchange of oxygen and carbon dioxide within the body's tissues; also called *breathing, pulmonary ventilation,* or *ventilation*

thoracic
thō-RĂS-ĭk
   thorac: chest
   -ic: pertaining to
	Pertaining to the thorax or thoracic cage (bony enclosure formed by the sternum, costal cartilages, ribs, and the bodies of the thoracic vertebrae)

vascular
VĂS-kū-lăr
   vascul: vessel (usually blood or lymph)
   -ar: pertaining to
	Pertaining to a blood vessel

Pronunciation Help	Long Sound	ā in rāte	ē in rēbirth	ī in īsle	ō in ōver	ū in ūnite
	Short Sound	ă in ălone	ĕ in ĕver	ĭ in ĭt	ŏ in nŏt	ŭ in cŭt

MEDICAL SPECIALTY OF PULMONOLOGY

The respiratory system is associated with the medical specialty of **pulmonology,** also known as **pulmonary medicine.** This branch of medicine focuses on treatment of diseases involving the structures of the lower respiratory tract, including the lungs, their airways, and the chest wall (**thoracic** cage).

Medical doctors who treat respiratory disorders are called **pulmonologists.** Pulmonologists treat pulmonary disorders such as asthma, **emphysema,** chronic **bronchitis,** occupational and industrial lung disease, and **pulmonary vascular** disease. Pulmonologists also care for patients who require specialized ventilator support and lung transplantation.

In general, pulmonologists diagnose and manage pulmonary disorders and acute and chronic respiratory failure. **Diagnosis** and management of pulmonary disorders may include administering pulmonary function tests, arterial blood gas analysis, chest x-rays, and chemical or microbiological tests.

RESPIRATORY SYSTEM QUICK STUDY

The **respiratory system** consists of the nose, pharynx, larynx, trachea, bronchial tubes, lungs, and breathing muscles. All of these organs work together to perform the mechanical and, for the most part, unconscious mechanism of **respiration**. Respiration, or breathing, consists of external and internal processes:

- In **external respiration,** oxygen (O_2) is inhaled into the lungs and absorbed into the bloodstream. Carbon dioxide (CO_2) leaves the bloodstream and enters the lungs where it is expelled during exhalation.
- In internal respiration, O_2 and CO_2 are exchanged at the cellular level. O_2 leaves the bloodstream and is delivered to the tissue cells where it is used for energy. In exchange, CO_2 enters the bloodstream from the tissues and is transported back to the lungs for removal. (See Respiratory System, page 78)

    ALERT: An extensive self-paced anatomy and physiology multimedia review is included in *TermPlus,* a powerful, interactive CD-ROM program that can be purchased separately from F.A. Davis Company.

MEDICAL WORD BUILDING

Constructing medical words using word elements (combining forms, suffixes, and prefixes) related to the respiratory system will enhance your understanding of those terms and reinforce your ability to use terms correctly.

Combining Forms

Begin your study of respiratory terminology by reviewing the organs and their associated combining forms (CFs), which are illustrated in the figure *Respiratory System* that follows.

Respiratory System

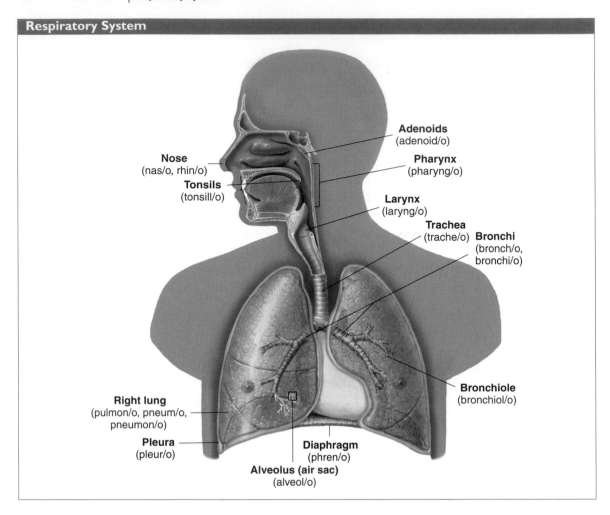

In the table that follows, CFs are listed alphabetically, and other word parts are defined as needed. Review the medical word and study the elements that make up the term. Then complete the meaning of the medical words in the right-hand column. The first one is completed for you. You may also refer to *Appendix A: Glossary of Medical Word Elements* to complete this exercise.

Combining Form	Meaning	Medical Word	Meaning
Upper Respiratory Tract			
adenoid/o	adenoids	**adenoid**/ectomy (ăd-ĕ-noyd-ĚK-tō-mē) *-ectomy:* excision, removal	*excision of the adenoids*

Combining Form	Meaning	Medical Word	Meaning
Upper Respiratory Tract			
laryng/o	larynx (voice box)	**laryng/o**/scope (lăr-ĬN-gō-skōp) *-scope:* instrument for examining	
nas/o	nose	**nas**/al (NĀ-zl) *-al:* pertaining to	
rhin/o		**rhin/o**/rrhea (rī-nō-RĒ-ă) *-rrhea:* discharge, flow	
pharyng/o	pharynx (throat)	**pharyng/o**/spasm (far-ĬN-gō-spăzm) *-spasm:* involuntary contraction, twitching	
tonsill/o	tonsils	**tonsill**/ectomy (tŏn-sĭl-ĔK-tō-mē) *-ectomy:* excision, removal	
trache/o	trachea (windpipe)	**trache/o**/tomy (trā-kē-ŎT-ō-mē) *-tomy:* incision	
Lower Respiratory Tract			
alveol/o	alveolus; air sac	**alveol**/ar (ăl-VĒ-ō-lăr) *-ar:* pertaining to	
bronch/o	bronchus (plural, bronchi)	**bronch/o**/scopy (brŏng-KŎS-kō-pē) *-scopy:* visual examination Get a closer look at bronchoscopy on page 95.	
bronchi/o		**bronchi**/ectasis (brŏng-kē-ĔK-tă-sĭs) *-ectasis:* expansion, dilation	

(Continued)

Combining Form	Meaning	Medical Word	Meaning
Lower Respiratory Tract			
bronchiol/o	bronchiole	**bronchiol**/itis (brŏng-kē-ō-LĪ-tĭs) *-itis:* inflammation	
phren/o	diaphragm	**phren**/algia (frĕ-NĂL-jē-ă) *-algia:* pain	
pleur/o	pleura	**pleur**/o/dynia (ploo-rō-DĬN-ē-ă) *-dynia:* pain	

pneum/o	air; lung	**pneum**/o/melan/osis
		(nū-mō-mĕl-ăn-Ō-sĭs)
		melan: black
		   -osis: abnormal condi-
		      tion; increase
		      (used primarily
		      with blood cells)	

pneumon/o		**pneumon**/ia (nū-MŌ-nē-ă) *-ia:* condition	
pulmon/o	lung	**pulmon**/o/logist (pŭl-mŏ-NŌL-ŏ-jĭst) *-logist:* specialist in the study of	
thorac/o	chest	**thorac**/o/pathy (thō-răk-ŎP-ă-thē) *-pathy:* disease	
Other Related Combining Forms			
aer/o	air	**aer**/o/phagia (ĕr-ō-FĂ-jē-ă) *-phagia:* swallowing, eating	

cyan/o	blue	**cyan**/osis
		(sī-ă-NŌ-sĭs)
		-osis: abnormal condi-
		      tion; increase (used
		      primarily with
		      blood cells)	

Combining Form	Meaning	Medical Word	Meaning
Other Related Combining Forms			
muc/o	mucus	muc/oid (MŪ-koyd) *-oid:* resembling	
myc/o	fungus	myc/osis (mī-KŌ-sĭs) *-osis:* abnormal condition; increase (used primarily with blood cells	
orth/o	straight	orth/o/pnea (or-THŎP-nē-ă) *-pnea:* breathing	
py/o	pus	py/o/thorax (pī-ō-THŌ-răks) *-thorax:* chest	

Suffixes and Prefixes

In the table that follows, suffixes and prefixes are listed alphabetically, and other word parts are defined as needed. Review the medical word and study the elements that make up the term. Then complete the meaning of the medical words in the right-hand column. You may also refer to *Appendix A: Glossary of Medical Word Elements* to complete this exercise.

Word Element	Meaning	Medical Word	Meaning
Suffixes			
-oma	tumor	chondr/oma (kŏn-DRŌ-mă) *chondr/o:* cartilage	
-plasty	surgical repair	rhin/o/plasty (RĪ-nō-plăs-tē) *rhin/o:* nose	
-plegia	paralysis	laryng/o/plegia (lă-rĭn-gō-PLĒ-jē-ă) *laryng/o:* larynx (voice box)	

(Continued)

Word Element	Meaning	Medical Word	Meaning
Prefixes			
a-	without, not	**a**/pnea (ăp-NĒ-ă) *-pnea:* breathing Get a closer look at apnea on page 93.	
brady-	slow	**brady**/pnea (brād-ĭp-NĒ-ă) *-pnea:* breathing	
dys-	bad; painful; difficult	**dys**/pnea (dĭsp-NĒ-ă) *-pnea:* breathing	
eu-	good, normal	**eu**/pnea (ūp-NĒ-ă) *-pnea:* breathing	
tachy-	rapid	**tachy**/pnea (tăk-ĭp-NĒ-ă) *-pnea:* breathing	

 Competency Verification: Check your answers in Appendix B, Answer Key, pages 368–369. If you are not satisfied with your level of comprehension, review the terms in the table and retake the review.

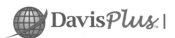 Visit the *Medical Terminology Express* online resource center at *DavisPlus* for an audio exercise of the terms in this table. Other activities are also available to reinforce content.

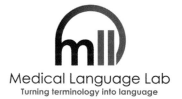

Medical Language Lab
Turning terminology into language

Visit the Medical Language Lab at *medicallanguagelab.com* to enhance your study and reinforce this chapter's word elements with the flash-card activity. We recommend you complete the flash-card activity before continuing with the next section.

Medical Terminology Word Building

In this section, combine the word parts you have learned to construct medical terms related to the respiratory system.

Use *rhin/o* (nose) to build words that mean:

1. surgical repair of the nose _____

2. watery discharge from the nose _____

Use *laryng/o* (voice box) to build words that mean:

3. paralysis of the larynx _____

4. inflammation of the larynx _____

Use *bronch/o* or *bronchi/o* (bronchus) to build words that mean:

5. dilation or expansion of the bronchus _____

6. visual examination of the bronchus _____

Use *pleur/o* (pleura) to build words that mean:

7. pain in the pleura _____

8. inflammation of the pleura _____

Use *cyan/o* (blue) to build a word that means:

9. abnormal condition of blue (skin) _____

Use *-pnea* (breathing) to build words that mean:

10. difficult or painful breathing _____

11. slow breathing _____

12. rapid breathing _____

13. good or normal breathing _____

Use *-thorax* (chest) to build a word that means:

14. pus in the thorax _____

Use *-phagia* (swallowing) to build a word that means:

15. swallowing air _____

 Competency Verification: Check your answers in Appendix B, Answer Key, on page 369. Review material that you did not answer correctly.

Correct Answers: _____ × **6.67** = _____ %

MEDICAL VOCABULARY

The following tables consist of selected terms that pertain to diseases and conditions of the respiratory system. Terms related to diagnostic, medical, and surgical procedures are included as well as pharmacological agents used to treat diseases. Recognizing and learning these terms will help you understand the connection between diseases and their treatments. Word analyses for selected terms are also provided.

Diseases and Conditions

abnormal breath sounds	Abnormal sounds heard during inhalation or expiration, with or without a stethoscope
crackles KRĂK-ălz	Fine crackling or bubbling sounds, commonly heard during inspiration when there is fluid in the alveoli; also called *rales*
friction rub	Dry, grating sound heard with a stethoscope during auscultation (listening for sounds within the body)
rhonchi RŎNG-kī	Loud coarse or snoring sounds heard during inspiration or expiration; caused by obstructed airways
stridor STRĪ-dor	High-pitched, musical sound made on inspiration; caused by an obstruction in the trachea or larynx
wheezes HWĒZ-ĕz	Continuous high-pitched whistling sounds, usually during expiration; caused by narrowing of an airway
acidosis ăs-ĭ-DŌ-sĭs *acid:* acid *-osis:* abnormal condition; increase (used primarily with blood cells)	Excessive acidity of blood as a result of an accumulation of acids or an excessive loss of bicarbonate caused by abnormally high levels of carbon dioxide (CO_2) in the body
acute respiratory distress syndrome (ARDS) ă-KŪT RĔS-pĭ-ră-tō-rē dĭs-TRĔS SĬN-drōm	Life-threatening build-up of fluid in the air sacs (alveoli), caused by vomit into the lungs (aspiration), inhaling chemicals, pneumonia, septic shock, or trauma, that prevents enough oxygen from passing into the bloodstream; also called *adult respiratory distress syndrome (ARDS)*
anosmia ăn-ŎZ-mē-ă *an-:* without, not *-osmia:* smell	Absence or decrease in the sense of smell
anoxia ăn-ŎK-sē-ă *an-:* without, not *-oxia:* oxygen	Total absence of O_2 in body tissues; caused by a lack of O_2 in inhaled air or by obstruction that prevents O_2 from reaching the lungs

asphyxia ăs-FĬK-sē-ă *a-:* without, not *-sphyxia:* pulse	Condition of insufficient intake of oxygen as a result of choking, toxic gases, electric shock, drugs, drowning, smoke, or trauma
asthma ĂZ-mă	Inflammatory airway disorder that results in attacks of wheezing, short-ness of breath that gets worse with exercise or activity, and coughing (with or without sputum) Get a closer look at COPD and asthma on page 94.

atelectasis
ăt-ĕ-LĔK-tă-sĭs
   atel: incomplete;
      imperfect
-ectasis: dilation,
      expansion
	Collapse of lung tissue, which prevents the respiratory exchange of oxy-gen and carbon dioxide and is caused by various conditions including obstruction of foreign bodies, excessive secretions, or pressure on the lung from a tumor

bronchitis
brŏng-KĪ-tĭs
bronch: bronchus (plural,
      bronchi)
  -itis: inflammation
	Acute or chronic inflammation of mucous membranes of the bronchial airways caused by irritation, infection, or both
	
	 Get a closer look at COPD and bronchitis on page 94.

coryza kŏ-RĪ-ză	Acute inflammation of the nasal passages accompanied by profuse nasal discharge; also called a *cold*
croup croop	Acute respiratory syndrome that occurs primarily in children and infants and is characterized by laryngeal obstruction and spasm, barking cough, and stridor

cystic fibrosis (CF)
SĬS-tĭk fĭ-BRŌ-sĭs
-cyst: bladder
  -ic: pertaining to
fibr: fiber, fibrous tissue
-osis: abnormal condition;
     increase (used
     primarily with
     blood cells)
	Genetic disease that is one of the most common types of chronic lung disease in children and young adults and causes thick, sticky mucus to build up in the lungs and digestive tract, possibly resulting in early death

emphysema ĕm-fĭ-SĒ-mă	Chronic obstructive pulmonary disease (COPD) that makes it difficult to breathe and is characterized by loss of elasticity of the lung tissue that causes the small airways to collapse during forced exhalation Get a closer look at COPD and emphysema on page 94.

epistaxis
ĕp-ĭ-STĂK-sĭs
  epi-: above, upon
  -staxis: dripping, oozing
    (of blood)
	Hemorrhage from the nose; also called *nosebleed*

hypercapnia
hī-pĕr-KĂP-nē-ă
  hyper-: excessive, above
    normal
  -capnia: carbon dioxide
    (CO_2)
	Greater than normal amounts of carbon dioxide in the blood

hypoxemia
hī-pŏks-Ē-mē-ă
  hyp-: under, below,
    deficient
  ox: oxygen
  -emia: blood condition
	Deficiency of oxygen in the blood; usually a sign of respiratory impairment

hypoxia
hī-PŎKS-ē-ă
  hyp-: under, below,
    deficient
  -oxia: oxygen
	Deficiency of oxygen in body tissues; usually a sign of respiratory impairment

influenza ĭn-floo-ĔN-ză	Acute, contagious respiratory infection characterized by sudden onset of fever, chills, headache, and muscle pain

otitis media (OM)
ō-TĪ-tĭs MĒ-dē-ă
  ot: ear
  -itis: inflammation
  med: middle
  -ia: condition
	Inflammation of the middle ear, commonly the result of an upper respiratory infection (URI) with symptoms of otodynia; may be treated with myringotomy or tympanostomy tubes

exudative ĔKS-ū-dă-tĭv	OM with the presence of fluid, such as pus or serum
pertussis pĕr-TŬS-ĭs	Acute infectious disease characterized by a "whoop"-sounding cough; also called *whooping cough*
pleurisy PLOO-rĭs-ē *pleur:* pleura *-isy:* state of; condition	Inflammation of the pleural membrane characterized by a stabbing pain that is intensified by deep breathing or coughing

pneumothorax nū-mō-THŌ-răks *pneum/o:* air, lung *-thorax:* chest	Collection of air or gas in the pleural cavity, causing the complete or partial collapse of a lung (See Figure 4-1.)
sudden infant death syndrome (SIDS)	Completely unexpected and unexplained death of an apparently well, or virtually well, infant; also called *crib death*

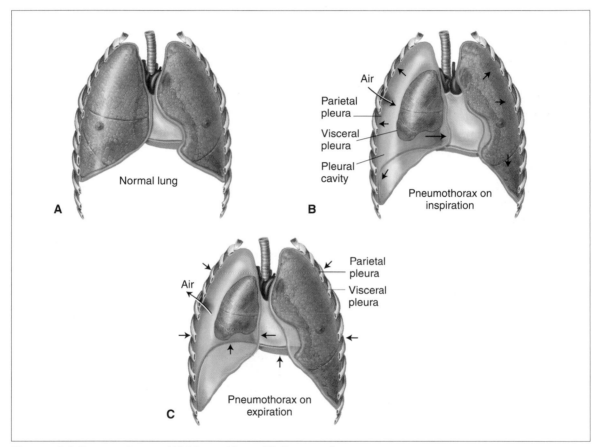

Figure 4-1 Pneumothorax. (A) Normal lung. (B) Pneumothorax on inspiration. (C) Pneumothorax on expiration.

Diagnostic Procedures

arterial blood gases (ABGs) ăr-TĒ-rē-ăl *arteri:* artery *-al:* pertaining to	Group of tests that measure the oxygen and carbon dioxide concentration in an arterial blood sample
Mantoux test măn-TŪ	Intradermal test to determine recent or past exposure to tuberculosis (TB)
polysomnography (PSG) pŏl-ē-sŏm-NŎG-ră-fē *poly-:* many, much *somn/o:* sleep *-graphy:* process of recording	Sleep study test monitored by a technician while the patient sleeps; used to evaluate physical factors affecting sleep, such as heart rate and activity, breathing, eye and muscle movements, snoring, kicking during sleep, and sleep cycles and stages (See Figure 4-2.)
pulmonary function tests (PFTs) PŬL-mō-nĕ-rē *pulmon:* lung *-ary:* pertaining to	Various tests used to determine the capacity of the lungs to exchange O_2 and CO_2 efficiently
spirometry spī-RŎM-ĕ-trē *spir/o:* to breathe *-metry:* act of measuring	Common lung function test that measures and records the volume and rate of inhaled and exhaled air; used to assess pulmonary function by means of a spirometer and to assess obstructive lung diseases, especially asthma and chronic obstructive pulmonary disease (COPD) (See Figure 4-3.)

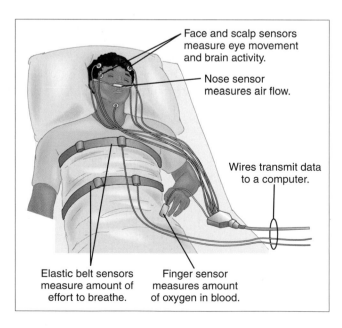

Face and scalp sensors measure eye movement and brain activity.

Nose sensor measures air flow.

Wires transmit data to a computer.

Elastic belt sensors measure amount of effort to breathe.

Finger sensor measures amount of oxygen in blood.

Figure 4-2 Polysomnography (PSG).

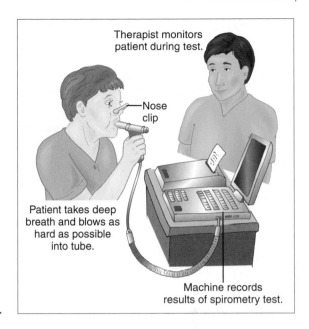

Therapist monitors
patient during test.

Nose
clip

Patient takes deep
breath and blows as
hard as possible
into tube.

Machine records
results of spirometry test.

Figure 4-3 Spirometry.

Medical and Surgical Procedures

cardiopulmonary resuscitation (CPR) kăr-dē-ō-PŬL-mō-nĕr-ē rĕ-sŭs-ĭ-TĀ-shŭn *cardi/o:* heart *pulmon:* lung *-ary:* pertaining to	Basic emergency procedure for life support, consisting of artificial respiration and manual external cardiac massage
endotracheal intubation ĕn-dō-TRĀ-kē-ăl ĭn-tū-BĀ-shŭn *endo-:* in, within *trache:* trachea (windpipe) *-al:* pertaining to	Procedure in which an airway catheter is inserted through the mouth or nose into the trachea just above the bronchi in patients who are unable to breathe on their own; also used to administer oxygen, medication, or anesthesia (See Figure 4-4.)
postural drainage	Use of body positioning to assist in the removal of secretions from specific lobes of the lung, bronchi, or lung cavities
thoracocentesis thō-ră-cō-sĕn-TĒ-sĭs *thorac/o:* chest *-centesis:* surgical puncture	Use of a needle to collect pleural fluid for laboratory analysis or to remove excess pleural fluid or air from the pleural space; also called *thoracentesis* (See Figure 4-5.)

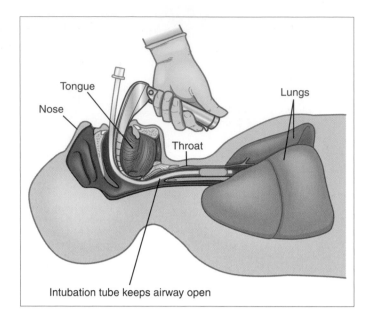

Figure 4-4 Endotracheal intubation. A lighted laryngoscope is used to hold the airway open and helps visualize the vocal cords.

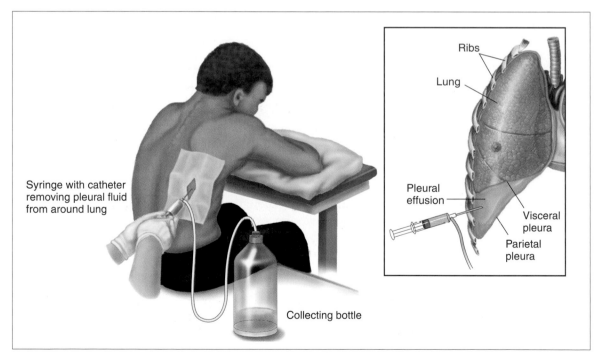

Figure 4-5 Thoracentesis.

tracheostomy tra-ke-ŎS-tŏ-mē *trache/o:* trachea (windpipe) *-stomy:* forming an opening (mouth)	Incision into the trachea (tracheotomy) and creation of a permanent opening through which a tracheostomy tube is inserted to keep the opening patent (accessible or wide open) (See Figure 4-6.)

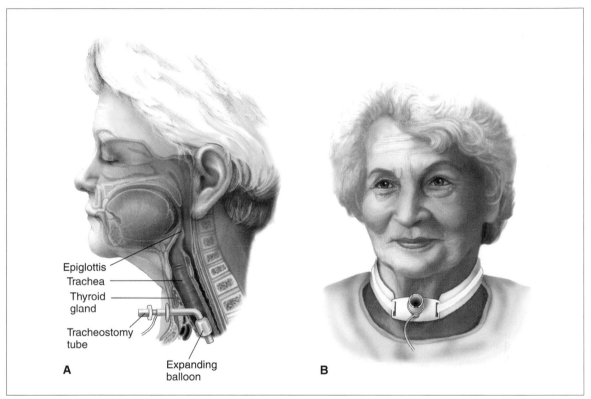

Epiglottis
Trachea
Thyroid gland
Tracheostomy tube
A
Expanding balloon
B

Figure 4-6 Tracheostomy. (A) Lateral view with tracheostomy tube in place. (B) Frontal view.

Pharmacology

bronchodilators brŏng-kō-DĪ-lā-tŏrs	Dilate constricted airways by relaxing muscle spasms in the bronchial tubes through oral administration or inhalation via a metered-dose inhaler (MDI)
corticosteroids kōr-tĭ-kō-STĔR-oyds	Suppress the inflammatory reaction that causes swelling and narrowing of the bronchi

expectorants ĕk-SPĔK-tō-rănts	Improve the ability to cough up mucus from the respiratory tract
metered-dose inhaler (MDI)	Device that enables the patient to self-administer a specific amount of medication into the lungs through inhalation (See Figure 4-7.)
nebulized mist treatment (NMT) NĔB-ū-līzd	Method of administering medication directly into the lungs using a device (nebulizer) that produces a fine spray; also called *aerosol therapy* (See Figure 4-8.)

Pronunciation Help	Long Sound	ā in rāte	ē in rēbirth	ī in īsle	ō in ōver	ū in ūnite
	Short Sound	ă in ălone	ĕ in ĕver	ĭ in ĭt	ŏ in nŏt	ŭ in cŭt

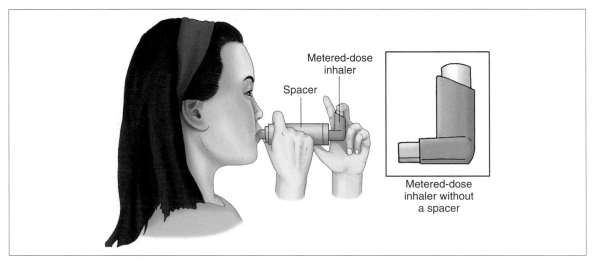

Figure 4-7 Metered-dose inhaler.

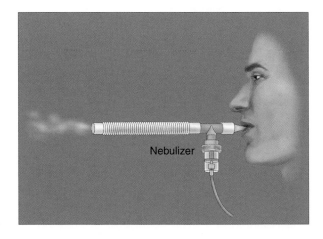

Figure 4-8 Nebulizer.

A Closer Look

Take a closer look at these respiratory disorders and endoscopic procedures to enhance your understanding of the medical terminology associated with them.

Apnea

Apnea is a temporary cessation of breathing. **Sleep apnea** refers to a sudden cessation of breathing during sleep that can result in hypoxia and lead to cognitive impairment, **hypertension,** and **arrhythmias. Obstructive sleep apnea (OSA)** involves a physical obstruction in the upper airways. The condition is usually marked by recurrent sleep interruptions, choking and gasping spells on awakening, and drowsiness caused by loss of normal sleep. **Continuous positive airway pressure (CPAP)** is a gentle ventilator support used to keep the airways open. Uncorrected, OSA commonly leads to central sleep apnea, pulmonary failure, and cardiac abnormalities. The following illustration shows the airway obstruction caused by enlarged tonsils that eventually leads to obstructive sleep apnea (A) and the CPAP machine used to treat sleep apnea (B).

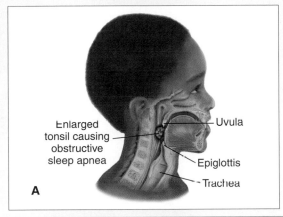

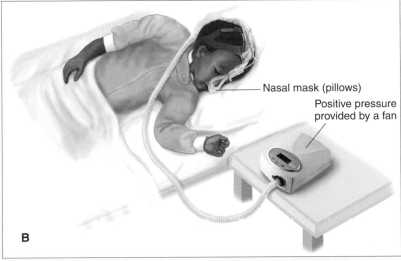

Apnea. (A) Obstructive sleep apnea. (B) CPAP machine used to treat sleep apnea.

(Continued)

A Closer Look—cont'd

COPD

Chronic obstructive pulmonary disease (COPD) refers to a group of respiratory disorders characterized by chronic, partial obstruction of the bronchi and lungs that makes it difficult to breathe. The three major disorders included in COPD are asthma, chronic bronchitis, and emphysema. In COPD, the airway passages become clogged with mucus. Although air reaches the alveoli in the lungs during inhalation, it may not be able to escape during exhalation. COPD tends to be progressive and irreversible. Smoking, prolonged exposure to polluted air, **respiratory infections,** and allergies are predisposing factors to the disease. **Bronchodilators** and **corticosteroids** are commonly prescribed to help alleviate the symptoms of COPD. The following illustration shows the inflamed airways and excessive mucus involved in chronic bronchitis (A), the distended bronchioles and alveoli associated with emphysema (B), and the narrowed bronchial tubes and swollen mucous membranes associated with asthma (C).

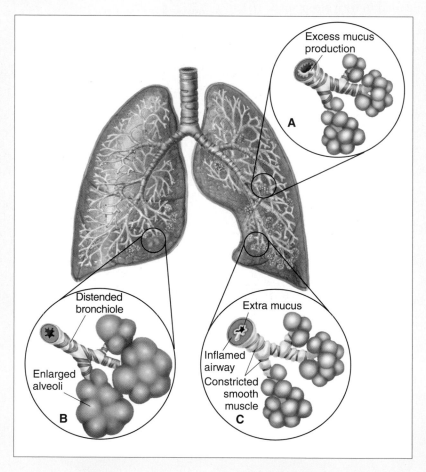

COPD.

A Closer Look—cont'd

Bronchoscopy

Bronchoscopy, a type of endoscopic procedure, is the visual examination of the interior bronchi using a flexible fiberoptic instrument with a light **(bronchoscope).** It is inserted either through the nose **(transnasally)** or through the mouth. This procedure may be performed to remove obstructions, obtain a **biopsy specimen,** or observe directly for pathological changes. In children, this procedure may be used to remove foreign objects that have been inhaled. In adults, the procedure is most commonly performed to obtain samples of suspicious lesions **(biopsy)** and for culturing specific areas in the lung. The cavity, organ, or canal being examined dictates the name of the endoscopic procedure, such as **cystoscopy, gastroscopy,** or **bronchoscopy.** The following illustration shows bronchoscopy of the left bronchus.

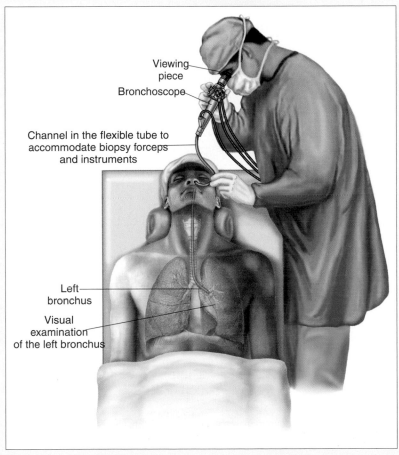

Bronchoscopy.

Medical Vocabulary Recall

Match the medical terms below with the definitions in the numbered list.

ABGs	atelectasis	corticosteroids	hypoxemia	pleurisy
anosmia	bronchodilators	croup	Mantoux	pneumothorax
asthma	CF	epistaxis	PFT	stridor

1. _____ is an inflammation of the pleura.

2. _____ is an acute respiratory syndrome of childhood characterized by laryngeal obstruction and spasm, barking cough, and stridor.

3. _____ is a deficiency of oxygen in the blood.

4. _____ are hormonal agents that reduce edema and inflammation.

5. _____ is a disease that causes severe congestion within the lungs and digestive system as a result of production of thick mucus.

6. _____ is a high-pitched musical sound made on inspiration resulting from an obstruction of air passages.

7. _____ is a respiratory disorder marked by recurrent attacks of difficult or labored breathing accompanied by wheezing.

8. _____ are drugs that dilate the bronchioles and bronchi to increase airflow.

9. _____ refers to a collection of air or gas in the pleural cavity.

10. _____ involve analyzing oxygen and carbon dioxide concentrations in an arterial blood sample.

11. _____ is a hemorrhage from the nose; also called *nosebleed.*

12. _____ is an absence or decrease in the sense of smell.

13. _____ refers to any of several tests used to evaluate respiratory function.

14. _____ is an intradermal test to determine recent or past exposure to tuberculosis.

15. _____ is a collapse of lung tissue, preventing the respiratory exchange of oxygen and carbon dioxide.

Competency Verification: Check your answers in Appendix B, Answer Key, on page 369. Review material that you did not answer correctly.

Correct Answers: _____ × 6.67 = _____ %

Pronunciation and Spelling

Use the following list to practice correct pronunciation and spelling of medical terms. Practice the pronunciation aloud, and then write the correct spelling of the term. The first word is completed for you.

Pronunciation	Spelling
1. ăs-ĭ-DŌ-sĭs	*acidosis*
2. ĕr-ō-FĂ-jē-ă	
3. ăn-ŎZ-mē-ă	
4. ăs-FĬK-sē-ă	
5. ĂZ-mă	
6. ăt-ĕ-LĔK-tă-sĭs	
7. brăd-ĭp-NĒ-ă	
8. brŏng-kē-ĔK-tă-sĭs	
9. brŏng-kō-DĬ-lā-tŏrz	
10. brŏng-KŎS-kō-pē	
11. ĕm-fĭ-SĒ-mă	
12. kor-tĭ-kō-STĒR-oydz	
13. kŏ-RĪ-ză	
14. KRĂK-ăl	
15. dĭsp-NĒ-ă	
16. hī-pŏks-Ē-mē-ă	
17. hī-PŎKS-ē-ă	
18. pĕr-TŬS-ĭs	
19. PLOO-rĭs-ē	
20. RŎNG-kī	

 Competency Verification: Check your answers in Appendix B, Answer Key, on page 370. Review material that you did not answer correctly.

Correct Answers: _____ × 5 = _____ %

ABBREVIATIONS

The following table introduces abbreviations associated with the respiratory system.

Abbreviation	Meaning	Abbreviation	Meaning
ABG	arterial blood gas(es)	NMT	nebulized mist treatment
ARDS	adult respiratory distress syndrome; acute respiratory distress syndrome	OM	otitis media
CF	cystic fibrosis	O_2	oxygen
CO_2	carbon dioxide	OSA	obstructive sleep apnea
COPD	chronic obstructive pulmonary disease	PFT	pulmonary function test
CPAP	continuous positive airway pressure	TB	tuberculosis
CPR	cardiopulmonary resuscitation	UPP	uvulopalatopharyngoplasty
MDI	metered-dose inhaler	URI	upper respiratory infection

CHART NOTES

Chart notes make up part of the medical record and are used in various types of health care facilities. The chart notes that follow were dictated by the patient's physician and reflect common clinical events using medical terminology to document the patient's care. Studying and completing the terminology and chart note analysis sections below will help you learn and understand terms associated with the medical specialty of pulmonary medicine.

Terminology

The following terms are linked to chart notes in the medical specialty of pulmonology, also called *pulmonary medicine*. Practice pronouncing each term aloud, and then use a medical dictionary such as *Taber's Cyclopedic Medical Dictionary; Appendix A: Glossary of Medical Word Elements,* page xxx; or other resources to define each term.

Term	Meaning
anesthesia ăn-ĕs-THĒ-zē-ă	
biopsy BĪ-ŏp-sē	
carcinoma kăr-sĭ-NŌ-mă	
diagnosis dī-ăg-NŌ-sĭs	
expired	
fascia FĂSH-ē-ă	
hemorrhage HĔM-ĕ-rĭj	
lymph node lĭmf nōd	
meatus mē-Ā-tŭs	
metastatic mĕt-ă-STĂT-ĭk	
necropsy NĔK-rŏp-sē	
papillary PĂP-ĭ-lăr-ē	
pathological păth-ō-LŎJ-ĭk-ăl	
pneumonia nū-MŌ-nē-ă	
polypectomy pŏl-ĭ-PĔK-tō-mē	
polypoid PŎL-ē-poyd	
pulmonary PŬL-mō-nĕ-rē	
snare SNĀR	
submaxillary sŭb-MĂK-sĭ-lĕr-ē	

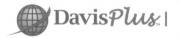

Airway Obstruction

Read the following chart note aloud. Underline any term you have trouble pronouncing or cannot define. If needed, refer to the Terminology section above for correct pronunciations and meanings of terms.

This 45-year-old white man was seen 2 years ago because of upper airway obstruction as a result of large polyps in the right nasal cavity. On examination, a large polypoid mass filled most of the right nasal cavity. The mass originated in the middle meatus. With use of a nasal snare, polypectomy was performed to remove several sections. There was a slight hemorrhage. On the next day, with the patient under local anesthesia, a 4-cm × 3-cm oval soft mass was excised from beneath the left submaxillary region. The mass was just beneath the superficial fascia and appeared to be an enlarged lymph node unconnected with the nasal disease.

Pathological diagnosis of the nasal growth was low-grade papillary carcinoma. The diagnosis of the lymph node was metastatic carcinoma. A chest film was taken that indicated the presence of pulmonary densities attributed to unresolved pneumonia. Also, a needle biopsy of the enlarged liver nodes yielded no results.

The patient expired at home after discharge from the hospital, and no necropsy was obtained.

Chart Note Analysis

From the preceding chart note, select the medical word that means

1. resembling a polyp: _____

2. an opening: _____

3. removal of a small piece of tissue for microscopic examination: _____

4. pertaining to a carcinoma that has spread to a distant site: _____

5. excision of a polyp: _____

6. wire loop instrument used for excision of polyps: _____

7. abnormal bursting forth of blood: _____

8. administered substance that results in a loss of feeling sensation: _____

9. metric abbreviation that refers to a unit of length: _____

10. tumor that is cancerous: _____

Competency Verification: Check your answers in Appendix B, Answer Key, on page 370. Review material that you did not answer correctly.

Correct Answers: _____ × 10 = _____ %

Demonstrate What You Know!

To evaluate your understanding of how medical terms you have studied in this and previous chapters are used in a clinical environment, complete the numbered sentences by selecting an appropriate term from the words below.

alveoli	diaphragm	laryngectomy	pharyngitis	rhonchi
apnea	emphysema	laryngoscope	phrenalgia	tachypnea
bronchioles	hypoxia	O₂	pneumonia	tracheotomy

1. An incision of the trachea to allow for oxygen exchange is called _____.

2. The exchange of oxygen and carbon dioxide takes place in the lungs in small sacs called _____.

3. A person with cancer of the voice box may undergo the surgery called _____.

4. _____ is one of the major disorders included in COPD.

5. To view the voice box of a patient with nodules on the vocal cords, the physician uses a(n) _____.

6. A patient with streptococcal infection of the throat has a condition called _____.

7. Patients with asthma have spasms of the _____.

8. Temporary cessation of breathing is known as _____.

9. _____ is a snoring sound heard during inspiration or expiration that is caused by obstructed airways.

10. The chemical symbol for oxygen is _____.

11. Acute inflammation of the lungs, caused by a bacterium, is called _____.

12. The diagnosis of a pain in the diaphragm is charted as _____.

13. _____ is a deficiency of oxygen in body tissues.

14. The muscle that separates the lungs from the abdominal cavity is called the _____.

15. The diagnosis of a patient who is breathing rapidly is charted as _____.

✓ **Competency Verification:** Check your answers in Appendix B, Answer Key, on page 370. Review material that you did not answer correctly.

Correct Answers: _____ × **6.67** = _____ %

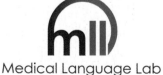
Medical Language Lab
Turning terminology into language

If you are not satisfied with your retention level of the respiratory chapter, visit *DavisPlus* Student Online Resource Center and the Medical Language Lab to complete the website activities linked to this chapter.

Cardiovascular System

Objectives

Upon completion of this chapter, you will be able to:

- Describe types of medical treatment provided by cardiologists.
- Name five structures of the cardiovascular system.
- Discuss the primary function of the cardiovascular system.
- Identify combining forms, suffixes, and prefixes associated with the cardiovascular system.
- Recognize, pronounce, build, and spell medical terms and abbreviations associated with the cardiovascular system.
- Demonstrate your knowledge by successfully completing the activities in this chapter.

VOCABULARY PREVIEW

Term	Meaning
angioplasty ĂN-jē-ō-plăs-tē *angi/o:* vessel (usually blood or lymph) *-plasty:* surgical repair	Surgical procedure that opens a blocked artery by inflating a small balloon within a catheter to widen and restore blood flow in the artery
arteries ĂR-tĕr-ēz	Large blood vessels that carry oxygenated blood away from the heart
capillaries KĂP-ĭ-lār-ēz	Microscopic blood vessels joining arterioles and venules
congenital kŏn-JĔN-ĭ-tăl	Pertaining to presence of a disorder at the time of birth, which may result from genetic or environmental causes
metabolism mĕ-TĂB-ō-lĭzm	Sum of all physical and chemical changes that take place within an organism
veins vānz	Vessels that return deoxygenated blood to the heart

Pronunciation Help	Long Sound Short Sound	ā in rāte ă in ălone	ē in rēbirth ĕ in ĕver	ī in īsle ĭ in ĭt	ō in ōver ŏ in nŏt	ū in ūnite ŭ in cŭt

MEDICAL SPECIALTY OF CARDIOLOGY

The medical specialty of **cardiology** focuses on medical, surgical, and therapeutic treatments of heart diseases. Generally, three types of cardiology specialists provide medical care: **cardiologists, pediatric cardiologists,** and **cardiac surgeons.** The cardiologist specializes in treating adults, and the pediatric cardiologist specializes in treating infants, children, and adolescents. Surgeries performed by the cardiac surgeon include, but are not limited to, coronary artery bypass, **angioplasty**, pacemaker insertion, valve replacement or repair, heart transplantation, and repairs of **congenital** heart diseases.

CARDIOVASCULAR SYSTEM QUICK STUDY

The **cardiovascular (CV) system** is composed of the heart, which is essentially a muscular pump, and an extensive network of blood vessels. The main purpose of the CV system, also called the *circulatory system,* is to deliver oxygen, nutrients, and other essential substances to body cells and remove waste products of cellular **metabolism**. This process is carried out by a complex network of blood vessels that includes **arteries**, **capillaries**, and **veins**—all of which are connected to the heart. Circulation of blood through the heart and body depends on contraction of the heart, or the heartbeat. The heart also contracts and relaxes in a regular rhythm that is coordinated by a series of nodes and nerve tissues in the conduction system of the heart. A contraction is known as **systole,** and the resting period between contractions when the heart fills with blood is known as **diastole.** A healthy CV system is vital to a person's survival. A CV system that does not provide adequate circulation deprives tissues of oxygen and nutrients and fails to remove waste products. These problems result in irreversible cell changes that could be life-threatening. (See *Cardiovascular System,* page 106.)

   ALERT: An extensive self-paced anatomy and physiology multimedia review is included in *TermPlus,* a powerful, interactive CD-ROM program that can be purchased separately from F.A. Davis Company.

MEDICAL WORD BUILDING

Constructing medical words using word elements (combining forms, suffixes, and prefixes) related to the cardiovascular system will enhance your understanding of those terms and reinforce your ability to use terms correctly.

Combining Forms

Begin your study of cardiovascular terminology by reviewing the organs and their associated combining forms (CFs), which are illustrated in the figure *Cardiovascular System* that follows.

Cardiovascular System: Systemic and Pulmonary Circulation

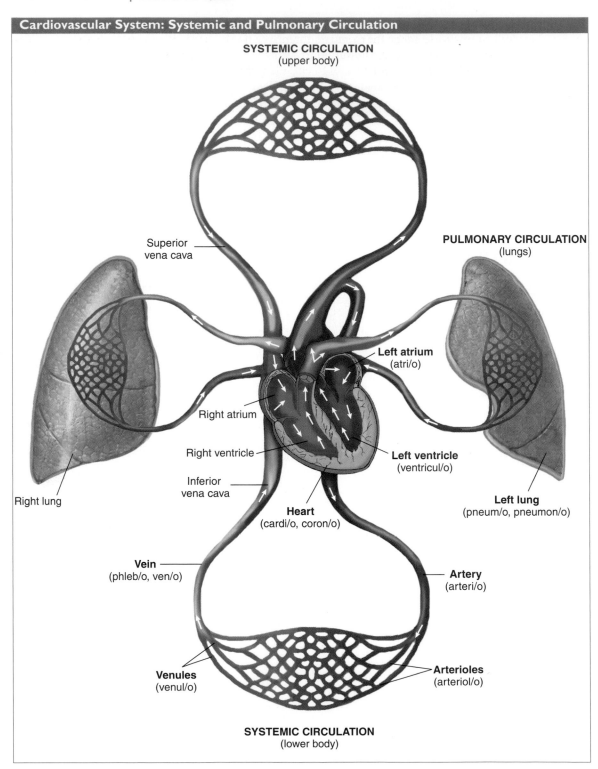

In the table that follows, CFs are listed alphabetically, and other word parts are defined as needed. Review the medical word and study the elements that make up the term. Then complete the meaning of the medical words in the right-hand column. The first one is completed for you. You may also refer to *Appendix A: Glossary of Medical Word Elements* to complete this exercise.

Combining Form	Meaning	Medical Word	Meaning
Cardiovascular System			
aneurysm/o	widening, widened blood vessel	**aneurysm**/ectomy (ăn-ū-rĭz-MĔK-tō-mē) -*ectomy:* excision, removal Get a closer look at abdominal aortic aneurysm on page 123.	*excision of an aneurysm (to repair a weak area in the aorta that is likely to rupture if left in place)*
aort/o	aorta	**aort/o/stenosis** (ā-or-tō-stĕ-NŌ-sĭs) -*stenosis:* narrowing, stricture	
arter/o	artery	**arter**/itis (ăr-tĕ-RĪ-tĭs) -*itis:* inflammation	
arteri/o		**arteri/o/scler/osis** (ăr-tē-rē-ō-sklĕ-RŌ-sĭs) *scler:* hardening; sclera (white of eye) -*osis:* abnormal condition; increase (used primarily with blood cells) Get a closer look at coronary artery disease (CAD) on page 122.	
ather/o	fatty plaque	**ather**/oma (ăth-ĕr-Ō-mă) -*oma:* tumor	
atri/o	atrium	**atri**/um (Ā-trē-ŭm) -*um:* structure, thing	

(Continued)

Combining Form	Meaning	Medical Word	Meaning
Cardiovascular System			
cardi/o	heart	**cardi/o**/megaly (kăr-dē-ō-MĔG-ă-lē) *-megaly:* enlargement	
coron/o		**coron**/ary (KOR-ō-nă-rē) *-ary:* pertaining to	
phleb/o	vein	**phleb**/itis (flĕb-Ī-tĭs) *-itis:* inflammation	
ven/o		**ven**/ous (VĒ-nŭs) *-ous:* pertaining to	
thromb/o	blood clot	**thromb**/o/lysis (thrŏm-BŎL-ĭ-sĭs) *-lysis:* separation; destruction; loosening	
varic/o	dilated vein	**varic**/ose (VĂR-ĭ-kōs) *-ose:* pertaining to; sugar Get a closer look at varicose veins on pages 124–125.	
vas/o	vessel; vas defer- ens; duct	**vas**/o/spasm (VĂS-ō-spăzm) *-spasm:* involuntary contraction, twitching	
vascul/o	vessel	**vascul**/ar (VĂS-kū-lăr) *-ar:* pertaining to	
ventricul/o	ventricle (of heart or brain)	inter/**ventricul**/ar (ĭn-tĕr-vĕn-TRĬK-ū-lăr) *inter-:* between *-ar:* pertaining to	

Suffixes and Prefixes

In the table that follows, suffixes and prefixes are listed alphabetically, and other word parts are defined as needed. Review the medical word and study the elements that make up the term. Then complete the meaning of the medical words in the right-hand column. You may also refer to *Appendix A: Glossary of Medical Word Elements* to complete this exercise.

Word Element	Meaning	Medical Words	Meaning
Suffixes			
-cardia	heart condition	tachy/**cardia** (tăk-ē-KĂR-dē-ă) *tachy-:* rapid	
-gram	record, writing	electr/o/cardi/o/**gram** (ē-lĕk-trō-KĂR-dē-ō-grăm) *electr/o:* electricity *cardi/o:* heart	
-graph	instrument for recording	electr/o/cardi/o/**graph** (ē-lĕk-trō-KĂR-dē-ŏ-grăf) *electr/o:* electricity *cardi/o:* heart	
-graphy	process of recording	angi/o/**graphy** (ăn-jē-ŎG-ră-fē) *angi/o:* vessel (usually blood or lymph)	
-stenosis	narrowing, stricture	aort/o/**stenosis** (ā-or-tō-stĕn-Ō-sĭs) *aort/o:* aorta	
Prefixes			
brady-	slow	**brady**/cardi/ac (brăd-ē-KĂR-dē-ăk) *cardi:* heart *-ac:* pertaining to	
endo-	in, within	**endo**/cardi/um (ĕn-dō-KĂR-dē-ŭm) *cardi:* heart *-um:* structure, thing	

(Continued)

Word Element	Meaning	Medical Words	Meaning
Prefixes			
epi-	above, upon	**epi**/cardi/um (ĕp-ĭ-KĂR-dē-ŭm) *cardi:* heart *-um:* structure, thing	
peri-	around	**peri**/cardi/um (pĕr-ĭ-KĂR-dē-ŭm) *cardi:* heart *-um:* structure, thing	

 Competency Verification: Check your answers in Appendix B, Answer Key, pages 370–371. If you are not satisfied with your level of comprehension, review the terms in the table and retake the review.

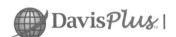 Visit the *Medical Terminology Express* online resource center at *DavisPlus* for an audio exercise of the terms in this table. Other activities are also available to reinforce content.

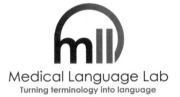

Visit the Medical Language Lab at *medicallanguagelab.com* to enhance your study and reinforce this chapter's word elements with the flash-card activity. We recommend you complete the flash-card activity before continuing with the next section.

Medical Terminology Word Building

In this section, combine the word parts you have learned to construct medical terms related to the cardiovascular system.

Use **ather/o** (fatty plaque) to build words that mean:

1. tumor of fatty plaque _____

2. hardening of fatty plaque _____

Use **phleb/o** (vein) to build words that mean:

3. inflammation of a vein (wall) _____

4. abnormal condition of a blood clot in a vein _____

Use **ven/o** (vein) to build words that mean:

5. pertaining to a vein _____

6. spasm of a vein _____

Use *cardi/o* (heart) to build words that mean:

7. specialist in the study of the heart _____

8. instrument for recording the electrical activity of the heart _____

9. enlargement of the heart _____

Use *angi/o* (vessel) to build words that mean:

10. disease of blood vessels _____

11. tumor of a vessel _____

Use *-stenosis* (narrowing, stricture) to build words that mean:

12. narrowing of the aorta _____

13. stricture of an artery _____

Use *-cardia* (heart condition) to build words that mean:

14. rapid heart rate _____

15. slow heart rate _____

✓ **Competency Verification:** Check your answers in Appendix B, Answer Key, on page 371. Review material that you did not answer correctly.

Correct Answers: _____ × **6.67** = _____ %

MEDICAL VOCABULARY

The following tables consist of selected terms that pertain to diseases and conditions of the cardiovascular (CV) system. Terms related to diagnostic, medical, and surgical procedures are included as well as pharmacological agents used to treat diseases. Recognizing and learning these terms will help you understand the connection between diseases and their treatments. Word analyses for selected terms are also provided.

Diseases and Conditions

aneurysm ĂN-ū-rĭzm	abnormal widening (ballooning) of a portion of an artery as a result of weakness in its wall, or it may be present at birth (congenital)—the larger the aneurysm becomes, the greater the risk of rupture (See Figure 5-1.) Get a closer look at abdominal aortic aneurysm on page 123.
angina pectoris ăn-JĪ-nă PĔK-tō-rĭs	Mild to severe pain or pressure in the chest caused by ischemia; also called *angina*

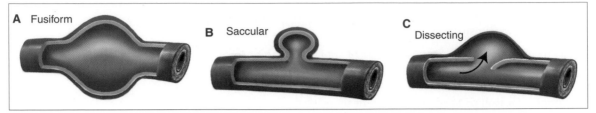

Figure 5-1 Aneurysms. (A) Fusiform aneurysm with dilation of entire circumference of the artery. (B) Saccular aneurysm with bulging on only one side of the artery wall. (C) Dissecting aneurysm with tear (dissection) in the wall of an artery because of bleeding into the weakened wall, which splits the wall (more common in the aorta).

arrhythmia
ă-RĬTH-mē-ă
   a-: without, not
rrhythm: rhythm
   -ia: condition
	Irregularity or loss of rhythm of the heartbeat; also called *dysrhythmia*

fibrillation fĭ-brĭl-Ā-shŭn	Arrhythmia in which there is rapid, uncoordinated quivering of the myocardium that can affect the atria or ventricles; usually described by the part that is contracting abnormally, such as atrial fibrillation or ventricular fibrillation

arteriosclerosis
ăr-tē-rē-ō-sklĕ-RŌ-sĭs
arteri/o: artery
   scler: hardening, sclera
   (white of eye)
	Thickening, hardening, and loss of elasticity of arterial walls; also called *hardening of the arteries*
	
	Get a closer look at coronary artery disease on page 122.

atherosclerosis
ăth-ĕ-rō-sklĕ-RŌ-sĭs
ather/o: fatty plaque
   scler: hardening, sclera
   (white of eye)
   -osis: abnormal
   condition;
   increase (used
   primarily with
   blood cells)
	Most common form of arteriosclerosis caused by accumulation of fatty substances within the arterial walls, resulting in partial and, eventually, total blockage (See Figure 5-2.)

bruit brwē	Soft blowing sound heard on auscultation caused by turbulent blood flow
embolus ĔM-bō-lŭs *embol:* embolus (plug) *-us:* condition; structure	Mass of undissolved matter (commonly a blood clot, fatty plaque, or air bubble) that travels through the bloodstream and becomes lodged in a blood vessel

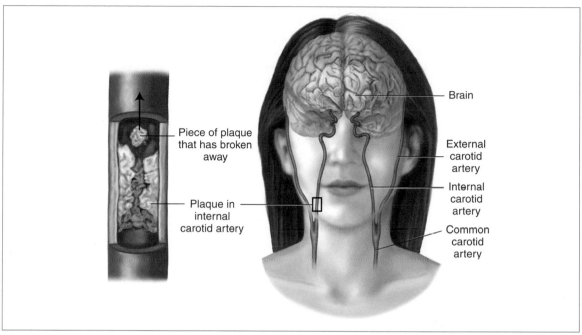

Figure 5-2 Atherosclerosis of the internal carotid artery.

heart block	Disease of the electrical system of the heart, which controls activity of heart muscle
first-degree	Atrioventricular (AV) block in which atrial electrical impulses are delayed by a fraction of a second before being conducted to the ventricles
second-degree	AV block in which only some atrial electrical impulses are conducted to the ventricles
third-degree	AV block in which no electrical impulses reach the ventricles; also called *complete heart block (CHB)*
heart failure (HF)	Occurs when the heart is unable to pump enough blood flow to meet the needs of the body and can cause a number of symptoms, such as shortness of breath, leg swelling, and exercise intolerance
hypertension (HTN) hī-pĕr-TĔN-shŭn *hyper:* excessive, above normal *-tension:* to stretch	Consistently elevated blood pressure, causing damage to the blood vessels and, ultimately, the heart

ischemia ĭs-KĒ-mē-ă *isch:* to hold back *-emia:* blood	Inadequate supply of oxygenated blood to a body part as a result of an interruption of blood flow Get a closer look at ischemia resulting from coronary artery disease on page 122.
mitral valve prolapse (MVP) MĪ-trăl vălv PRŌ-lăps	Structural abnormality in which the mitral (bicuspid) valve does not close completely, resulting in a backflow of blood into the left atrium with each contraction
murmur MĔR-mĕr	Abnormal sound heard on auscultation caused by defects in the valves or chambers of the heart
myocardial infarction (MI) mī-ō-KĂR-dē-ăl ĭn-FĂRK-shŭn *my/o:* muscle *cardi:* heart *-al:* pertaining to	Necrosis of a portion of cardiac muscle caused by partial or complete occlusion of one or more coronary arteries; also called *heart attack*
patent ductus arteriosus (PDA) PĂT-ĕnt DŬK-tŭs ăr-tē-rē-Ō-sĭs	Failure of the ductus arteriosus (which connects the pulmonary artery to the aortic arch in a fetus) to close after birth, resulting in an abnormal opening between the pulmonary artery and the aorta
Raynaud disease rā-NŌ	Severe, sudden vasoconstriction and spasm in fingers and toes followed by cyanosis after exposure to cold temperature or emotional stress; also called *Raynaud phenomenon*
rheumatic heart disease rū-MĂT-ĭk	Streptococcal infection that causes damage to the heart valves and heart muscle, most commonly in children and young adults
stroke STRŌK	Damage to part of the brain as a result of interruption of its blood supply caused by bleeding within brain tissue or, more commonly, blockage of an artery; also called *cerebrovascular accident (CVA)*
thrombus THRŎM-bŭs *thromb:* blood clot *-us:* condition; structure	A stationary blood clot formed within a blood vessel or within the heart, commonly causing vascular obstruction; also called *blood clot*

deep vein thrombosis (DVT)
  dēp vān thrŏm-BŌ-sĭs
  thromb: blood clot
    -osis: abnormal condition; increased (used primarily with blood cells)
	Formation of a blood clot in a deep vein of the body, occurring most commonly in the lower legs (See Figure 5-3.)

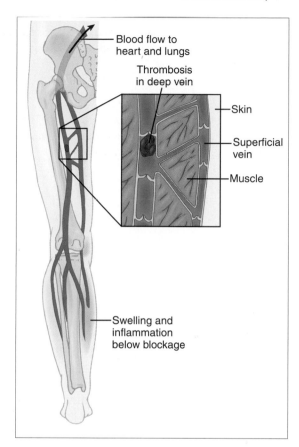

Figure 5-3 Deep vein thrombosis.

transient ischemic attack (TIA) TRĂN-zhĕnt ĭs-KĒ-mĭk	Blood supply to part of the brain is briefly interrupted but does not cause permanent brain damage and may be a warning sign of a more serious and debilitating stroke in the future; also called *ministroke*

Diagnostic Procedures

cardiac catheterization KĂR-dē-ăk kăth-ĕ-tĕr-ĭ-ZĀ-shŭn *cardi:* heart *-ac:* pertaining to	Insertion of a small tube (catheter) through a large vein or artery, usually of an arm (brachial approach) or leg (femoral approach), which is threaded through a blood vessel until it reaches the heart: used to inject a contrast medium for imaging, diagnosing abnormalities, obtaining blood samples, or measuring pressure within the heart, and often includes interventional procedures such as angioplasty and atherectomy (See Figure 5-4.)
cardiac enzyme studies KĂR-dē-ăk ĔN-zīm	Battery of blood tests performed to determine the presence of cardiac damage

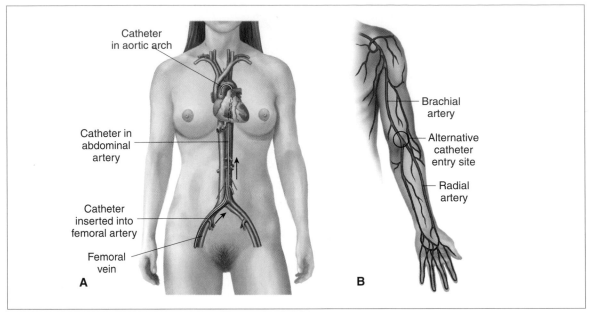

Figure 5-4 Cardiac catheterization. (A) Catheter insertion into a femoral vein or artery. (B) Catheter insertion into a brachial or radial artery.

Doppler ultrasonography ŭl-tră-sōn-ŎG-ră-fē	Ultrasound technique that records blood flow velocity (speed) to image major blood vessels (arteries or veins in arms, neck, legs, abdomen) to detect obstructions caused by atherosclerotic plaques in patients at risk for a stroke (See Figure 5-5.)
echocardiography (ECHO) ĕk-ō-kăr-dē-ŎG-ră-fē *echo-:* repeated sound *cardi/o:* heart *-graphy:* process of recording	Ultrasound technique used to image the heart and evaluate how the heart's chambers and valves are working and to diagnose and detect pathological conditions
electrocardiography (ECG, EKG) ē-lĕk-trō-kăr-dē-ŎG-ră-fē *electr/o:* electricity *cardi/o:* heart *-graphy:* process of recording	Creation and study of graphic recordings (electrocardiograms) produced by electrical activity generated by the heart muscle; also called *cardiography*
Holter monitor HŎL-tĕr MŎN-ĭ-tor	Monitoring device worn by a patient that records prolonged electrocardiograph readings (usually 24 hours) on a portable tape recorder while the patient conducts normal daily activities (See Figure 5-6.)

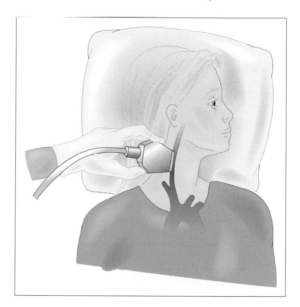

Figure 5-5 Doppler ultrasound of the carotid artery.

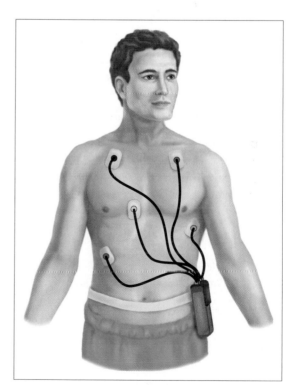

Figure 5-6 Holter monitor.

stress test	Electrocardiography (ECG) taken under controlled exercise stress conditions (typically using a treadmill) while measuring oxygen consumption
nuclear	ECG that uses a radioisotope to evaluate coronary blood flow
troponin I TRŌ-pō-nĭn	Blood test that measures protein released into the blood by damaged heart muscle (not skeletal muscle) and is a highly sensitive, specific indicator of recent myocardial infarction (MI)

Medical and Surgical Procedures

angioplasty ĂN-jē-ō-plăs-tē *angi/o:* vessel *-plasty:* surgical repair	Surgery that opens a blocked artery by inflating a small balloon within a catheter to widen and restore blood flow in the artery (See Figure 5-7.)
cardioversion căr-dē-ō-VĔR-zhŭn *cardi/o:* heart *-version:* turning	Restoration of normal heart rhythm by applying an electrical counter-shock to the chest using a device (defibrillator); also called *defibrillation*
coronary artery bypass graft (CABG) KOR-ō-nă-rē ĂR-tĕr-ē *coron:* heart *-ary:* pertaining to	Bypass surgery in which peripheral veins are removed, and each end of the vein is sutured onto the coronary artery to create new routes around narrowed and blocked arteries, allowing sufficient blood flow to deliver oxygen and nutrients to the heart muscle (See Figure 5-8.)
defibrillator dē-FĬB-rĭ-lā-tĕr	Device used to administer a defibrillating electrical shock to restore normal heart rhythm
automatic implantable cardioverter-defibrillator (AICD) căr-dē-ō-VĔR-tĕr dē-FĬB-rĭ-lā-tĕr	Surgically implanted electrical device that continuously monitors and corrects potentially fatal arrhythmias by delivering low-energy shocks to the heart; also called *implantable cardioverter defibrillator* (ICD) (See Figure 5-9.)
automatic external defibrillator (AED) dē-FĬB-rĭ-lā-tĕr	Portable computerized device that analyzes the patient's heart rhythm and delivers an electrical shock to stimulate a heart in cardiac arrest

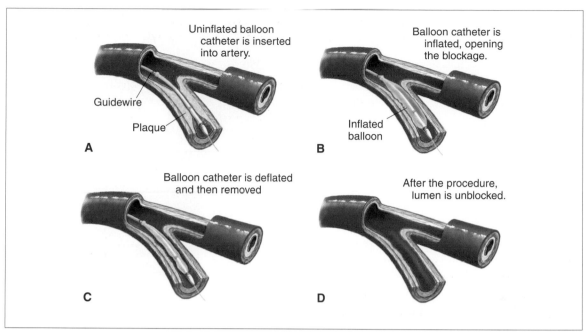

Figure 5-7 Balloon angioplasty.

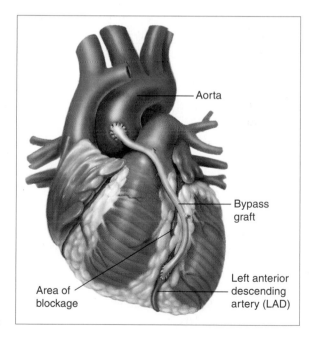

Figure 5-8 Coronary artery bypass graft.

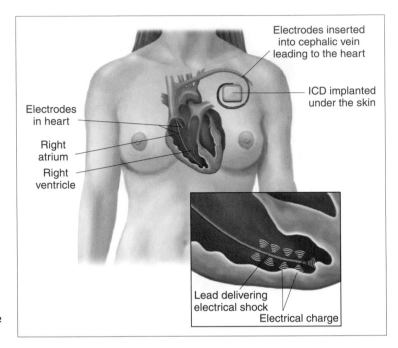

Electrodes inserted
into cephalic vein
leading to the heart

ICD implanted
under the skin

Electrodes
in heart

Right
atrium

Right
ventricle

Lead delivering
electrical shock

Electrical charge

Figure 5-9 Automatic implantable
cardioverter-defibrillator.

endarterectomy
ĕnd-ăr-tĕr-ĔK-tō-mē
   end-: in, within
   arter: artery
-ectomy: excision, removal
	Surgical removal of the lining of an artery

carotid endarterectomy
  kă-RŎT-ĭd
  ĕnd-ăr-tĕr-ĔK-tō-mē
	Removal of plaque (atherosclerosis) and thromboses from an occluded carotid artery to reduce the risk of stroke (See Figure 5-10.)

endovenous laser therapy (EVLT) ĕn-dō-VĒ-nŭs *endo:* in, within *ven:* vein *-ous:* pertaining to	Treatment of large varicose veins in the legs in which a laser fiber is inserted directly into the affected vein to heat the lining within the vein, causing it to collapse, shrink, and eventually disappear; also called *endovenous laser ablation (EVLA)* 🔍 Get a closer look at varicose veins, on pages 124–125.

sclerotherapy
sklĕr-ō-THĔR-ă-pē
  scler/o: hardening; sclera
     (white of eye)
-therapy: treatment
	Chemical injection into a varicose vein that causes inflammation and formation of fibrous tissue, which closes the vein
	
	🔍 Get a closer look at varicose veins, on pages 124–125.

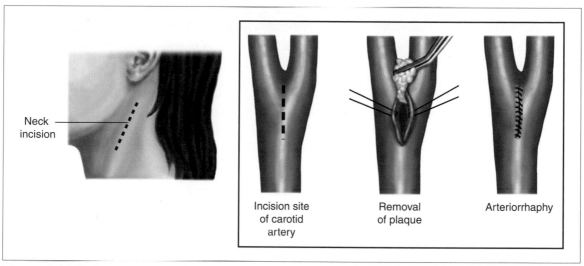

Figure 5-10 Endarterectomy of the common carotid artery.

valvuloplasty VĂL-vū-lō-plăs-tē	Insertion of a balloon catheter in a blood vessel in the groin through the aorta and into the heart to widen a stenotic (stiffened) heart valve and increase blood flow; also called *percutaneous valvuloplasty*

Pharmacology

anticoagulants ăn-tĭ-kō-ĂG-ū-lănts	Prevent clotting or coagulation of blood
beta blockers	Slow the heart rate and reduce the force with which the heart muscle contracts, lowering blood pressure
nitrates NĪ-trāts	Relieve chest pain associated with angina and ease symptoms of heart failure (HF)
statins STĂ-tĭnz	Reduce cholesterol levels in the blood and block production of an enzyme in the liver that produces cholesterol
thrombolytics thrŏm-bō-LĬT-ĭks	Dissolve (lyse) blood clots in a process known as *thrombolysis*

Pronunciation Help	Long Sound	ā in rāte	ē in rēbirth	ī in īsle	ō in ōver	ū in ūnite
	Short Sound	ă in ălone	ĕ in ĕver	ĭ in ĭt	ŏ in nŏt	ŭ in cŭt

A Closer Look

Take a closer look at the following cardiovascular disorders to enhance your understanding of the medical terminology associated with them.

Coronary Artery Disease

Coronary artery disease (CAD) is a narrowing of the coronary arteries that results in failure of the arteries to deliver an adequate supply of oxygenated blood to the heart muscle **(myocardium)**. Narrowing of arterial walls **(arteriostenosis),** usually caused by atherosclerosis, is a common form of arteriosclerosis. CAD causes the ordinarily smooth lining of the artery to become roughened as the atherosclerotic plaque collects in the artery. This accumulation causes partial and, eventually, total blockage **(occlusion)** of the artery. The following illustration shows a partial occlusion that results in a decreased supply of oxygenated blood to the myocardium, a condition known as **ischemia** (A). The illustration also shows a later stage of atherosclerosis with total occlusion (B). When the occlusion is total or almost total, the affected area of the heart muscle dies **(infarction)**, causing a heart attack, or **myocardial infarction (MI).** Surgical treatment for CAD includes angioplasty and coronary artery bypass graft (CABG), both of which are discussed on page 119.

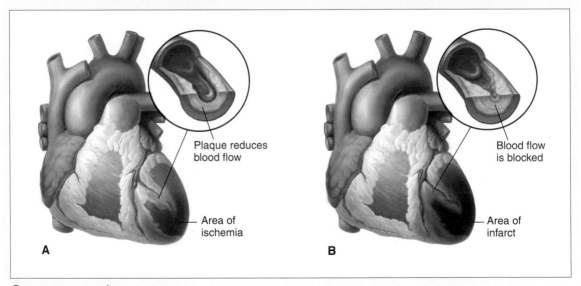

Coronary artery disease.

A Closer Look—cont'd

Abdominal Aortic Aneurysm (AAA)

The most common locations of cardiovascular aneurysms stem from a major artery from the heart (aortic aneurysm). One type, abdominal aortic aneurysm (AAA), forms as a localized dilation (ballooning) of the abdominal aorta exceeding its normal diameter by more than 50 percent. When an aneurysm reaches 5 cm in diameter, it is usually considered necessary to treat to prevent rupture. If an AAA ruptures, the chances of survival are low, with 80 to 90 percent of all ruptured AAAs resulting in death. These deaths can be avoided if an aneurysm is detected and treated before it ruptures. Most aortic aneurysms have no symptoms and are usually diagnosed on a chest x-ray or computed tomography (CT) scan performed for evaluation of another condition, such as lung disease, or during routine examinations. Large aortic aneurysms require repairing the aneurysm with a cylinder-like tube (synthetic graft) that is sewn to the aorta, connecting one end of the aorta at the site of the aneurysm to the other end. The blood flow then goes through the plastic graft and no longer allows the direct pulsation pressure of the blood to expand the weakened aortic wall further. The following illustration shows a synthetic graft repair of an AAA.

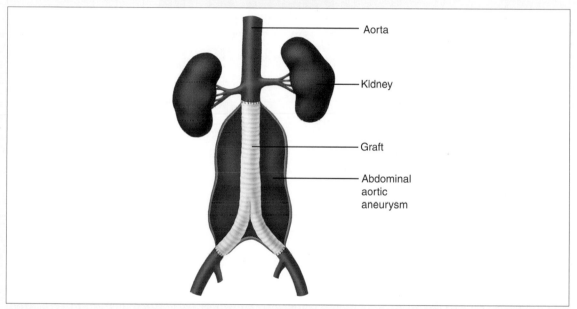

Graft repair of an abdominal aortic aneurysm.

(Continued)

A Closer Look—cont'd

A less invasive endovascular procedure may be performed in which a stent-graft is threaded into the blood vessel where the aneurysm is located. The stent-graft is expanded like a spring to hold tightly against the wall of the blood vessel and cut off the blood supply to the aneurysm. The following illustration shows the location of the AAA (fusiform) with dilation of the entire circumference of the artery (A) and a stent-graft in place to repair the AAA (B).

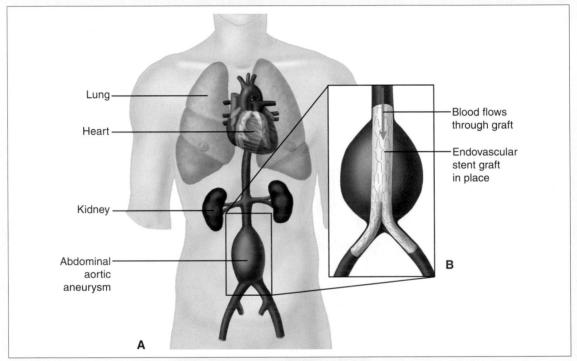

Abdominal aortic aneurysm (A) and stent-graft in place (B).

Varicose Veins

Normal veins are constructed with healthy (**competent**) valves. The venous walls are strong enough to withstand the lateral pressure of blood exerted on them. Blood flows through competent valves in one direction, toward the heart. In **varicose veins,** also known as *varicosities,* dilation of veins from long periods of pressure prevents complete closure of the valves. Unhealthy or damaged (**incompetent**) valves do not close completely. The incompetent valves result in a backflow and pooling of blood in the veins. This pooling causes varicosities that contribute to enlarged, twisted superficial veins, called **varicose veins.** Varicose veins commonly appear blue (contain deoxygenated blood), bulging, and twisted. If left untreated, varicose veins can cause aching and feelings of fatigue as well as skin changes. Because the blood pools, the risk of **thrombosis** is increased as well. Besides incompetent valves, varicose veins result from occupations that require prolonged standing or sitting, which causes pressure

A Closer Look—cont'd

on the valves in the veins of the lower legs. Varicosities may also occur during pregnancy as the enlarging uterus increases pressure on the leg veins, compromising the free flow of blood in the lower extremities. Lastly, there seems to be a family tendency to develop varicose veins. Treatment consists of **sclerotherapy** and surgical interventions such as **endovenous laser ablation (EVLA)** of the greater saphenous (large) veins in the legs and **microphlebectomies** of the lesser saphenous (small) veins. Stripping and ligation of varicose veins is less commonly performed. The following illustration shows valve function in competent and incompetent valves (A) and varicose veins (B).

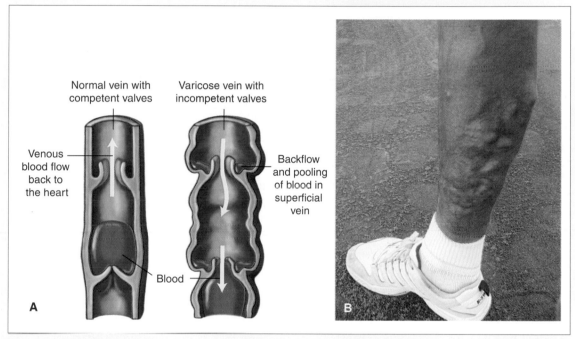

Varicose veins.

Medical Vocabulary Recall

Match the medical terms below with the definitions in the numbered list.

arrhythmia	embolus	HF	Raynaud disease	stroke
bruit	endarterectomy	Holter monitor	rheumatic heart disease	thrombolytics
DVT	fibrillation	HTN	statin	varicose veins

1. _____ are swollen, distended veins most commonly seen in the lower legs.

2. _____ means irregular, rapid, and uncoordinated contractions of the myocardium.

3. _____ are drugs used to dissolve a blood clot.

4. _____ is a mass of undissolved matter that travels through the bloodstream and becomes lodged in a blood vessel.

5. _____ is a condition in which the heart cannot pump enough blood to meet the metabolic requirement of body tissues.

6. _____ refers to formation of a blood clot in a deep vein of the body.

7. _____ refers to blood pressure that is consistently higher than normal.

8. _____ is irregularity or loss of heart rhythm.

9. _____ is an agent that reduces cholesterol levels in the blood and blocks production of cholesterol in the liver.

10. _____ is a soft blowing sound caused by turbulent blood flow.

11. _____ refers to partial brain damage as a result of interruption of blood supply to the brain, commonly caused by blockage of an artery.

12. _____ is a streptococcal infection that causes damage to heart valves and heart muscle.

13. _____ is a device worn by a patient that records prolonged electrocardiograph readings, usually for 24 hours.

14. _____ is numbness in fingers or toes caused by intermittent constriction of arterioles in the skin.

15. _____ is the excision of the lining of an artery.

 Competency Verification: Check your answers in Appendix B, Answer Key, on page 371. Review material that you did not answer correctly.

Correct Answers: _____ × **6.67** = _____ %

Pronunciation and Spelling

Use the following list to practice correct pronunciation and spelling of medical terms. Practice the pronunciation aloud, and then write the correct spelling of the term. The first word is completed for you.

Pronunciation	Spelling
1. ĂN-ū-rĭzm	*aneurysm*
2. ă-RĬTH-mē-ă	
3. ăth-ĕ-rō-sklĕ-RŌ-sĭs	
4. brwē	
5. kăr-dē-ō-MĔG-ă-lē	
6. dī-ĂS-tō-lē	
7. ē-lĕk-trō-kăr-dē-ŎG-ră-fē	
8. fĭ-brĭl-Ā-shŭn	
9. ĭn-FĂRK-shŭn	
10. hī-p ĕr-TĔN-shŭn	
11. ĭs-KĒ-mē-ă	
12. mī-ō-KĂR-dē-ăl	
13. tăk-ē-KĂR-dē-ă	
14. THRŎM-bŭs	
15. VĂR-ĭ-kōs	

Competency Verification: Check your answers in Appendix B, Answer Key, page 372. Review material that you did not answer correctly.

Correct Answers: _____ × **6.67** = _____ **%**

ABBREVIATIONS

The following table introduces abbreviations associated with the cardiovascular system.

Abbreviation	Meaning	Abbreviation	Meaning
AAA	abdominal aortic aneurysm	EVLT	endovenous laser therapy; endoluminal laser therapy
AED	automatic external defibrillator	HDL	high-density lipoprotein
AICD	automated implantable cardioverter-defibrillator	HF	heart failure
ASHD	arteriosclerotic heart disease	HTN	hypertension
BP	blood pressure	ICD	implantable cardioverter-defibrillator
CABG	coronary artery bypass graft	MI	myocardial infarction
CAD	coronary artery disease	MVP	mitral valve prolapse
CT	computed tomography	PDA	patent ductus arteriosus
CV	cardiovascular	TIA	transient ischemic attack
CVA	cerebrovascular accident; costovertebral angle	US	ultrasound, ultrasonography

CHART NOTES

Chart notes comprise part of the medical record and are used in various types of health care facilities. The chart notes that follow were dictated by the patient's physician and reflect common clinical events using medical terminology to document the patient's care. Studying and completing the terminology and chart notes sections below will help you learn and understand terms associated with the medical specialty of cardiology.

Terminology

The following terms are linked to chart notes in the specialty of cardiology. Practice pronouncing each term aloud, and then use a medical dictionary such as *Taber's Cyclopedic Medical Dictionary; Appendix A: Glossary of Medical Word Elements,* or other resources to define each term.

Term	Meaning
apnea ăp-NĒ-ă	
desiccated DĔS-ĭ-kā-tĕd	
dyspnea dĭsp-NĒ-ă	
EKG	
fibrillation fĭ-brĭl-Ā-shŭn	
malaise mă-LĀZ	
myocardial infarction mī-ō-KĂR-dē-ăl ĭn-FĂRK-shŭn	
ST segment–T wave	
syncope SĬN-kō-pē	
tachycardia tăk-ē-KĂR-dē-ă	
thyroidectomy thī-royd-ĔK-tō-mē	

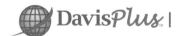

Visit *Medical Terminology Express* at *DavisPlus* Online Resource Center. Use it to practice pronunciations and reinforce the meanings of the terms in this chart note.

Myocardial Infarction

Read the chart note that follows aloud. Underline any term you have trouble pronouncing or cannot define. If needed, refer to the Terminology section on pages 128 and 129 for correct pronunciations and meanings of terms.

This 65-year-old woman presents at the hospital for evaluation of a syncopal episode. She states that most recently she has experienced generalized malaise, increased shortness of breath while at rest, and dyspnea followed by periods of apnea and syncope. Her past history includes recurrent episodes of thyroiditis, which led her to have a thyroidectomy 6 years ago while she was under the care of Dr. Knopp. At the time of surgery, the results of her EKG were interpreted as sinus tachycardia with nonspecific ST segment—T wave changes. The tachycardia was attributed to preoperative anxiety and thyroiditis. Postoperatively, under the direction of Dr. Knopp, the patient was treated with a daily dose of 50 mg of desiccated thyroid and has been symptom-free until this admission.

On clinical examination, the patient's radial pulse was found to be irregular, and the EKG showed uncontrolled atrial fibrillation with evidence of a recent myocardial infarction.

Chart Note Analysis

From the preceding chart note, select the medical word that means

1. temporary cessation of breathing: _____

2. occurring after an operation: _____

3. feeling of apprehension, worry, uneasiness, or dread: _____

4. inflammation of the thyroid gland: _____

5. fainting: _____

6. dried up: _____

7. rapid and irregular contractions of the myocardium: _____

8. discomfort or indisposition, commonly indicating infection: _____

9. tachycardia that originates with the sinoatrial node: _____

10. abbreviation for a test that provides a recording of electrical impulses of the heart: _____

11. difficult breathing: _____

12. abbreviation for metric unit of one one-thousandth of a gram: _____

Competency Verification: Check your answers in Appendix B, Answer Key, on page 372. Review material that you did not answer correctly.

Correct Answers: _____ × 8.34 = _____ %

Demonstrate What You Know!

To evaluate your understanding of how medical terms you have studied in this and previous chapters are used in a clinical environment, complete the numbered sentences by selecting an appropriate term from the words below.

aneurysm	arteriosclerosis	cardiomegaly	nitrate	statin
angioplasty	arteriostenosis	ischemia	oxygen	tachycardia
arteriole	cardiologist	MI	phlebitis	tricuspid

1. The _____ provides nonsurgical treatment to detect, prevent, and treat heart and vascular disease.

2. A small artery is called a(n) _____.

3. An endovascular procedure that reopens a narrowed, blocked vessel by balloon dilation is called _____.

4. To reduce plaque build-up in arteries and lower blood cholesterol levels, the cardiologist prescribes a drug called a(n) _____.

5. The valve that contains three leaflets is the _____ valve.

6. Without CV circulation, body tissues are deprived of nutrients and _____.

7. Disorder characterized by thickening and calcification of arterial walls is _____.

8. A patient with an enlarged heart has _____.

9. The diagnosis of inflammation of a vein is charted as _____.

10. A drug that treats chest pain associated with angina is called a(n) _____.

11. Decreased supply of oxygenated blood to a body part or organ is called _____.

12. When performing an angiogram, the surgeon notes a narrowing of an artery, which is charted as _____.

13. A widened, stretched-out portion of a blood vessel that forms a bulge is called a(n) _____.

14. A patient arrives at the emergency department with a rapid heart rate, a condition called _____.

15. When heart tissue dies as a result of lack of oxygen, the patient has had a(n) _____.

Competency Verification: Check your answers in Appendix B, Answer Key, on page 372. Review material that you did not answer correctly.

Correct Answers: _____ × 6.67 = _____ %

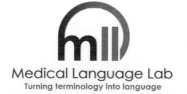

Medical Language Lab
Turning terminology into language

If you are not satisfied with your retention level of the cardiovascular chapter, visit *DavisPlus* Student Online Resource Center and the Medical Language Lab to complete the website activities linked to this chapter.

Blood, Lymphatic, and Immune Systems

Objectives

Upon completion of this chapter, you will be able to:

- Describe types of medical treatment provided by hematologists and immunologists.
- Discuss the main components of blood and their functions.
- Understand the four different types of blood groups.
- Name five structures of the lymphatic system.
- List three primary functions of the lymphatic system.
- Explain the relationship between the lymphatic and the immune systems in the immune response.
- Identify combining forms, suffixes, and prefixes associated with the blood, lymphatic, and immune systems.
- Recognize, pronounce, build, and spell medical terms and abbreviations associated with the blood, lymphatic, and immune systems.
- Demonstrate your knowledge by successfully completing the activities in this chapter.

VOCABULARY PREVIEW

Term	Meaning
antigen ĂN-tĭ-jĕn *anti-:* against *gen:* forming, producing, origin	Substance that, when entering the body, prompts the generation of antibodies, causing an immune response
autoimmune aw-tō-ĭ-MŪN	Type of immune response by the body against its own cells or tissues
capillaries KĂP-ĭ-lār-ēz	Microscopic blood vessels that connect the ends of the smallest arteries (arterioles) with the smallest veins (venules) of the circulatory system
hematopoiesis hē-mă-tō-poy-Ē-sĭs *hemat/o:* blood *-poiesis:* formation, production	Production and development of blood cells, normally in the bone marrow; also called *hemopoiesis*
immune response ĭm-MŪN	Defense function of the body that protects it against invading pathogens, foreign tissues, and malignancies
immunodeficiency ĭm-ū-nō-dĕ-FĬSH-ĕn-sē	Decreased or compromised ability to fight disease or a condition resulting from a defective immune mechanism
interstitial fluid ĭn-tĕr-STĬSH-ăl	Fluid between cells and in tissue spaces
lymphocyte LĬM-fō-sīt *lymph/o:* lymph *-cyte:* cell	Type of white blood cell (WBC) found in the lymph nodes, spleen, bloodstream, and lymph that functions in the body's immune system by recognizing and deactivating foreign substances (antigens)
monocytes MŎN-ō-sīts *mono-:* one *-cyte:* cell	Large WBCs formed in the bone marrow that circulate in the bloodstream and destroy pathogenic bacteria through phagocytosis
oncology ŏn-KŎL-ō-jē *onc/o:* tumor *-logy:* study of	Branch of medicine concerned with the study of cancerous growths (malignancies)

Term	Meaning
pathogens PĂTH-ō-jĕns *path/o*: disease -*gen*: forming, producing, origin	Any microorganism capable of producing disease
transfusion trăns-FŪ-zhŭn	Collection of blood or a blood component from a donor followed by its infusion into a recipient

Pronunciation Help	Long Sound	ā in rāte	ē in rēbirth	ī in īsle	ō in ōver	ū in ūnite
	Short Sound	ă in ălone	ĕ in ĕver	ĭ in ĭt	ŏ in nŏt	ŭ in cŭt

MEDICAL SPECIALTIES OF HEMATOLOGY AND IMMUNOLOGY

Hematology

Hematology is the study of the blood and blood-forming tissues and the diseases associated with these tissues. Physicians who specialize in the study and treatment of blood and blood disorders are called **hematologists.** Hematologists treat malignant (cancerous) and nonmalignant blood diseases. Historically, hematologists were the first to use chemical therapies (chemotherapy) to treat hematological malignancies. With time, it was discovered that these treatments could also be effective on so-called solid tumors, such as breast, lung, and stomach cancers (previously treated only with surgery). Consequently, hematology became closely associated with the medical specialty of **oncology**. Oncological terms are included throughout all body system chapters. In addition, *Appendix G, Index of Oncological Terms* provides a summary of these terms.

Immunology

Immunology is the study of the body's protection from invading organisms and its responses to them. These invaders include viruses, bacteria, protozoa, and even larger parasites. Anything that causes an **immune response** is called an **antigen**. An antigen may be harmless, such as grass pollen, or harmful, such as the flu virus. Disease-causing antigens are called **pathogens**. The immune system is designed to protect the body from pathogens. The body's ability to fight disease and protect itself depends on an adequately functioning **immune response**. An **immunologist** is a medical specialist who studies and treats the body's defense mechanism against invasion of foreign substances that cause disease. The immunologist is consulted when the immune system breaks down and the body loses its ability to recognize antigens or its ability to mount an attack against them. The immune system also has the ability to react in a manner disadvantageous to the body by way of allergic and **autoimmune** diseases. Immunologists treat patients with **immunodeficiency** diseases, such as acquired immune deficiency syndrome (AIDS); immune complex diseases, such as malaria and viral hepatitis; autoimmune diseases, such as lupus; transplanted cells and organs; allergies; and various cancer types related to the immune system.

BLOOD, LYMPHATIC, AND IMMUNE SYSTEMS QUICK STUDY

Blood

The major function of blood is to transport oxygen and nutrients to the cells of the body and remove carbon dioxide and metabolic waste products from the cells. The two main components of blood are plasma and **formed elements,** such as erythrocytes (red blood cells), leukocytes (white blood cells), and platelets (clotting cells). Erythrocytes deliver oxygen to the body tissues via the circulatory system. Leukocytes provide a line of defense against **pathogens**. Platelets have a clotting ability that prevents excessive loss of blood. Erythrocytes, leukocytes, and platelets are produced in the bone marrow by a process called **hematopoiesis**.

Blood Types

The four main blood types, or groups, are A, B, AB, and O. The groups are based on the presence or absence of A or B antigens on the red blood cells (RBCs). The antigens, also known as **markers,** stimulate production of antibodies.

Safe administration of blood from donor to recipient requires careful typing and crossmatching to ensure a compatible **transfusion**. Incompatible transfusions can result in serious, possibly fatal, reactions. For example, antibodies contained in type A blood and type B blood can cause each other to **agglutinate** (clump together). Because type O blood does not contain A or B antigens, type O blood may be given to a person with any of the other blood type. A person with type O blood is called a **universal donor.** Similarly, a person with type AB blood is a universal recipient because type AB blood has no antibodies against the other blood types. For a summary of compatible donors and recipients, see Table 6-1.

Rh Factor

In addition to ABO antigens, blood may contain other antigens, called Rh factors. When these antigens are present on RBCs, the blood type is further classified as **Rh-positive** (Rh+). When these antigens are not present, the blood type is classified as **Rh-negative** (Rh–). A person with Rh+ blood may receive a transfusion with Rh+ or Rh– blood. However, a person with Rh– blood can receive a transfusion with only Rh– blood.

TABLE 6-1 **Blood Types, Donors, and Recipients**				
Blood Type	**Antigen on RBC**	**Antigen on Plasma**	**Donate to**	**Receive From**
A	A	anti-B antibodies	A or AB	A or O
B	B	anti-A antibodies	B or AB	B or O
AB (universal recipient)	A and B	none	AB only	A, B, AB, O
O (universal donor)	none	anti-A and anti-B antibodies	A, B, AB, O	O

Lymphatic and Immune Systems

The **lymphatic system** consists of lymph, lymph vessels, lymph nodes, and three organs: the tonsils, thymus, and spleen, as shown in the figure Lymphatic System on page 139. The lymph circulating through the lymphatic system comes from the blood. It contains white blood cells (leukocytes) responsible for immunity, **monocytes**, and **lymphocytes**. **Interstitial fluid** is created when certain components of blood plasma filter through tiny **capillaries** into the spaces between cells, called **interstitial** (or **intercellular**) **spaces.** Thin-walled vessels called **lymph capillaries** absorb most interstitial fluid from the interstitial spaces. At this point of absorption, interstitial fluid becomes lymph and passes through lymphatic tissue called **lymph nodes.** The nodes are located in clusters in areas such as the neck (cervical lymph nodes), under the arm (axillary lymph nodes), pelvis (iliac lymph nodes), and groin (inguinal lymph nodes). These nodes act as filters against foreign materials. Eventually, lymph reaches large lymph vessels in the upper chest and re-enters the bloodstream.

The lymphatic and immune systems are closely involved with the **immune response**. They work together to protect the body against invasion of foreign organisms such as viruses and bacteria.

ALERT: An extensive anatomy and physiology review is included in *TermPlus*, a powerful, interactive CD-ROM program that can be purchased separately from F.A. Davis Company.

MEDICAL WORD BUILDING

Constructing medical words using word elements (combining forms, suffixes, and prefixes) related to the blood, lymphatic, and immune systems will enhance your understanding of those terms and reinforce your ability to use terms correctly.

Combining Forms

Begin your study of the blood, lymphatic, and immune systems by reviewing their associated combining forms (CFs) and other word elements. These are illustrated in the figures *Blood Components* and *Lymphatic System*, which follow.

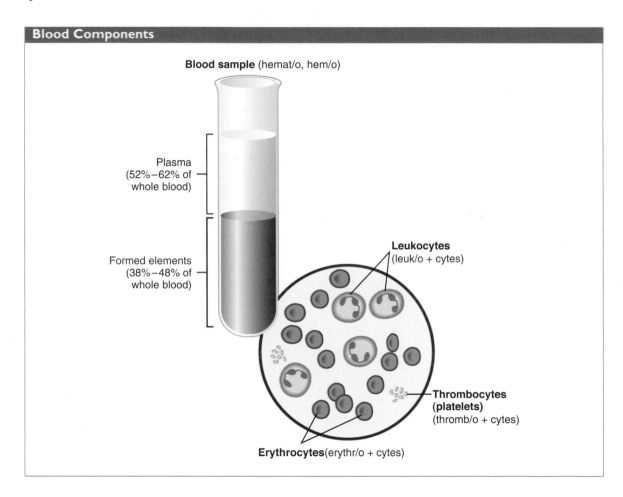

Blood Components

Blood sample (hemat/o, hem/o)

Plasma (52%–62% of whole blood)

Formed elements (38%–48% of whole blood)

Leukocytes (leuk/o + cytes)

Thrombocytes (platelets) (thromb/o + cytes)

Erythrocytes (erythr/o + cytes)

Lymphatic System

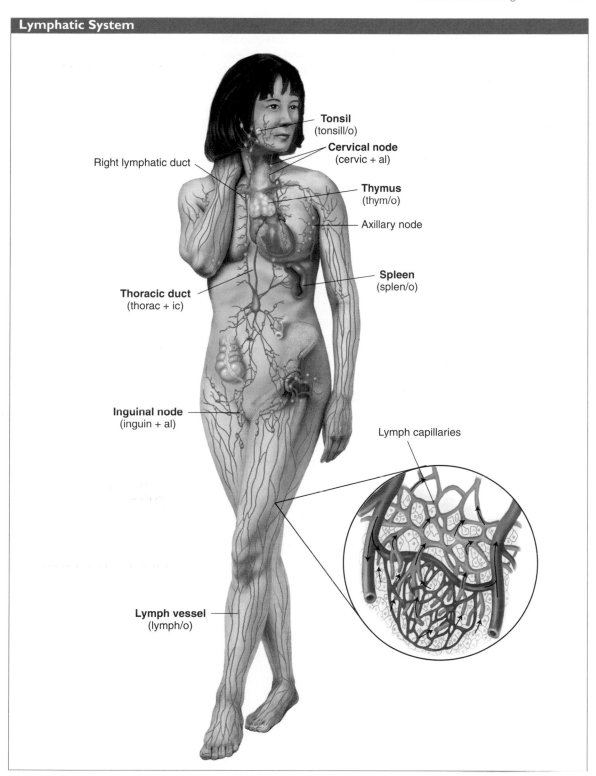

Tonsil
(tonsill/o)

Cervical node
(cervic + al)

Right lymphatic duct

Thymus
(thym/o)

Axillary node

Spleen
(splen/o)

Thoracic duct
(thorac + ic)

Inguinal node
(inguin + al)

Lymph capillaries

Lymph vessel
(lymph/o)

In the table that follows, CFs are listed alphabetically, and other word parts are defined as needed. Review the medical word and study the elements that make up the term. Then complete the meaning of the medical words in the right-hand column. The first one is completed for you. You may also refer to *Appendix A: Glossary of Medical Word Elements* to complete this exercise.

Combining Form	Meaning	Medical Word	Meaning
Blood System			
agglutin/o	clumping, gluing	**agglutin**/ation (ă-gloo-tĭ-NĀ-shŭn) -*ation*: process (of)	*process by which particles are caused to adhere and form into clumps*
embol/o	embolus (plug)	**embol**/ectomy (ĕm-bō-LĔK-tō-mē) -*ectomy*: excision, removal	removal of an embolus
erythr/o	red	**erythr/o**/cyte (ĕ-RĬTH-rō-sīt) -*cyte*: cell	red blood cell
hem/o hemat/o	blood	**hem/o**/phobia (hē-mō-FŌ-bē-ă) -*phobia*: fear **hemat**/oma (hēm-ă-TŌ-mă) -*oma*: tumor	fear of blood
leuk/o	white	**leuk/o**/cyte (LOO-kō-sīt) -*cyte*: cell	white blood cell
myel/o	bone marrow; spinal cord	**myel/o**/gen/ic (mī- ĕ-lō-JĔN-ĭk) *gen*: forming, producing, origin -*ic*: pertaining to	pertaining to forming bone marrow
thromb/o	blood clot	**thromb/o**/lysis (thrŏm-BŌL-ĭ-sĭs) -*lysis*: separation; destruction; loosening	destruction of blood clot
ven/o	vein	**ven**/ous (VĒ-nŭs) -*ous*: pertaining to	pertaining to veins

Combining Form	Meaning	Medical Word	Meaning
Lymphatic and Immune Systems			
aden/o	gland	**aden/o**/pathy (ă-dĕ-NŎP-ă-thē) *-pathy:* disease	gland disease
immun/o	immune, immunity, safe	**immun/o**/gen (ĭ-MŪ-nō-jĕn) *-gen:* forming, producing, origin	forming immunity
lymph/o	lymph	**lymph/o**/poiesis (lĭm-fō-poy-Ē-sĭs) *-poiesis:* formation, production	production of lymph
lymphaden/o	lymph gland (node)	**lymphaden**/itis (lĭm-făd-ĕn-Ī-tĭs) *-itis:* inflammation	inflammation of lymph gland
lymphangi/o	lymph vessel	**lymphangi**/oma (lĭm-făn-jē-Ō-mă) *-oma:* tumor	lymph tumor
phag/o	swallowing, eating	**phag/o**/cyte (FĂG-ō-sīt) *-cyte:* cell	swallowing cell
splen/o	spleen	**splen/o**/megaly (splĕ-nō-MĔG-ă-lē) *-megaly:* enlargement	spleen enlargement
thym/o	thymus gland	**thym**/oma (thī-MŌ-mă) *-oma:* tumor	thymus gland tumor

Suffixes and Prefixes

In the table that follows, suffixes and prefixes are listed alphabetically, and other word parts are defined as needed. Review the medical word and study the elements that make up the term. Then complete the meaning of the medical words in the right-hand column. You may also refer to *Appendix A: Glossary of Medical Word Elements* to complete this exercise.

Word Element	Meaning	Medical Word	Meaning
Suffixes			
-emia	blood condition	leuk/**emia** (loo-KĒ-mē-ă) *leuk/o:* white	*white blood cell condition*
-phage	swallowing, eating	macro/**phage** (MĂK-rō-făj) *macro-:* large	*large swallowing*
-phylaxis	protection	ana/**phylaxis** (ăn-ă-fĭ-LĂK-sĭs) *ana-:* against; up; back	*protection against*
-poiesis	formation, production	hem/o/**poiesis** (hē-mō-poy-Ē-sĭs) *hem/o:* blood	*blood production*
-stasis	standing still	hem/o/**stasis** (hē-mō-STĀ-sĭs) *hem/o:* blood	*blood standing still*
Prefixes			
macro-	large	**macro**/cyte (MĂK-rō-sīt) *-cyte:* cell	*large cell*
micro-	small	**micro**/cyte (MĪ-krō-sīt) *-cyte:* cell	*small cell*
mono-	one	**mono**/nucle/osis (mŏn-ō-nū-klē-Ō-sĭs) *nucle:* nucleus *-osis:* abnormal condition; increase (used primarily with blood cells)	*abnormal condition or one cell*

 Competency Verification: Check your answers in Appendix B, Answer Key, pages 372–373. If you are not satisfied with your level of comprehension, review the terms in the table and retake the review.

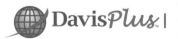 Visit the *Medical Terminology Express* online resource center at *DavisPlus* for an audio exercise of the terms in this table. Other activities are also available to reinforce content.

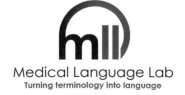

Visit the Medical Language Lab at *medicallanguagelab.com* to enhance your study and reinforce this chapter's word elements with the flash-card activity. We recommend you complete the flash-card activity before continuing with the next section.

Medical Terminology Word Building

In this section, combine the word parts you have learned to construct medical terms related to the blood, lymphatic, and immune systems.

Use **hemat/o** (blood) to build words that mean:

1. tumor (composed) of blood _hematoma_
2. production and development of blood cells _hematopoiesis_
3. specialist in the study of blood _hematologist_

Use **thromb/o** (blood clot) to build words that mean:

4. excision or removal of a thrombus _thrombectomy_
5. resembling a thrombus _thromboid_
6. separation, destruction, loosening of a blood clot _thrombolysis_

Use **-cytes** (cells) to build words that mean:

7. cells that are red _erythrocytes_
8. cells that are white _leukocytes_
9. cells that swallow or eat _phagocytes_

Use **lymph/o** (lymph) to build words that mean:

10. formation or production of lymph _lymphopoiesis_
11. lymph cells _lymphocytes_
12. disease of lymph glands _lymphadenopathy_

Use **immun/o** (immune, immunity, safe) to build words that mean:

13. study of immunity _immunology_
14. producing immunity _immunogen_

Use **agglutin/o** (clumping, gluing) to build words that mean:

15. process of cells clumping together _agglutination_
16. forming, producing, or origin of clumping or gluing _agglutination_

Use **splen/o** (spleen) to build words that mean:

17. enlargement of the spleen _splenomegaly_
18. enlargement of the liver and spleen _hepatosplenomegaly_

Use **myel/o** (bone marrow, spinal cord) to build a word that means:

19. pertaining to forming, producing, or origin in bone marrow _myelogenic_

Use **-phylaxis** (protection) to build a word that means:

20. against protection _anaphylaxis_

Competency Verification: Check your answers in Appendix B, Answer Key, on page 374. Review material that you did not answer correctly.

Correct Answers: _____ × 5 = _____ %

MEDICAL VOCABULARY

The following tables consist of selected terms that pertain to diseases and conditions of the blood, lymphatic, and immune systems. Terms related to diagnostic, medical, and surgical procedures are included as well as pharmacological agents used to treat diseases. Recognizing and learning these terms will help you understand the connection between diseases and their treatments. Word analyses for selected terms are also provided.

Diseases and Conditions

Blood System

anemia ă-NĒ-mē-ă *an:* without, not *-emia:* blood condition	Blood disorder characterized by a deficiency of red blood cell production and hemoglobin, increased red blood cell destruction, or blood loss (See Figure 6-1.) Get a closer look at sickle cell anemia on pages 148–150.
aplastic ă-PLĂS-tĭk	Failure of bone marrow to produce stem cells because it has been damaged by disease, cancer, radiation, or chemotherapy drugs; rare but serious form of anemia
pernicious pĕr-NĬSH-ŭs	Deficiency of erythrocytes resulting from inability to absorb vitamin B_{12} into the body, which plays a vital role in hematopoiesis
thalassemia thăl-ă-SĒ-mē-ă *thalass/o:* sea *-emia:* blood condition	Group of hereditary anemias caused by an inability to produce hemoglobin; usually seen in people of Mediterranean origin
hemophilia hē-mō-FĬL-ē-ă *hem/o:* blood *-philia:* attraction for	Group of hereditary bleeding disorders characterized by a deficiency of one of the factors necessary for coagulation of blood
leukemia loo-KĒ-mē-ă *leuk/o:* white *-emia:* blood condition	Malignant disease of the bone marrow characterized by excessive production of leukocytes

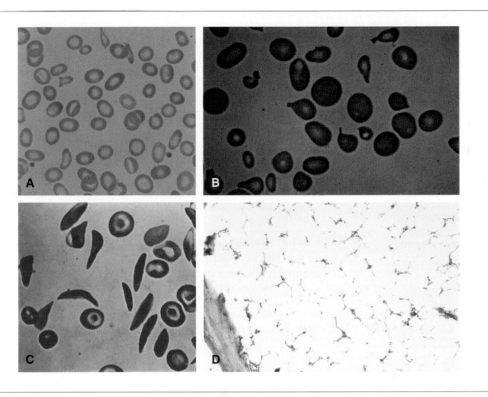

Figure 6-1 Anemias. (A) Iron-deficiency anemia; notice the pale, oval RBCs (magnification × 400). (B) Pernicious anemia, with large, misshapen RBCs (magnification × 400). (C) Sickle cell anemia (magnification × 400). (D) Aplastic anemia, bone marrow (magnification × 200) (From Harmening, DM: *Clinical Hematology and Fundamentals of Hemostasis,* ed 3. FA Davis, Philadelphia, 1997, with permission.)

Lymphatic and Immune System

acquired immune deficiency syndrome (AIDS) ă-KWĪRD ĭm-ŪN dē-FĬSH-ĕn-sē SĬN-drōm	Transmissible infection caused by human immunodeficiency virus (HIV) and associated with suppression of the immune system; characterized by increasing susceptibility to infections, malignancies, and neurological diseases
Hodgkin lymphoma HŎJ-kĭn	Malignant disease originating in the lymphocytes (part of the body's immune system) that occurs most often in young adults and characterized by the presence of unique Reed-Sternberg cells (malignant cells) in the lymph nodes; also called *Hodgkin disease*

immunodeficiency disease ĭm-ū-nō-dĕ-FĬSH-ĕn-sē	Any of a group of diseases caused by a defect in the immune system and generally characterized by susceptibility to infections and chronic diseases

Kaposi sarcoma
KĂP-ō-sē săr-KŌ-mă
   sarc: flesh (connective
       tissue)
  -oma: tumor
	Malignancy of connective tissue, including bone, fat, muscle, and fibrous tissue, that is commonly fatal (because the tumors readily metastasize to various organs) and closely associated with AIDS

lymphadenitis
lĭm-făd-ĕn-Ī-tĭs
lymph: lymph
  aden: gland
   -itis: inflammation
	Inflammation and enlargement of the lymph nodes, usually as a result of infection

lymphedema lĭmf-ĕ-DĒ-mă *lymph:* lymph *-edema:* swelling	Debilitating condition of localized fluid retention and tissue swelling caused by a blockage in the lymphatic system that prevents lymph fluid in the upper limbs from draining adequately

mononucleosis
mŏn-ō-nū-klē-Ō-sĭs
mono-: one
  nucle: nucleus
   -osis: abnormal condition;
     increase (used
     primarily with
     blood cells)
	Acute infection caused by Epstein-Barr virus (EBV) and characterized by a sore throat, fever, fatigue, and enlarged lymph nodes

multiple myeloma mī-ĕ-LŌ-mă	Malignant disease of bone marrow plasma cells (antibody-producing B lymphocytes)
non-Hodgkin lymphoma nŏn-HŎJ-kĭn lĭm-FŌ-mă *lymph:* lymph *-oma:* tumor	A group of more than 20 different types of lymphomas (except Hodgkin lymphoma) that occur in older adults but are not characterized by Reed-Sternberg cells (malignant cells)
opportunistic infection	Any infection that results from a defective immune system that cannot defend against pathogens normally found in the environment
stroke	Sudden loss of neurological function, caused by vascular injury (loss of blood flow) to an area of the brain; also known as *CVA*

Diagnostic Procedures

bone marrow aspiration ăs-pĭ-RĀ-shŭn	Removal of a small amount of tissue (bone marrow biopsy) to diagnose blood disorders (e.g., anemias), cancers, or infectious diseases or to gather cells for later infusion into a patient (bone marrow transplantation) (See Figure 6-2.)
complete blood count (CBC)	Series of blood tests to determine general health status as well as screening for infection, anemias, and other diseases; also called *CBC*
ELISA	Test to screen blood for presence of HIV antibodies or for other disease-causing substances

lymphangiography
lĭm-făn-jē-ŎG-ră-fē
   lymph: lymph
   angi/o: vessel (usually
        blood or lymph)
   -graphy: process of recording
	Radiographic examination of lymph glands and lymphatic vessels after an injection of a contrast medium to view the path of lymph flow as it moves into the chest region

tissue typing	Technique used to determine the histocompatibility of tissues; used in grafts and transplants with the recipient's tissues and cells; also known as *histocompatibility testing*
Western blot	Test to detect presence of viral DNA in the blood and used to confirm the diagnosis of AIDS as well as detecting other viruses

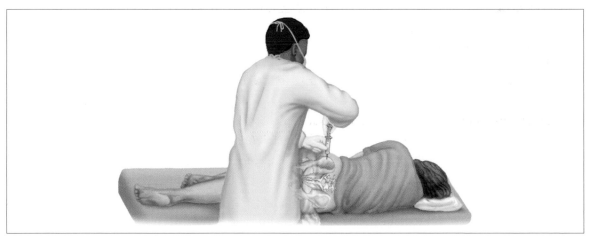

Figure 6-2 Bone marrow aspiration.

Medical and Surgical Procedures

blood transfusion	Administration of whole blood or a component, such as packed red cells, to replace blood lost through trauma, surgery, or disease
bone marrow transplant	Diseased bone marrow is destroyed by irradiation and chemotherapy and replaced from a healthy donor to simulate production of normal blood cells; used to treat aplastic anemia, leukemia, and certain cancers
lymphangiectomy lĭm-făn-jē-ĔK-tō-mē *-ectomy:* excision	Removal of a lymph vessel

Pharmacology

anticoagulants ăn-tĭ-kō-ĂG-ū-lăntz	Prevent or delay blood coagulation
immunizations ĭm-ū-nĭ-ZĀ-shŭns	Vaccination or injection of immune globulins to induce immunity to a particular infectious disease
immunosuppressants ĭm-ū-nō-sū-PRĔS-ănts	Suppress the immune response to prevent organ rejection after transplantation or slow the progression of autoimmune disease
thrombolytics thrŏm-bō-LĬT-ĭks	Dissolve a blood clot
vaccinations văk-sĭ-NĀ-shŭnz	Introduction of altered antigens (viruses or bacteria) into the body to produce an immune response and protect against disease

Pronunciation Help	Long Sound	ā in rāte	ē in rēbirth	ī in īsle	ō in ōver	ū in ūnite
	Short Sound	ă in ălone	ě in ěver	ĭ in ĭt	ŏ in nŏt	ŭ in cŭt

A Closer Look

Take a closer look at the following disorders to enhance your understanding of the medical terminology associated with them.

Sickle Cell Anemia

Sickle cell anemia is a hereditary form of **anemia** in which there is a deficiency of healthy RBCs to carry adequate oxygen throughout the body. RBCs, also called **erythrocytes,** are flexible and round and move easily through blood vessels. Sickle cell anemia is characterized by crescent- or sickle-shaped erythrocytes that become rigid and sticky. These irregularly shaped cells have a tendency to get stuck in small blood vessels, which slows down or blocks blood flow and oxygen to various parts of the body. The illustration that follows shows sickle cell anemia with (A) normal RBCs passing easily through

A Closer Look—cont'd

capillaries and (B) sickle cells becoming trapped and obstructing blood flow. Because sickle cells impair circulation, chronic ill health (**fatigue, dyspnea** on exertion, swollen joints), periodic crises, long-term complications, and premature death can result. The incidence of sickle cell anemia is highest among African Americans and people of Mediterranean ancestry. There is no cure for sickle cell anemia. Treatment is palliative and relieves pain and prevents further exacerbations associated with this disease. The illustration below shows the most common clinical signs and symptoms of sickle cell anemia.

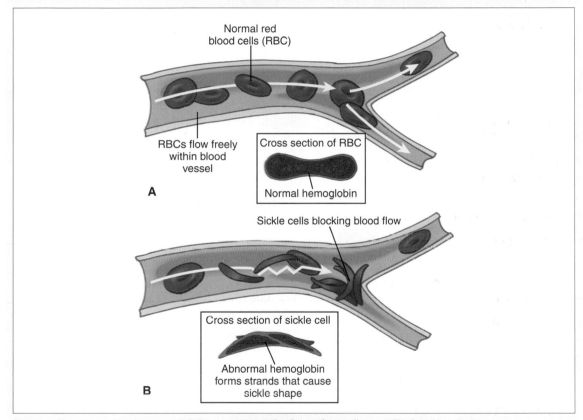

Sickle cell anemia. (A) Normal RBCs passing easily through capillaries. (B) Sickle cells becoming trapped and obstructing normal blood flow.

(Continued)

A Closer Look—cont'd

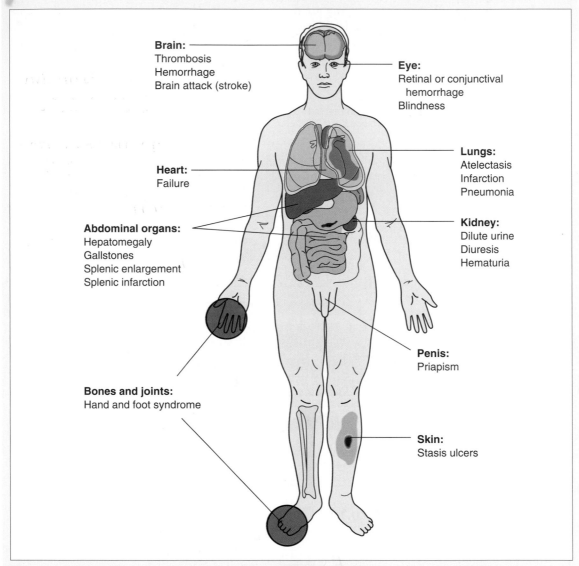

Brain:
Thrombosis
Hemorrhage
Brain attack (stroke)

Eye:
Retinal or conjunctival
hemorrhage
Blindness

Lungs:
Atelectasis
Infarction
Pneumonia

Heart:
Failure

Kidney:
Dilute urine
Diuresis
Hematuria

Abdominal organs:
Hepatomegaly
Gallstones
Splenic enlargement
Splenic infarction

Penis:
Priapism

Bones and joints:
Hand and foot syndrome

Skin:
Stasis ulcers

Clinical manifestations of sickle cell anemia. (From Williams and Hopper: *Understanding Medical-Surgical Nursing,* ed 2. FA Davis, 2002, page 381, with permission.)

A Closer Look—cont'd

Systemic Lupus Erythematosus

Systemic lupus erythematosus (SLE), also called **lupus,** is an autoimmune disease characterized by unusual antibodies in the blood that inflame and damage connective tissues anywhere in the body. It occurs in the skin, joints, nervous system, kidneys, and lungs and typically results in a butterfly rash that appears on the face. This autoimmune disease affects women more often than men and is usually diagnosed between ages of 15 and 45. Although the exact cause of SLE is unknown, it is thought that genetic, environmental, and hormonal factors may predispose a person to this disease. Events that can precipitate SLE include stress, immunization reactions, pregnancy, and overexposure to ultraviolet light. Symptoms of SLE include fatigue, low-grade fever, anorexia, and weight loss. Additional symptoms include photosensitivity, arthralgia, myalgia, hair loss, splenomegaly, lymphadenopathy, and Raynaud phenomenon (circulatory disorder of the fingers and toes). Treatment includes anti-inflammatory agents, including aspirin, antimalarial drugs, and immune suppressants. Other treatments include rest, stress reduction, avoiding the sun, regular exercise to prevent fatigue and joint stiffness, and smoking cessation. The illustration shows the characteristic butterfly-shaped, erythematous rash over the bridge of the nose that spreads out over the cheeks.

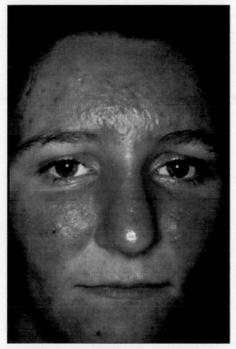

Butterfly rash of SLE. (From Goldsmith & Tharp: Adult & Pediatric Dermatology, FAD 1997, Philadelphia, p. 230.)

Medical Vocabulary Recall

Match the medical terms below with the definitions in the numbered list.

AIDS	ELISA	Hodgkin lymphoma	lymphangiography	SLE
anemia	hemophilia	leukemia	lymphedema	thrombolytics
anticoagulants	HIV	lymphadenitis	mononucleosis	tissue typing

1. _anemia_ is a disease characterized by deficiency of RBCs or hemoglobin.

2. _mononucleosis_ is an acute infection caused by Epstein-Barr virus (EBV) and characterized by a sore throat, fever, fatigue, and enlarged lymph nodes.

3. _thrombolytics_ are drugs that dissolve a blood clot.

4. _SLE_ is a chronic autoimmune inflammatory disease that affects many body systems.

5. _lymphadenitis_ is inflammation and enlargement of the lymph nodes.

6. _HIV_ is the retrovirus that causes AIDS.

7. _lymphangiography_ is a radiographic examination of lymph glands and lymphatic vessels after an injection of a contrast medium.

8. _tissue typing_ is also known as *histocompatibility testing*.

9. _Hodgkins disease_ refers to malignant tumors of the lymphatic system with presence of Reed-Sternberg cells.

10. _AIDS_ is induced by infection with HIV.

11. _leukemia_ is a malignant disease of the bone marrow characterized by excessive production of leukocytes.

12. _ELISA_ is a test to detect HIV antibodies.

13. _lymphedema_ is a debilitating condition of localized fluid retention and tissue swelling caused by blockage.

14. _hemophilia_ is a hereditary bleeding disorder.

15. _anticoagulants_ are agents that prevent formation of blood clots.

Competency Verification: Check your answers in Appendix B, Answer Key, on page 374. Review material that you did not answer correctly.

Correct Answers: _____ × 5 = _____ %

Pronunciation and Spelling

Use the following list to practice correct pronunciation and spelling of medical terms. Practice the pronunciation aloud, and then write the correct spelling of the term. The first word is completed for you.

Pronunciation	Spelling
1. ă-dĕ-NŎP-ă-thē	*adenopathy*
2. ă-gloo-tĭ-NĀ-shŭn	agglutination
3. ăn-ă-fĭ-LĂK-sĭs	anaphylaxis
4. ăn-tĭ-kō-ĂG-ū-lănt	anticoagulant
5. ĕ-RĬTH-rō-sīt	erythrocyte
6. hēm-ă-TŌ-mă	hematoma
7. hē-mō-STĀ-sĭs	hemostasis
8. ĭ-MŪ-nō-jĕn	immunogen
9. loo-KĒ-mē-ă	leukemia
10. lĭm-făn-jē-ŎG-ră-fē	lymphangiography
11. MĂK-rō-sīt	macrocyte
12. mŏn-ō-nū-klē-Ō-sĭs	mononucleosis
13. FĂG-ō-sīt	phagocyte
14. splĕ-nō-MĔG-ă-lē	splenomegaly
15. văk-sĭ-NĀ-shŭn	vaccination

Competency Verification: Check your answers in Appendix B, Answer Key, on page 374. Review material that you did not answer correctly.

Correct Answers: _____ × 6.67 = _____ %

ABBREVIATIONS

The following table introduces abbreviations associated with the blood, lymphatic, and immune systems.

Abbreviation	Meaning	Abbreviation	Meaning
A, B, AB, O	blood types in ABO blood group	HIV	human immunodeficiency virus
AIDS	acquired immune deficiency syndrome	KS	Kaposi sarcoma
CA	cancer	PCP	*Pneumocystis* pneumonia; primary care physician; phencyclidine (hallucinogen)
DNA	deoxyribonucleic acid	RBC, rbc	red blood cell
CBC	complete blood count	SLE	systemic lupus erythematosus
EBV	Epstein-Barr virus	WBC, wbc	white blood cell
ELISA	enzyme-linked immunosorbent assay	WNL	within normal limits

CHART NOTES

Chart notes comprise part of the medical record and are used in various types of health care facilities. The chart notes that follow were dictated by the patient's physician and reflect common clinical events using medical terminology to document the patient's care. Studying and completing the terminology and chart notes sections below will help you learn and understand terms associated with the medical specialty of immunology.

Terminology

The following terms are linked to chart notes in the specialty of immunology. Practice pronouncing each term aloud, and then use a medical dictionary such as *Taber's Cyclopedic Medical Dictionary; Appendix A: Glossary of Medical Word Elements,* or other resources to define each term.

Term	Meaning
AIDS	*aquirred immune deficiency Syndrome*
antiretroviral ăn-tĭ-rĕt-rō-VĪ-răl	
CD4	
dyspnea dĭsp-NĒ-ă	
hemoglobin HĒ-mō-glō-bĭn	
platelets PLĀT-lĕts	
Pneumocystis pneumonia nū-mō-SĬS-tĭs nū-MŌ- nē-ă	
sputum SPŪ-tŭm	
WNL	

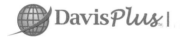 **DavisPlus** | Visit *Medical Terminology Express* at *DavisPlus* Online Resource Center. Use it to practice pronunciations and reinforce the meanings of the terms in this chart note.

Acquired Immune Deficiency Syndrome

Read the chart note that follows aloud. Underline any term you have trouble pronouncing or cannot define. If needed, refer to the Terminology section on this page for correct pronunciations and meanings of terms.

SUBJECTIVE: Patient returns to clinic today for continued evaluation and treatment of his AIDS diagnosis. He has completed 2 weeks of antiretroviral therapy. He is tolerating this quite well. Today, he complains of chills, night sweats, and persistent cough with clear productive sputum along with some dyspnea.

OBJECTIVE: Vital Signs: T 99.9°F. P 100. B/P 135/70. WEIGHT: 150 pounds. Lungs: diminished breath sounds in right middle lower lobe.

Laboratory data from today: CD4: 190. White count: 3.3. Hemoglobin: 12.8. Platelets: 123. Liver function tests are WNL.

ASSESSMENT: A 40-year-old man with a 2-year diagnosis of AIDS and possible complications of secondary infection in the lungs, rule out *Pneumocystis* pneumonia.

PLAN:
1. Chest x-ray.
2. Sputum culture.
3. Continue antiretroviral therapy.
4. Tylenol as needed for fever.
5. Return to the clinic in 2 weeks.

Chart Note Analysis

From the preceding chart note, select the medical word that means

1. difficult breathing: _dyspnea_
2. drug treatment for a viral infection: _antiretroviral therapy_
3. symptoms of a fever: _chills, night sweats_
4. medication used to control fever: _Tylenol_
5. laboratory test to measure oxygen carrying capacity of the blood: _hemoglobin_
6. a frequent cough: _persistent_
7. a type of pneumonia seen in patients with AIDS: _Pneumocytes_
8. abbreviation for a normal test result: _WNL_
9. laboratory test performed on T lymphocytes: _CD4_
10. mucus or phlegm coughed up from the respiratory tract: _Sputum_

> **Competency Verification:** Check your answers in Appendix B, Answer Key, on page 374. Review material that you did not answer correctly.
>
> **Correct Answers:** _____ × 10 = _____ %

Demonstrate What You Know!

To evaluate your understanding of how medical terms you have studied in this and previous chapters are used in a clinical environment, complete the numbered sentences by selecting an appropriate term from the words below.

agglutination	hematology	immunodeficiency	lymphocytes	pernicious
antigen	hemopoiesis	immunosuppressants	oncology	phagocytes
aplastic	HIV	lymphadenitis	pathogen	splenomegaly

1. __hematology__ is the study of blood and the diseases associated with it.

2. The formation or production of blood is known as __hemopoiesis__.

3. The branch of medicine concerned with study of malignancies is __oncology__.

4. Immune cells known as __lymphocytes__ are located in the lymph nodes, spleen, blood, and lymph.

5. __phagocytes__ are cells that ingest bacteria.

6. __aplastic__ anemia is a failure of bone marrow to produce stem cells.

7. __immunosuppressants__ are used to prevent organ rejection after a transplantation.

8. The retrovirus that causes AIDS is known as __HIV__.

9. __pernicious__ anemia is a deficiency of RBCs resulting from inability to absorb vitamin B$_{12}$ into the body.

10. A toxin, bacterium, or foreign cell that is introduced into the body and stimulates the production of antibodies is known as a(n) __antigen__.

11. __splenomegaly__ is a pathological condition in which the spleen is enlarged.

12. __lymphadenitis__ is an inflammation and enlargement of the lymph nodes.

13. An inability to fight disease is a condition known as __immunodeficiency__.

14. __pathogen__ refers to any microorganism capable of producing disease.

15. The process of cells clumping together is called __agglutination__.

 Competency Verification: Check your answers in Appendix B, Answer Key, on page 374. Review material that you did not answer correctly.

Correct Answers: _____ × **6.67 =** _____ %

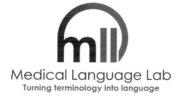
Medical Language Lab
Turning terminology into language

If you are not satisfied with your retention level of the blood, lymphatic, and immune systems chapter, visit *DavisPlus* Student Online Resource Center and the Medical Language Lab to complete the website activities linked to this chapter.

Digestive System

Objectives

Upon completion of this chapter, you will be able to:

- Describe types of medical treatment provided by gastroenterologists.
- Name the primary structures of the digestive system and discuss their functions.
- Identify combining forms, suffixes, and prefixes associated with the digestive system.
- Recognize, pronounce, build, and spell medical terms associated with the digestive system.
- Demonstrate your knowledge of this chapter by successfully completing the activities in this chapter.

VOCABULARY PREVIEW

Terms	Meanings
biopsy BĪ-ŏp-sē *bi:* two *-opsy:* view of	Removal of a small portion of tissue from the body for microscopic examination
endoscopic ĕn-dō-SKŎ-pĭk	Pertains to the use of an endoscope (flexible fiberoptic tube with a light source and magnifying lens) to examine the interior of a hollow organ or body cavity, such as the gastrointestinal (GI) tract; used for various medical purposes

Pronunciation Help	Long Sound	ā in rāte	ē in rēbirth	ī in īsle	ō in ōver	ū in ūnite
	Short Sound	ă in ălone	ĕ in ĕver	ĭ in ĭt	ŏ in nŏt	ŭ in cŭt

MEDICAL SPECIALTY OF GASTROENTEROLOGY

Gastroenterology is the branch of medicine concerned with disorders of the digestive system and its accessory organs. The **gastroenterologist,** usually an internist, specializes in the diagnosis and treatment of diseases of the gastrointestinal (GI) system, which includes its accessory organs, the liver, gallbladder, and pancreas.

The gastroenterologist is not a surgeon, but under the broad classification of surgery, the gastroenterologist performs **endoscopic** procedures to remove polyps (polypectomy) in the colon and to obtain tissue samples for a **biopsy**. Other endoscopic procedures are commonly performed to inspect the esophagus, stomach, and small and large intestines. These procedures help detect pathological conditions, including cancers, at an early stage. Additional diagnostic tests, x-rays, drugs, and medical and surgical procedures are also used to diagnose and treat GI diseases.

DIGESTIVE SYSTEM QUICK STUDY

Food is essential for our survival and is required for the chemical reactions that occur in every cell of the body. However, the foods we eat must be broken down physically and chemically into nutrients so that they can be absorbed by cell membranes. This process is known as digestion, and the organs of the digestive system collectively perform these functions.

The digestive system consists of the digestive tract, also called the **alimentary canal** or **GI tract,** and the accessory organs of digestion. The digestive tract is a tube that starts at the mouth, where food enters the body, and ends at the anus, where solid waste products are excreted from the body. The digestive tube is twisted, swollen, and shaped along its length into several distinct regions: mouth, pharynx (throat), esophagus, stomach, small intestine, large intestine, rectum, and anus. These structures are separated into two sections: the **upper GI tract** (mouth, pharynx, esophagus, and stomach) and the **lower GI tract** (large and small intestines, rectum, and anus). (See *Digestive System,* page 162.) Food passing through the digestive tract mixes with many chemicals that break it down into nutrient molecules. The digestive system absorbs the molecules into the bloodstream. The body eliminates the indigestible remains after this process of absorption in a process called **defecation.** The accessory organs of digestion (liver, gallbladder, and pancreas) contribute to, but are not physically involved in, the process of digestion. Although food does not pass through these organs, their secretions play an important role in the processing of food and nutrients.

ALERT: An extensive self-paced anatomy and physiology multimedia review is included in *TermPlus,* a powerful, interactive CD-ROM program that can be purchased separately from F.A. Davis Company.

MEDICAL WORD BUILDING

Constructing medical words using word elements (combining forms, suffixes, and prefixes) related to the digestive system will enhance your understanding of those terms and reinforce your ability to use terms correctly.

Combining Forms

Begin your study of digestive terminology by reviewing the organs and their associated combining forms (CFs), which are illustrated in the figure *Digestive System* that follows.

Digestive System

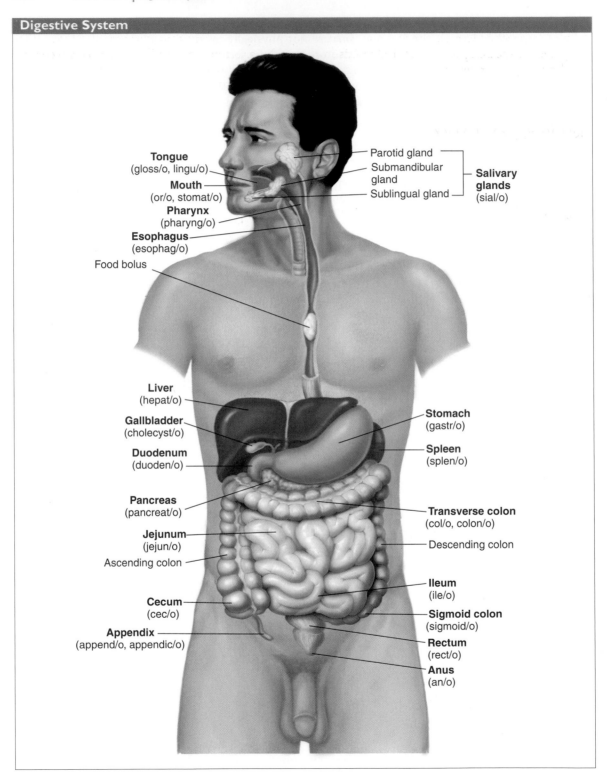

Tongue
(gloss/o, lingu/o)

Mouth
(or/o, stomat/o)

Pharynx
(pharyng/o)

Esophagus
(esophag/o)

Food bolus

Parotid gland

Submandibular
gland

Sublingual gland

**Salivary
glands**
(sial/o)

Liver
(hepat/o)

Gallbladder
(cholecyst/o)

Duodenum
(duoden/o)

Pancreas
(pancreat/o)

Jejunum
(jejun/o)

Ascending colon

Cecum
(cec/o)

Appendix
(append/o, appendic/o)

Stomach
(gastr/o)

Spleen
(splen/o)

Transverse colon
(col/o, colon/o)

Descending colon

Ileum
(ile/o)

Sigmoid colon
(sigmoid/o)

Rectum
(rect/o)

Anus
(an/o)

In the table that follows, CFs are listed alphabetically and highlighted, and other word parts are defined as needed. Review the medical word and study the elements that make up the term. Then complete the meaning of the medical words in the right-hand column. The first one is completed for you. You may also refer to *Appendix A: Glossary of Medical Word Elements* to complete this exercise.

Combining Form	Meaning	Medical Word	Meaning
Oral Cavity			
dent/o	teeth	**dent**/ist (DĔN-tĭst) *-ist:* specialist	*specialist in treatment of the teeth*
odont/o	teeth	orth/**odont**/ist (ŏr-thō-DŎN-tĭst) *orth:* straight *-ist:* specialist	Specialist in Straightening teeth
gingiv/o	gum(s)	**gingiv**/itis (jĭn-jĭ-VĪ-tĭs) *-itis:* inflammation	inflammation of the gums
gloss/o	tongue	hypo/**gloss**/al (hī-pō-GLŎS-ăl) *hypo-:* under, below, deficient *-al:* pertaining to	Pertaining to below the tongue
lingu/o	tongue	sub/**lingu**/al (sŭb-LĬNG-gwăl) *sub-:* under, below *-al:* pertaining to	Pertaining to below the tongue
or/o	mouth	**or**/al (OR-ăl) *-al:* pertaining to	pertaining to mouth
stomat/o	mouth	**stomat**/o/pathy (stō-mă-TŎP-ă-the) *-pathy:* disease	disease of the mouth
ptyal/o	saliva	**ptyal**/ism (TĪ-ă-lĭzm) *-ism:* condition	Saliva condition
sial/o	saliva, salivary gland	**sial**/o/rrhea (sī-ă-lō-RĒ-ă) *-rrhea:* discharge, flow	discharge of salivary gland

(Continued)

Combining Form	Meaning	Medical Word	Meaning
Oral Cavity			
esophag/o	esophagus	**esophag/o**/scope (ē-SŎF-ă-gō-skōp) *–scope:* instrument for examining	*instrument for examining esophagus*
gastr/o	stomach	**gastr/o**/scopy (găs-TRŎS-kō-pē) *–scopy:* visual examination	*visual examination of stomach*
pharyng/o	pharynx (throat)	**pharyng/o**/tonsill/itis (fă-rĭng-gō-tŏn-sĭ-LĪ-tĭs) *tonsill:* tonsils *–itis:* inflammation	*inflammation of pharynx + tonsils*
pylor/o	pylorus (sphincter in lower portion of stomach that opens into duodenum)	**pylor/o**/tomy (pī-lor-ŎT-ō-mē) *–tomy:* incision	*incision in pylorus*
Small Intestine			
duoden/o	duodenum (first part of small intestine)	**duoden/o**/scopy (dū-ŏd-ĕ-NŎS-kō-pē) *–scopy:* visual examination	*visual examination of duodenum*
enter/o	intestine (usually small intestine)	**enter/o**/pathy (ĕn-tĕr-ŎP-ă-thē) *–pathy:* disease	*disease of intestine*
jejun/o	jejunum (second part of small intestine)	**jejun/o**/rrhaphy (jĕ-joo-NOR-ă-fē) *–rrhaphy:* suture	*suture in the jejunum*
ile/o	ileum (third part of small intestine)	**ile/o**/stomy (ĭl-ē-ŎS-tō-mē) *–stomy*:* forming an opening (mouth)	*forming an opening in the ileum*
Large Intestine			
an/o	anus	peri/**an**/al (pĕr-ē-Ā-năl) *peri–:* around *–al:* pertaining to	*pertaining to around the anus*

*When the suffix -stomy is used with a CF that denotes an organ, it refers to a surgical opening to the outside of the body.

Combining Form	Meaning	Medical Word	Meaning
Large Intestine			
append/o	appendix	**append**/ectomy (ăp-ĕn-DĔK-tō-mē) -*ectomy*: excision, removal	removal of appendix
appendic/o	appendix	**appendic**/itis (ă-pĕn-dĭ-SĪ-tĭs) -*itis*: inflammation	inflammation of appendix
col/o	colon	**col/o**/stomy (kō-LŎS-tō-mē) -*stomy**: forming an opening (mouth)	forming an opening in the colon
colon/o	colon	**colon/o**/scopy (kō-lŏn-ŎS-kō-pē) -*scopy*: visual examination Get a closer look at colonoscopy on pages 179 and 180.	visual examination of colon
proct/o	anus, rectum	**proct/o**/logist (prŏk-TŎL-ō-jĭst) -*logist*: specialist in the study of	specialist in study of anus
rect/o	rectum	**rect/o**/cele (RĔK-tō-sēl) -*cele*: hernia, swelling	swelling in the rectum
sigmoid/o	sigmoid colon	**sigmoid/o**/tomy (sĭg-moyd-ŎT-ō-mē) -*tomy*: incision	incision in sigmoid colon
Accessory Organs of Digestion			
cholangi/o	bile vessel	**cholangi**/ole (kō-LĂN-jē-ōl) -*ole*: small, minute	small bile vessel
chol/e†	bile, gall	**chol/e**/lith (KŌ-lē-lĭth) -*lith*: stone, calculus Get a closer look at gallstones on page 178.	gall stone

†Using the combining vowel e instead of o is an exception to the rule.

(Continued)

Combining Form	Meaning	Medical Word	Meaning
Accessory Organs of Digestion			
cholecyst/o	gallbladder	**cholecyst**/itis (kō-lē-sĭs-TĪ-tĭs) *-itis:* inflammation Get a closer look at cholecystitis on page 178.	inflammation of the gallbladder
choledoch/o	bile duct	**choledoch/o**/tomy (kō-lĕd-ō-KŎT-ō-mē) *-tomy:* incision	incision in bile duct
hepat/o	liver	**hepat**/itis (hĕp-ă-TĪ-tĭs) *-itis:* inflammation	inflammation of liver
pancreat/o	pancreas	**pancreat/o**/lysis (păn-krē-ă-TŎL-ĭ-sĭs) *-lysis:* separation; destruction; loosening	destruction of pancreas

Suffixes and Prefixes

In the table that follows, suffixes and prefixes are listed alphabetically and highlighted, and other word parts are defined as needed. Review the medical word and study the elements that make up the term. Then complete the meaning of the medical words in the right-hand column. You may also refer to *Appendix A: Glossary of Medical Word Elements* to complete this exercise.

Word Element	Meaning	Medical Words	Meaning
Suffixes			
-algia	pain	gastr/**algia** (găs-TRĂL-jē-ă) *gastr:* stomach	Stomach pain
-dynia	pain	gastr/o/**dynia** (găs-trō-DĬN-ē-ă) *gastr/o:* stomach	Stomach pain
-emesis	vomiting	hyper/**emesis** (hī-pĕr-ĔM-ĕ-sĭs) *hyper-:* excessive, above normal	excessive vomiting

Word Element	Meaning	Medical Words	Meaning
Suffixes			
-iasis	abnormal condition (produced by something specified)	chol/e/lith/**iasis** (kō-lē-lĭ-THĪ-ă-sĭs) *chol/e:* bile, gall *lith/o:* stone, calculus ⌕ Get a closer look at cholelithiasis on page 178.	abnormal gall stone condition
-megaly	enlargement	hepat/o/**megaly** (hĕp-ă-tō-MĔG-ă-lē) *hepat/o:* liver	enlarged liver
-orexia	appetite	an/**orexia** (ăn-ō-RĔK-sē-ă) *an-:* without, not	loss of appetite
-osis	abnormal condition; increase (used primarily with blood cells)	cirrh/**osis** (sĭr-RŌ-sĭs) *cirrh:* yellow	abnormal yellowing condition
-pepsia	digestion	dys/**pepsia** (dĭs-PĔP-sē-ă) *dys-:* bad; painful; difficult	painful digestion
-phagia	swallowing, eating	dys/**phagia** (dĭs-FĀ-jē-ă) *dys-:* bad; painful; difficult	painful swallowing
-prandial	meal	post/**prandial** (pōst-PRĂN-dē-ăl) *post-:* after, behind	meal after
-rrhea	discharge, flow	dia/**rrhea** (dī-ă-RĒ-ă) *dia-:* through, across	discharge through

(Continued)

Word Element	Meaning	Medical Words	Meaning
Prefixes			
endo-	in, within	**endo**/scopy (ĕn-DŎS-kō-pē) -*scopy:* visual examination Get a closer look at endoscopy on pages 179 and 180.	*visual examination within*
hemat-	blood	**hemat**/emesis (hĕm-ăt-ĔM-ĕ-sĭs) -*emesis:* vomiting	*blood in vomit*
hypo-	under, below, deficient	**hypo**/gastr/ic (hī-pō-GĂS-trĭk) *gastr/o:* stomach -*ic:* pertaining to	*Pertaining to below the stomach*

✓ **Competency Verification:** Check your answers in Appendix B, Answer Key, pages 374–376. If you are not satisfied with your level of comprehension, review the terms in the table and retake the review.

🌐 **DavisPlus** | Visit the *Medical Terminology Express* online resource center at *DavisPlus* for an audio exercise of the terms in this table. Other activities are also available to reinforce content.

Medical Language Lab
Turning terminology into language

Visit the Medical Language Lab at *medicallanguagelab.com* to enhance your study and reinforce this chapter's word elements with the flash-card activity. We recommend you complete the flash-card activity before continuing with the next section.

Medical Terminology Word Building

In this section, combine the word parts you have learned to construct medical terms related to the digestive system.

Use **esophag/o** (esophagus) to build words that mean:

1. spasm of the esophagus <u>esophagospasm</u>

2. stricture or narrowing of the esophagus <u>esophagostenosis</u>

Use *gastr/o* (stomach) to build words that mean:

3. inflammation of the stomach _gastritis_

4. pain in the stomach _gastrodynia_

5. disease of the stomach _gastropathy_

Use *duoden/o* (duodenum), *jejun/o* (jejunum), or *ile/o* (ileum) to build words that mean:

6. excision of all or part of the jejunum _jejunectomy_

7. inflammation of the ileum _ileitis_

8. pertaining to the jejunum and ileum _jejunoileal_

Use *enter/o* (usually small intestine) to build words that mean:

9. inflammation of the small intestine _enteritis_

10. disease of the small intestine _enteropathy_

Use *col/o* (colon) to build words that mean:

11. pertaining to the colon and rectum _colorectal_

12. prolapse or downward displacement of the colon _coloptosis_

Use *proct/o* (anus, rectum) or *rect/o* (rectum) to build words that mean:

13. narrowing or constriction of the rectum _proctostenosis_

14. herniation of the rectum _proctocele_

15. paralysis of the anus (anal muscles) _proctoplegia_

Use *chol/e* (bile, gall) to build words that mean:

16. inflammation of the gallbladder _cholecystitis_

17. abnormal condition of a gallstone _cholelithiasis_

Use *hepat/o* (liver) or *pancreat/o* (pancreas) to build words that mean:

18. tumor of the liver _hepatoma_

19. enlargement of the liver _hepatomegaly_

20. inflammation of the pancreas _pancreatitis_

Competency Verification: Check your answers in Appendix B, Answer Key, on page 377. Review material that you did not answer correctly.

Correct Answers: _____ × **5** = _____ %

MEDICAL VOCABULARY

The following tables consist of selected terms that pertain to diseases and conditions of the digestive system. Terms related to diagnostic, medical, and surgical procedures are included as well as pharmacological agents used to treat diseases. Recognizing and learning these terms will help you understand the connection between diseases and their treatments. Word analyses for selected terms are also provided.

Diseases and Conditions

appendicitis ă-pĕn-dĭ-SĪ-tĭs *appendic:* appendix *-itis:* inflammation	Inflammation of the appendix, typically an acute condition caused by blockage of the appendix followed by infection that is treated with surgical removal of the inflamed appendix and antibiotic therapy (See Figure 7-1.)
ascites ă-SĪ-tēz	Pathological buildup of fluid in the abdominal (peritoneal) cavity as a result of liver disease, cancer, heart failure, or kidney failure (See Figure 7-2.)
borborygmus bŏr-bō-RĬG-mŭs	Gurgling or rumbling sound heard over the large intestine that is caused by gas moving through the intestines
cirrhosis sĭ-RŌ-sĭs *cirrh:* yellow *-osis:* abnormal condition; increase (used primarily with blood cells)	Chronic liver disease characterized by destruction of liver cells that eventually leads to ineffective liver function and jaundice

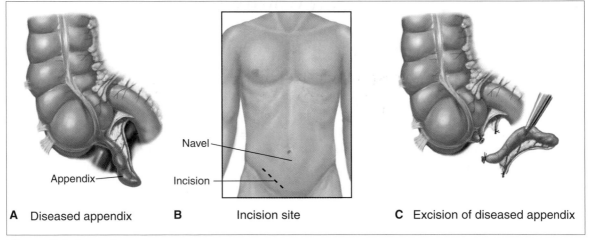

A Diseased appendix	**B** Incision site	**C** Excision of diseased appendix

Navel

Incision

Appendix

Figure 7-1 Appendectomy.

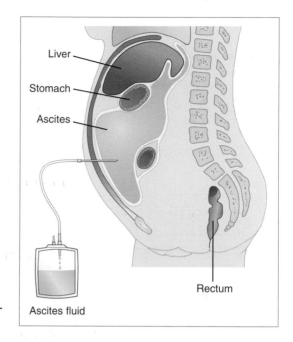

Figure 7-2 Ascites with removal of fluid from abdominal cavity using a catheter.

diverticular disease dī-vĕr-TĬK-ū-lăr	Formation of bulging pouches (diverticula) throughout the colon but most commonly in the lower portion of the colon (includes diverticulosis, diverticular bleeding, and diverticulitis) (See Figure 7-3.)

dysentery
DĬS-ĕn-tĕr-ē
  dys-: bad; painful; difficult
enter: intestine (usually
     small intestine)
  -y: condition; process
	Inflammation of the intestine, especially of the colon, caused by chemical irritants, bacteria, or parasites and characterized by diarrhea, colitis, and abdominal cramps

fistula FĬS-tū-lă	Abnormal tunnel connecting two body cavities, such as the rectum and the vagina (rectovaginal fistula), or a body cavity to the skin, such as the rectum to the outside of the body, caused by an injury, infection, or inflammation

gastroesophageal reflux disease (GERD)
găs-trō-ē-sŏf-ă-JĒ-ăl
RĒ-flŭks dĭ-ZĒZ
  gastr/o: stomach
esophag: esophagus
  -eal: pertaining to
	Backflow (reflux) of gastric contents into the esophagus as a result of malfunction of the lower esophageal sphincter (LES)

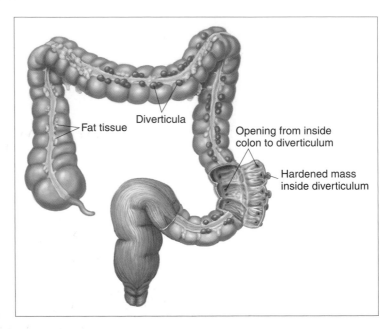

Figure 7-3 Diverticular disease.

hematochezia hĕm-ă-tō-KĒ-zē-ă	Passage of bright red, bloody stools (usually an indication that the colon is bleeding somewhere) commonly caused by diverticulitis or hemorrhoids but may be a symptom of cancer
hemorrhoid HĔM-ō-royd *hem/o:* blood *-oid:* resembling	Mass of enlarged, twisted varicose veins in the mucous membrane inside (internal) or just outside (external) the rectum; also called *piles*
hernia HĔR-nē-ă	Protrusion or projection of an organ or a part of an organ through the wall of the cavity that normally contains it (See Figure 7-4.)
strangulated	Hernia whose blood supply has been cut off, leading to necrosis with gangrene of the hernial sac and its contents; a condition that is life-threatening and requires immediate surgery
inflammatory bowel disease (IBD) ĭn-FLĂM-ă-tŏr-ē BŎ-wăl	Disorder that causes inflammation of the intestines
Crohn disease KRŌN	Chronic IBD that may affect any portion of the intestinal tract (usually the ileum) and is distinguished from closely related bowel disorders by its inflammatory pattern, which tends to be patchy or segmented; also called *regional colitis*
ulcerative colitis ŬL-sĕr-ā-tĭv kō-LĪ-tĭs *col:* colon *-itis:* inflammation	Chronic IBD of the colon characterized by ulcers, constant diarrhea mixed with blood, and pain

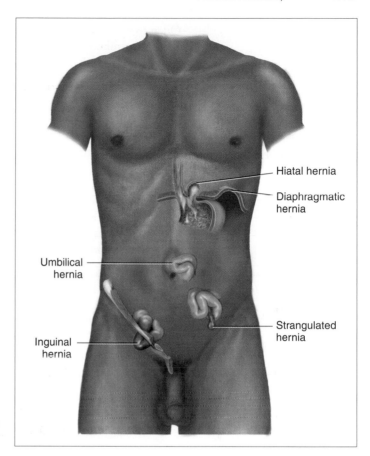

Figure 7-4 Common locations of hernia.

irritable bowel syndrome (IBS) ĬR-ĭ-tă-bl BŎ-wăl	Common colon disorder characterized by constipation, diarrhea, gas, and bloating that does not cause permanent damage to the colon; also called *spastic colon*
jaundice JAWN-dĭs *jaund:* yellow *-ice:* noun ending	Yellow discoloration of the skin, mucous membranes, and sclerae of the eyes caused by excessive levels of bilirubin in the blood; also called *hyperbilirubinemia*
obesity	Condition in which body weight exceeds the range of normal or healthy, which is characterized as a body mass index (BMI) greater than 25
morbid obesity	More severe obesity in which a person has a body mass index (BMI) of 40 or greater, which is generally 100 lb or more over ideal body weight

ulcer ŬL-sĕr	Open sore that may result from a perforation or lesion of the skin or mucous membrane accompanied by sloughing of inflamed necrotic (pathological death of a cell) tissue
volvulus VŎL-vū-lŭs	Twisting of the bowel on itself, causing obstruction

Diagnostic Procedures

barium enema (BE) BĂ-rē-ŭm ĔN-ĕ-mă	Radiographic examination of the rectum and colon after administration of barium sulfate (radiopaque contrast medium) into the rectum. BE is used for diagnosis of obstructions, tumors, or other abnormalities, such as ulcerative colitis (See Figure 7-5.)
barium swallow BĂ-rē-ŭm	Radiographic examination of the esophagus, stomach, and small intestine after oral administration of barium sulfate (radiopaque contrast medium); also called *upper GI series*
cholangiography kō-lăn-jē-ŎG-ră-fē	Radiographic examination of the bile ducts with a contrast medium to reveal gallstones or other obstruction in the bile ducts

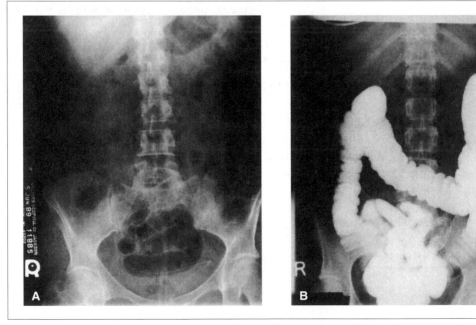

Figure 7-5 Barium enema done poorly (A) and done correctly (B).

esophagogastroduo-denoscopy (EGD) ĕ-sŏf-ă-gō-găs-trō-doo-ō-dĕn-ŎS-kō-pē *endo-:* in, within *-scopy:* visual examination	Visual examination of the esophagus (esophagoscopy), stomach (gastroscopy), and duodenum (duodenoscopy) using an endoscope; also called *upper GI endoscopy*
stool guaiac GWĪ-ăk	Test performed on feces using the reagent gum guaiac to detect presence of blood in feces that is not apparent on visual inspection; also called *Hemoccult test*

Medical and Surgical Procedures

bariatric surgery BĂR-ē-ă-trĭk	Any of a group of procedures used to treat morbid obesity
vertical banded gastroplasty GĂS-trō-plăs-tē *gastr/o:* stomach *-plasty:* surgical repair	Bariatric surgery in which the upper stomach near the esophagus is stapled vertically to reduce it to a small pouch and a band is inserted that restricts and delays food from leaving the pouch, causing a feeling of fullness (See Figure 7-6A.)
Roux-en-Y gastric bypass (RGB) rū-ĕn-WĪ GĂS-trĭk	Bariatric surgery in which the stomach is first stapled to decrease it to a small pouch and then the jejunum is shortened and connected to the small stomach pouch, causing the base of the duodenum leading from the nonfunctioning portion of the stomach to form a Y configuration, which decreases the pathway of food through the intestine, reducing absorption of calories and fats (See Figure 7-6B.)
colostomy kō-LŎS-tō-mē	Excision of a diseased part of the colon and relocation of the remaining end of the healthy colon through the abdominal wall to divert fecal flow to a colostomy bag (See Figure 7-7.)
lithotripsy LĬTH-ō-trĭp-sē *lith/o:* stone, calculus *-tripsy:* crushing	Eliminating a stone within the gallbladder or urinary system by crushing it surgically or using a noninvasive method, such as ultrasonic shock waves, to shatter it
extracorporeal shock-wave lithotripsy (ESWL) ĕks-tră-kor-POR-ē-ăl LĬTH-ō-trĭp-sē *extra-:* outside *corpor:* body *-eal:* pertaining to *lith/o:* stone, calculus *-tripsy:* crushing	Use of shock waves as a noninvasive method to destroy stones in the gallbladder and biliary ducts

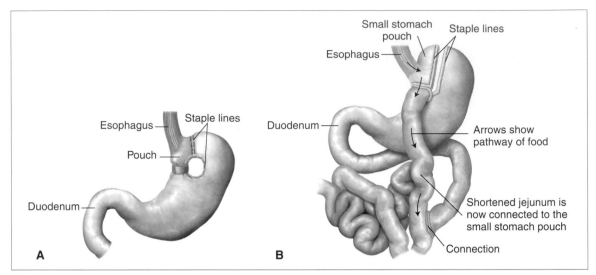

Figure 7-6 Bariatric surgery. (A) Vertical banded gastroplasty. (B) Roux-en-Y gastric bypass.

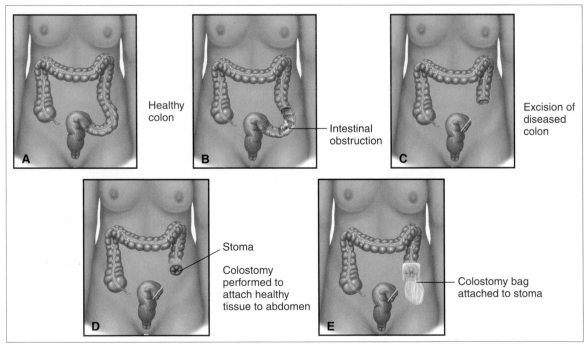

Figure 7-7 Colostomy.

nasogastric intubation nā-zō-GĂS-trĭk ĭn-tū-BĀ-shŭn *nas/o:* nose *gastr:* stomach *-ic:* pertaining to	Insertion of a soft plastic nasogastric tube through the nostrils, past the pharynx, and down the esophagus into the stomach to remove substances from the stomach; deliver medication, food, or fluids; or obtain a specimen for laboratory analysis
polypectomy pŏl-ĭ-PĔK-tō-mē *polyp:* small growth *ectomy:* excision, removal	Excision of small, tumorlike, benign growths (polyps) that project from a mucous membrane surface (See Figure 7-8.)

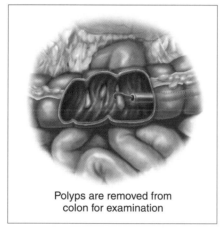

Polyps are removed from colon for examination

Figure 7-8 Polypectomy.

Pharmacology

antacids ănt-ĂS-ĭds	Neutralize acids in the stomach
antidiarrheals ăn-tĭ-dī-ă-RĒ-ăls	Control loose stools and relieve diarrhea by absorbing excess water in the bowel or slowing peristalsis in the intestinal tract
antiemetics ăn-tĭ-ē-MĔT-ĭks	Control nausea and vomiting by blocking nerve impulses to the vomiting center of the brain
laxatives LĂK-să-tĭvz	Relieve constipation and facilitate passage of feces through the lower GI tract

Pronunciation Help	Long Sound	ā in rāte	ē in rēbirth	ī in īsle	ō in ōver	ū in ūnite
	Short Sound	ă in ălone	ĕ in ĕver	ĭ in ĭt	ŏ in nŏt	ŭ in cŭt

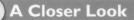

Take a closer look at the following digestive disorders and endoscopic procedures to enhance your understanding of the medical terminology associated with them.

Cholelithiasis and Cholecystitis

Cholelithiasis is a common condition in which there is an abnormal presence of gallstones **(choleliths)** or calculi **(cholelithiasis)** that form in the bile. Acute **cholecystitis** is a severe inflammation of the interior wall of the gallbladder. Most cases of acute cholecystitis are a consequence of the obstruction of bile ducts by gallstones.

When **calculi,** also called *stones,* are present in the common bile duct, the condition is known as **choledocholithiasis.** These stones may be formed of cholesterol or calcium-based compounds and range from a microscopic size to more than an inch. Most individuals with gallstones remain asymptomatic until the bile ducts become obstructed by the stones. The cause of cholelithiasis is not well understood. Any factors that cause the bile to become overloaded with cholesterol increase the likelihood of the formation of cholesterol-based gallstones. Such factors include obesity, high-calorie diets, certain drugs, oral contraceptives, multiple pregnancies, and increasing age.

Asymptomatic gallstones are neither removed nor treated. If a gallstone travels and obstructs the common bile duct or the cystic duct, pain can develop in the **epigastric** region, right upper quadrant, or both and sometimes radiate to the upper right back area. This discomfort is generally accompanied by **nausea** and vomiting. Symptomatic gallstone disease is treated by **laparoscopic cholecystectomy.** Surgery involves incisions in the abdomen so that a tiny video camera and surgical instruments can be inserted. The surgeon views the video pictures on a monitor and removes the gallbladder by manipulating the surgical instruments. The illustration that follows shows various sites of gallstones.

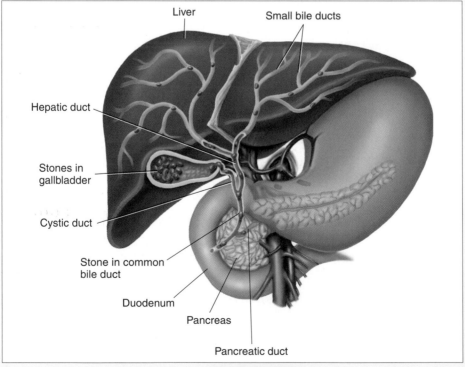

Sites of gallstones. Cholelithiasis and choledocholithiasis.

A Closer Look—cont'd

Endoscopy

Endoscopy is a minimally invasive diagnostic procedure that uses an endoscope (rigid or flexible fiberoptic tube and a lighted optical system) to visually examine the GI tract. Endoscopy can also be used to obtain samples for cytological and histological examination and to follow the course of a disease, such as assessment of healing of gastric and duodenal ulcers. A camera or video recorder is commonly used during endoscopic procedures to provide a permanent record for later reference. The organ being examined dictates the name of the endoscopic procedure. For example, visual examination of the esophagus is known as **esophagoscopy,** visual examination of the stomach is known as **gastroscopy,** and visual examination of the duodenum is known as **duodenoscopy.**

In the digestive system, endoscopies can be grouped into upper and lower GI endoscopies. An **upper GI endoscopy** uses an endoscope inserted through the nose or mouth. It includes endoscopy of the esophagus **(esophagoscopy);** stomach **(gastroscopy);** duodenum **(duodenoscopy);** and esophagus, stomach, and duodenum **(esophagogastroduodenoscopy).** Upper GI endoscopies help identify tumors, **esophagitis, gastroesophageal varices** (varicose veins or varicosities), peptic ulcers, and the source of upper GI bleeding. Endoscopy is also used to confirm the presence and extent of varices in the lower esophagus and stomach in patients with liver disease. Lower GI endoscopies consist of endoscopy of the colon **(colonoscopy),** sigmoid colon **(sigmoidoscopy),** and rectum and anal canal **(proctoscopy). Lower GI endoscopy** employs the use of an endoscope inserted through the rectum. Endoscopy of the lower GI tract helps identify pathological conditions of the colon, such as colorectal cancer. In the lower GI tract, endoscopy may be combined with a **polypectomy.** Detection of polyps in the colon requires their retrieval and testing for cancer. The illustration that follows shows the location of a colonoscopy and a sigmoidoscopy.

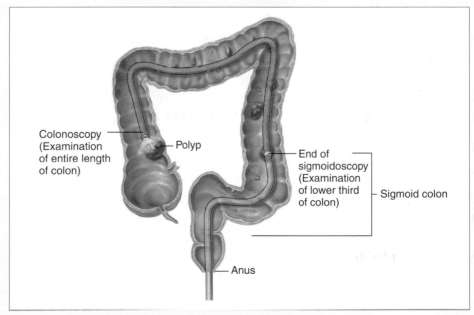

Sigmoidoscopy and colonoscopy.

(Continued)

A Closer Look—cont'd

Most endoscopic procedures are considered relatively painless but may be associated with moderate discomfort. For example, in esophagogastroduodenoscopy, most patients tolerate the procedure with only topical anesthesia of the oropharynx using lidocaine spray. Complications are rare but can include perforation of an organ under inspection with the endoscope or biopsy instrument. If such a complication occurs, surgery may be required to repair the injury.

Medical Vocabulary Recall

Match the medical terms below with the definitions in the numbered list.

ascites	cirrhosis	hematochezia	jaundice	polyp
barium enema	Crohn disease	IBD	lithotripsy	stool guaiac
barium swallow	fistula	IBS	nasogastric intubation	volvulus

1. **Stool guaiac** _____ is a test performed on feces that detects the presence of blood that is not apparent on visual inspection.

2. **nasogastric intubation** refers to insertion of a tube through the nose into the stomach for therapeutic and diagnostic purposes.

3. **polyp** _____ is a small benign growth that projects from the mucous membrane.

4. **ascites** _____ is an abnormal accumulation of serous fluid in the peritoneal cavity.

5. **Crohns disease** _____ refers to chronic inflammatory bowel disease, which usually affects the ileum.

6. **lithotripsy** _____ refers to surgical crushing of a stone.

7. **fistula** _____ is an abnormal passageway between two body cavities that normally do not connect.

8. **jaundice** _____ is a yellow discoloration of the skin caused by hyperbilirubinemia.

9. **barium enema** _____ is a radiographic examination of the rectum and colon after administration of barium sulfate.

10. **IBD** _____ refers to an inflammatory bowel disease, such as Crohn disease.

11. **hematochezia** _____ refers to passage of stools containing red blood.

12. **volvulus** _____ means twisting of the bowel on itself, causing obstruction.

13. **cirrhosis** _____ refers to a chronic liver disease characterized by destruction of liver cells and jaundice.

14. **barium swallow** _____ is a radiographic examination of the esophagus, stomach, and small intestine after oral administration of a contrast medium.

15. **IBS** _____ is a colon disorder characterized by constipation, diarrhea, gas, and bloating; also called *spastic colon*.

Competency Verification: Check your answers in Appendix B, Answer Key, on page 377. Review material that you did not answer correctly.

Correct Answers: _____ × **6.67** = _____ %

Pronunciation and Spelling

Use the following list to practice correct pronunciation and spelling of medical terms. First practice the pronunciation aloud. Then write the correct spelling of the term. The first word is completed for you.

Pronunciation	Spelling
1. ă-pĕn-dĭ-SĪ-tĭs	*appendicitis*
2. ă-SĪ-tēz	ascites
3. bĭl-ĭ-ROO-bĭn	bilirubin
4. bŏr-bō-RĬG-mŭs	borborygmus
5. kō-lăn-jē-ō-păn-krē-ă-TŎG-ră-fē	cholangiopancreatography
6. kō-lē-sĭs-TĔK-tō-mē	cholecystectomy
7. kō-LĔD ō kō plăs tē	choledochoplasty
8. kō-lē-lĭ-THĪ-ă-sĭs	cholelithiasis
9. sĭr-RŌ-sĭs	cirrhosis
10. kō-LŎS-tō-mē	colostomy
11. krōn dĭ-ZĒZ	Crohn disease
12. dū-ŏd-ĕ-NĪ-tĭs	duodenitis
13. ĕn-tĕr-ŎP-ă-thē	enteropathy
14. ĕ-sŏf-ă-gō-găs-trō-doo-ō-dĕn-ŎS-kō-pē	esophagogastroduodenoscopy
15. găs-trō-ē-sŏf-ă-Jē-ăl	gastroesophageal
16. glŏs-ĔK-tō-mē	glossectomy
17. hĕp-ă-TĪ-tĭs	hepatitis
18. ĭl-ē-ō-RĔK-tăl	ileorectal
19. JAWN-dĭs	jaundice
20. sĭg-moyd-ŎT-ō-mē	sigmoidotomy

 Competency Verification: Check your answers in Appendix B, Answer Key, on page 377. Review material that you did not answer correctly.

Correct Answers: _____ × 5 = _____ %

ABBREVIATIONS

The following table introduces abbreviations associated with the digestive system.

Abbreviation	Meaning	Abbreviation	Meaning
BE	barium enema; below the elbow	GERD	gastroesophageal reflux disease
Dx	diagnosis	GI	gastrointestinal
EGD	esophagogastroduodenoscopy	IBD	inflammatory bowel disease
ERCP	endoscopic retrograde cholangiopancreatography	IBS	irritable bowel syndrome
ESWL	extracorporeal shock-wave lithotripsy	RGB	Roux-en-Y gastric bypass
FBS	fasting blood sugar	UGI	upper gastrointestinal

CHART NOTES

Chart notes comprise part of the medical record and are used in various types of health care facilities. The chart notes that follow were dictated by the patient's physician and reflect common clinical events using medical terminology to document the patient's care. Studying and completing the terminology and chart notes sections below will help you learn and understand terms associated with the medical specialty of gastroenterology medicine.

Terminology

The following terms are linked to chart notes in the specialty of gastroenterology. Practice pronouncing each term aloud, and then use a medical dictionary such as *Taber's Cyclopedic Medical Dictionary; Appendix A: Glossary of Medical Word Elements,* or other resources to define each term.

Term	Meaning
angulation ăng-ū-LĀ-shŭn	
anorectal ā-nō-RĔK-tăl	
carcinoma kăr-sĭ-NŌ-mă	

Term	Meaning
cm	
diarrhea dī-ă-RĒ-ă	
diverticulum dī-vĕr-TĬK-ū-lŭm	
dysphagia dĭs-FĀ-jē-ă	
emesis ĔM-ĕ-sĭs	
enteritis ĕn-tĕr-Ī-tĭs	
hematemesis hĕm-ăt-ĔM-ĕ-sĭs	
ileostomy ĭl-ē-ŎS-tō-mē	
nausea NAW-sē-ă	
polyp PŎL-ĭp	
postprandial pōst-PRĂN-dē-ăl	
sigmoidoscopy sĭg-moy-DŎS-kō-pē	

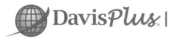

Visit *Medical Terminology Express* at *DavisPlus* Online Resource Center. Use it to practice pronunciations and reinforce the meanings of the terms in this chart note.

Rectal Bleeding

Read the chart note that follows aloud. Underline any term you have trouble pronouncing and any terms that you cannot define. If needed, refer to the Terminology section on page 182 for correct pronunciations and meanings of terms.

This 50-year-old white man has lost approximately 40 pounds since his last examination. The patient says he has had no dysphagia or postprandial distress, and there is no report of diarrhea, nausea, emesis, hematemesis, or constipation. The patient has had a history of regional enteritis, appendicitis, and colonic bleeding.

The regional enteritis resulted in an ileostomy with appendectomy about 6 months ago. On 5/30/xx, a sigmoidoscopy using a 10-cm scope showed no evidence of bleeding at the anorectal area. A 35-cm scope was then inserted to a level of 13 cm. Angulation prevented further passage of the scope. No abnormalities had been encountered, but dark blood was noted at that level.

Impression: Rectal bleeding caused by a polyp, bleeding diverticulum, or rectal carcinoma.

Chart Note Analysis

From the preceding chart note, select the medical word that means

1. following a meal: _Postprandial_
2. pertaining to the anus and rectum: _anorectal_
3. abnormal formation of an angle: _angulation_
4. tumor on a small stem: _polyp_
5. sac or pouch on the wall of a canal: _diverticulum_
6. painful or difficult swallowing: _dysphagia_
7. inflammation of the small intestine: _enteritis_
8. creation of a surgical passage through the abdominal wall to the last portion of the small intestine: _ileostomy_
9. vomiting blood: _hematemesis_
10. malignant tumor: _carcinoma_

Competency Verification: Check your answers in Appendix B, Answer Key, on page 377. Review material that you did not answer correctly.

Correct Answers: _____ × 10 = _____ %

Demonstrate What You Know!

To evaluate your understanding of how medical terms you have studied in this and previous chapters are used in a clinical environment, complete the numbered sentences by selecting an appropriate term from the words below.

bariatric	gastroesophagitis	hemorrhoids	pylorotomy	stones
bile ducts	GERD	nausea	sigmoidoscopy	stool
constipation	hematemesis	orthodontist	stomach	sublingually

1. When medication is placed under the tongue, it is administered *Sublingually*.

2. A specialist who straightens teeth is called a(n) *orthodontist*.

3. Inflammation of the stomach and esophagus is a condition known as *gastroesophagitis*.

4. Obese patients who fail to lose weight may consider *bariatric* surgery.

5. Visual examination of the last section of the colon is a procedure called *Sigmoidoscopy*.

6. A mass of dilated, tortuous veins in the anorectal area is charted as *hemrrhoids*.

7. An incision into the upper sphincter of the stomach is a surgical procedure known as *pylorotomy*.

8. A person with *constipation* experiences infrequent passage of hard, dry feces.

9. The Dx in a patient who vomits blood is diagnosed a condition known as *hematemesis*.

10. Cholangiography is a radiographic examination of the *bile ducts* to identify or confirm gallstones or other obstructions.

11. *nausea* is an unpleasant sensation that precedes vomiting.

12. A test performed using the reagent "guaiac" requires a *Stool* sample.

13. ESWL uses shock waves to destroy *Stones* in the gallbladder and biliary ducts.

14. A nasogastric tube is inserted through the nose into the *Stomach*.

15. *GERD* may cause heartburn as a result of malfunction of the lower esophageal sphincter, which allows gastric acid to reflux into the esophagus.

✓ **Competency Verification:** Check your answers in Appendix B, Answer Key, on page 377. Review material that you did not answer correctly.

Correct Answers: _____ × **6.67** = _____ %

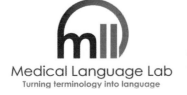

Medical Language Lab
Turning terminology into language

If you are not satisfied with your retention level of the digestive system chapter, visit *DavisPlus* Student Online Resource Center and the Medical Language Lab to complete the website activities linked to this chapter.

Urinary System

Objectives

Upon completion of this chapter, you will be able to:

- Describe types of medical treatment provided by urologists and nephrologists.
- Name the primary structures of the urinary system and discuss their functions.
- Identify combining forms, suffixes, and prefixes associated with the urinary system.
- Recognize, pronounce, build, and spell medical terms and abbreviations associated with the urinary system.
- Demonstrate your knowledge by successfully completing the activities in this chapter.

VOCABULARY PREVIEW

Term	Meaning
dialysis dī-ĂL-ĭ-sĭs *dia-:* through, across *-lysis:* separation; destruction; loosening	Mechanical filtering process used to remove metabolic waste products from blood, draw off excess fluids, and regulate body chemistry when kidneys fail to function properly
electrolytes ē-LĔK-trō-līts	Solutions that conduct electricity, such as acids, bases, and salts (sodium, potassium)
metabolism mĕ-TĂB-ō-lĭzm	Sum of all physical and chemical changes that take place within an organism
pH	Symbol for degree of acidity or alkalinity of a substance

Pronunciation Help	Long Sound	ā in rāte	ē in rēbirth	ī in īsle	ō in ōver	ū in ūnite
	Short Sound	ă in ălone	ĕ in ĕver	ĭ in ĭt	ŏ in nŏt	ŭ in cŭt

MEDICAL SPECIALTIES OF UROLOGY AND NEPHROLOGY

Urology

Physicians who specialize in diagnosis and treatment of disorders of the female and the male urinary systems are called **urologists.** Because some urinary structures in the male perform a dual role (both urinary functions and reproductive functions), the urologist also treats male reproductive disorders. These male disorders include, but are not limited to, treatment of bladder cancer, infertility, and sexual dysfunctions. Generally, the urologist performs surgery and treats urination problems, such as difficulty holding urine (**incontinence**) or obstruction of urinary flow as a result of tumors, stones, or other pathological conditions in the urinary organs. Also, urologists manage male reproductive disorders, such as impotence (erectile dysfunction). Other types of urologists include the **urogynecologist,** who specializes in treating urinary problems involving the female reproductive system, and the **pediatric urologist,** who specializes in diagnosing and treating urinary problems in children.

Nephrology

The medical specialty of **nephrology** is a subspecialty or branch of internal medicine. A **nephrologist** is a physician who specializes in the care of patients with diseases and conditions that affect the kidneys. They commonly treat chronic kidney disease (CKD), polycystic kidney disease (PKD), acute renal failure, kidney stones, and high blood pressure. Nephrologists are also educated on all aspects of kidney transplantation and dialysis. Their medical responsibilities include prescribing and coordinating **dialysis** treatments that are tailored to the needs of the individual patient, many of whom have been diagnosed with end-stage renal disease (ESRD).

URINARY SYSTEM QUICK STUDY

The primary function of the **urinary system** is to remove waste products of **metabolism** from the blood by excreting them in the urine. Organs of the urinary system are the kidneys, ureters, bladder, and urethra. Formation of urine is performed by the function of the kidneys. Other important functions of the kidneys include regulating the body's tissue fluid and maintaining a balance of **electrolytes** and an acid-base balance **(pH)** in the blood. The other urinary structures store and eliminate urine. (See *Urinary System*, page 190.)

    ALERT: An extensive self-paced anatomy and physiology multimedia review is included in *TermPlus*, a powerful, interactive CD-ROM program that can be purchased separately.

MEDICAL WORD BUILDING

Constructing medical words using word elements (combining forms, suffixes, and prefixes) related to the urinary system will enhance your understanding of those terms and reinforce your ability to use terms correctly.

Combining Forms

Begin the study of urology terminology by reviewing the organs of the urinary system and their associated combining forms (CFs). These are illustrated in the figure *Urinary System* that follows.

Urinary System

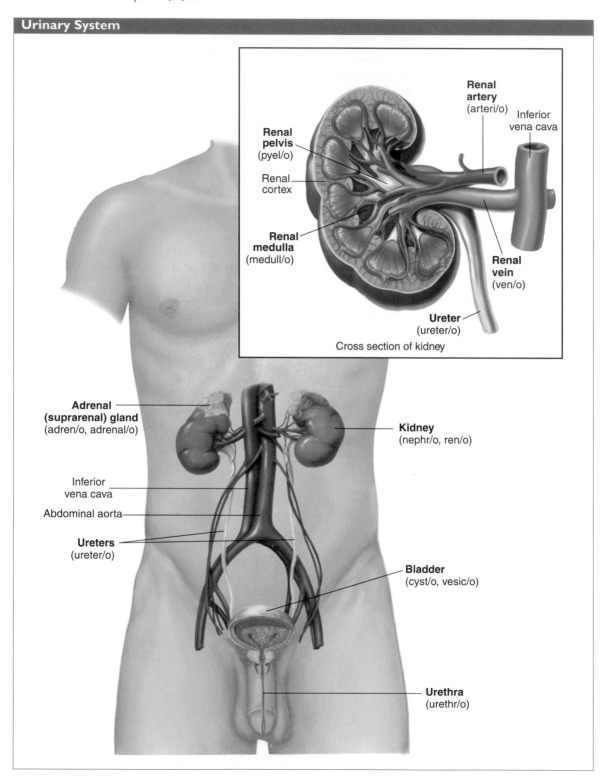

Renal pelvis (pyel/o)

Renal cortex

Renal medulla (medull/o)

Renal artery (arteri/o)

Inferior vena cava

Renal vein (ven/o)

Ureter (ureter/o)

Cross section of kidney

Adrenal (suprarenal) gland (adren/o, adrenal/o)

Kidney (nephr/o, ren/o)

Inferior vena cava

Abdominal aorta

Ureters (ureter/o)

Bladder (cyst/o, vesic/o)

Urethra (urethr/o)

In the table that follows, CFs are listed alphabetically, and other word parts are defined as needed. Review the medical word and study the elements that make up the term. Then complete the meaning of the medical word in the right-hand column. The first one is completed for you. You may also refer to *Appendix A: Glossary of Medical Word Elements* to complete this exercise.

Combining Form	Meaning	Medical Word	Meaning
cyst/o	bladder	cyst/o/scopy (sĭs-TŎS-kō-pē) *-scopy:* visual examination	*visual examination of the bladder*
vesic/o		vesic/o/cele (VĔS-ĭ-kō-sēl) *-cele:* hernia, swelling	
glomerul/o	glomerulus	glomerul/o/pathy (glō-mĕr-ū-LŎP-ă-thē) *-pathy:* disease	
meat/o	opening, meatus	meat/us (mē-Ā-tŭs) *-us:* condition, structure	
nephr/o	kidney	hydr/o/nephr/osis (hī-drō-nĕf-RŌ-sĭs) *hydr/o:* water *-osis:* abnormal condition (used primarily with blood cells) Get a closer look at hydronephrosis on page 204.	
ren/o		ren/al (RĒ-năl) *-al:* pertaining to	
pyel/o	renal pelvis	pyel/o/plasty (PĪ-ĕ-lō-plăs-tē) *-plasty:* surgical repair	
ur/o	urine, urinary tract	ur/emia (ū-RĒ-mē-ă) *-emia:* blood condition	
urin/o		urin/ary (Ŭ-rĭ-nār-ē) *-ary:* pertaining to	

(Continued)

Combining Form	Meaning	Medical Word	Meaning
ureter/o	ureter	**ureter/o**/stenosis (ū-rē-tĕr-ō-stĕ-NŌ-sĭs) *-stenosis:* narrowing, stricture	
urethr/o	urethra	**urethr/o**/cele (ū-RĒ-thrō-sēl) *-cele:* hernia, swelling	

Suffixes and Prefixes

In the table that follows, suffixes and prefixes are listed alphabetically, and other word parts are defined as needed. Review the medical word and study the elements that make up the term. Then complete the meaning of the medical word in the right-hand column. You may also refer to *Appendix A: Glossary of Medical Word Elements* to complete this exercise.

Word Element	Meaning	Medical Word	Meaning
Suffixes			
-emia	blood condition	azot/**emia** (ăz-ō-TĒ-mē-ă) *azot:* nitrogenous compounds	
-iasis	abnormal condition (produced by something specified)	lith/**iasis** (lĭth-Ī-ă-sĭs) *lith:* stone, calculus	
-lysis	separation; destruction; loosening	dia/**lysis** (dī-ĂL-ĭ-sĭs) *dia-:* through, across Get a closer look at dialysis on pages 205 and 206.	
-pathy	disease	nephr/o/**pathy** (nĕ-FRŎP-ă-thē) *nephr/o:* kidney	
-pexy	fixation (of an organ)	nephr/o/**pexy** (NĔF-rō-pĕks-ē) *nephr/o:* kidney	

Word Element	Meaning	Medical Word	Meaning
Suffixes			
-ptosis	prolapse, down-ward displacement	nephr/o/**ptosis** (nĕf-rŏp-TŌ-sĭs) *nephr/o:* kidney	
-tripsy	crushing	lith/o/**tripsy** (LĬTH-ō-trĭp-sē) *lith/o:* stone, calculus	
-uria	urine	olig/**uria** (ōl-ĭg-Ū-rē-ă) *olig:* scanty	
Prefixes			
an-	without, not	**an**/uria (ăn-Ū-rē-ă) *-uria:* urine	
poly-	many, much	**poly**/uria (pŏl-ē-Ū-rē-ă) *-uria:* urine	
supra-	above; excessive; superior	**supra**/ren/al (soo-pră-RĒ-năl) *ren:* kidney *-al:* pertaining to	

 Competency Verification: Check your answers in Appendix B, Answer Key, pages 377–378. If you are not satisfied with your level of comprehension, review the terms in the table and retake the review.

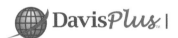 Visit the *Medical Terminology Express* online resource center at *DavisPlus* for an audio exercise of the terms in this table. Other activities are also available to reinforce content.

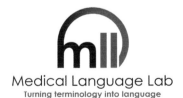
Medical Language Lab
Turning terminology into language

Visit the Medical Language Lab at *medicallanguagelab.com* to enhance your study and reinforce this chapter's word elements with the flash-card activity. We recommend you complete the flash-card activity before continuing with the next section.

Medical Terminology Word Building

In this section, combine the word parts you have learned to construct medical terms related to the urinary system.

Use **nephr/o** (kidney) to build words that mean:

1. stone or calculus in the kidney _____

2. disease of the kidney _____

3. abnormal condition of water in the kidney _____

Use **pyel/o** (renal pelvis) to build words that mean:

4. dilation of the renal pelvis _____

5. disease of the renal pelvis _____

Use **ureter/o** (ureter) to build words that mean:

6. hernia or swelling of the ureter _____

7. surgical repair of the ureter _____

Use **cyst/o** (bladder) to build words that mean:

8. inflammation of the bladder _____

9. instrument to view the bladder _____

Use **azot/o** (nitrogenous compounds) to build words that mean:

10. nitrogenous compounds in the urine _____

11. nitrogenous compounds in the blood _____

Use **urethr/o** (urethra) to build words that mean:

12. narrowing or stricture of the urethra _____

13. instrument used to incise the urethra _____

Use **ur/o** (urine, urinary tract) to build words that mean:

14. radiography of the urinary tract _____

15. disease of the urinary tract _____

Competency Verification: Check your answers in Appendix B, Answer Key, on page 379. Review material that you did not answer correctly.

Correct Answers: _____ × **6.67** = _____ %

MEDICAL VOCABULARY

The following tables consist of selected terms that pertain to diseases and conditions of the urinary system. Terms related to diagnostic, medical, and surgical procedures are included as well as pharmacological agents used to treat diseases. Recognizing and learning these terms will help you understand the connection between diseases and their treatments. Word analyses for selected terms are also provided.

Diseases and Conditions

azoturia
ăz-ō-TŪ-rē-ă
  azot: nitrogenous
      compounds
 -uria: urine
	Increase of nitrogenous substances, especially urea, in urine

cystocele SĬS-tō-sēl *cyst/o:* bladder *-cele:* hernia, swelling	Bulging of the urinary bladder through the wall of the vagina as a result of weakening of supportive tissue between the bladder and the vagina; also called *prolapsed bladder* (See Figure 8-1.)

diuresis
dī-ū-RĒ-sĭs
  di-: double
   ur: urine
-esis: condition
	Increased formation and secretion of urine

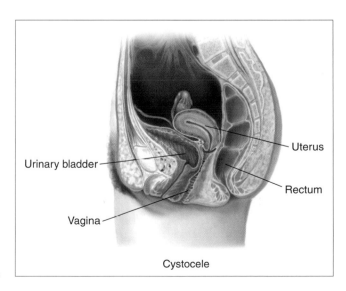

Figure 8-1 Cystocele.

dysuria
dĭs-Ū-rē-ă
  dys-: bad; painful; difficult
  -uria: urine
	Painful or difficult urination, typically caused by a urinary tract condition, such as *cystitis*

edema ĕ-DĒ-mă	Abnormal accumulation of fluids in the cells, tissues, or other parts of the body that may be a sign of kidney failure or other disease

end-stage renal disease (ESRD)
RĒ-năl
  ren: kidney
  -al: pertaining to
	Kidney disease that has advanced to the point that the kidneys can no longer adequately filter blood and eventually requires dialysis or renal transplantation for survival; also called *chronic renal failure* (CRF)
	
	Get a closer look at dialysis, on pages 205 and 206.

enuresis
ĕn-ū-RĒ-sĭs
  en-: in, within
  ur: urine
  -esis: condition
	Involuntary discharge of urine after the age at which bladder control should be established; also called *night-time bed-wetting* or *nocturnal enuresis*

hypospadias
hī-pō-SPĀ-dē-ăs
  hyp/o: under, below; deficient
  -spadias: slit, fissure
	Abnormal congenital opening of the male urethra on the undersurface of the penis

interstitial nephritis
ĭn-tĕr-STĬSH-ăl
nĕf-RĪ-tĭs
  nephr: kidney
  -itis: inflammation
	Form of nephritis in which pathological changes in renal interstitial tissue result in destruction of nephrons and severe impairment in renal function

nephrolithiasis
nĕf-rō-lĭth-Ī-ă-sĭs
  nephr/o: kidney
    lith: stone, calculus
  -iasis: abnormal condition (produced by something specified)
	Formation of calculi in the kidney that results when substances that are normally dissolved in the urine (such as calcium and acid salts) solidify (See Figure 8-2.)

renal hypertension
RĒ-năl hī-pĕr-TĔN-shŭn
  ren: kidney
  -al: pertaining to
  hyper-: excessive, above normal
  -tension: to stretch
	High blood pressure that results from kidney disease

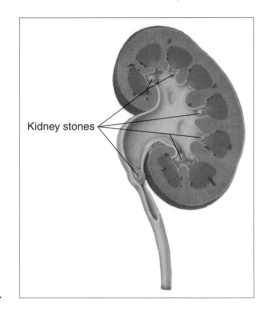

Figure 8-2 Kidney stones in the calyces and ureter.

uremia ū-RĒ-mē-ă *ur:* urine *-emia:* blood	Elevated level of urea and other nitrogenous waste products in the blood; also called *azotemia*
urinary tract infection (UTI)	Infection of the kidneys, ureters, or bladder by microorganisms that either ascend from the urethra or spread to the kidney from the bloodstream
Wilms tumor VĬLMZ	Malignant neoplasm of the kidney that occurs in young children, usually before age 5, and includes common early signs such as hypertension, a palpable mass, pain, and hematuria

Diagnostic Procedures

blood urea nitrogen (BUN) ū-RĒ-ă NĪ-trō-jĕn	Laboratory test that measures the amount of urea (nitrogenous waste product) in the blood and demonstrates the kidneys' ability to filter urea from the blood for excretion in urine
culture & sensitivity (C&S)	Laboratory test that isolates and grows colonies of microorganisms to identify a pathogen and to determine which drugs might be effective for combating an infection
kidneys, ureters, bladder (KUB)	Radiographic examination to determine the location, size, shape, and possible malformation of the kidneys, ureters, and bladder

pyelography pī-ĕ-LŎG-ră-fē *pyel/o:* renal pelvis *-graphy:* process of recording	Radiographic study of the kidneys, ureters, and, usually, the bladder after injection of a contrast agent
intravenous pyelography (IVP) ĭn-tră-VĒ-nŭs pī-ĕ-LŎG-ră-fē *intra-:* in, within *ven:* vein *-ous:* pertaining to *pyel/o:* renal pelvis *-graphy:* process of recording	Radiographic imaging in which a contrast medium is injected intravenously and serial x-ray films are taken to provide visualization of the entire urinary tract
retrograde pyelography (RP) RĔT-rō-grād pī-ĕ-LŎG-ră-fē *retro-:* backward, behind *-grade:* to go *pyel/o:* renal pelvis *-graphy:* process of recording	Radiographic imaging in which a contrast medium is introduced through a cystoscope directly into the bladder and ureters to provide detailed visualization of the urinary structures and to locate urinary tract obstruction
renal scan RĒ-năl *ren:* kidney *-al:* pertaining to	Nuclear medicine imaging procedure that determines renal function and shape through measurement of a radioactive substance injected intravenously that concentrates in the kidney
urinalysis (UA) ū-rĭ-NĂL-ĭ-sĭs	Physical, chemical, and microscopic analysis of urine
voiding cystourethrography (VCUG) sĭs-tō-ū-rē-THRŎG-ră-fē *cyst/o:* bladder *urethr/o:* urethra *-graphy:* process of recording	Radiography of the bladder and urethra during the process of voiding urine after filling the bladder with a contrast medium

Medical and Surgical Procedures

catheterization kăth-ĕ-tĕr-ĭ-ZĀ-shŭn	Insertion of a catheter (hollow flexible tube) into a body cavity or organ to instill a substance or remove fluid, most commonly through the urethra into the bladder to withdraw urine (See Figure 8-3.)
cystoscopy (cysto) sĭs-TŎS-kō-pē *cyst/o:* bladder *-scopy:* visual examination	Insertion of a rigid or flexible cystoscope through the urethra to examine the urinary bladder, obtain biopsy specimens of tumors or other growths, and remove polyps (See Figure 8-4.)

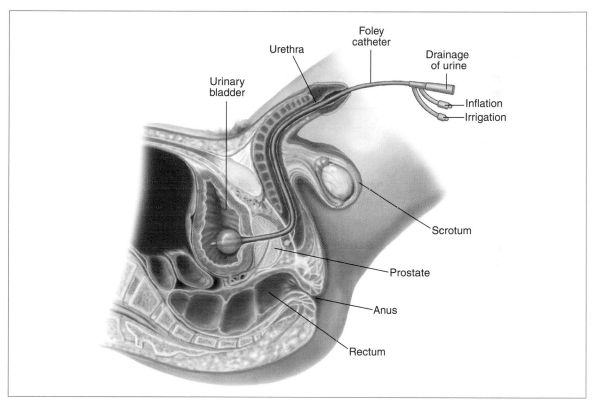

Figure 8-3 Catheterization.

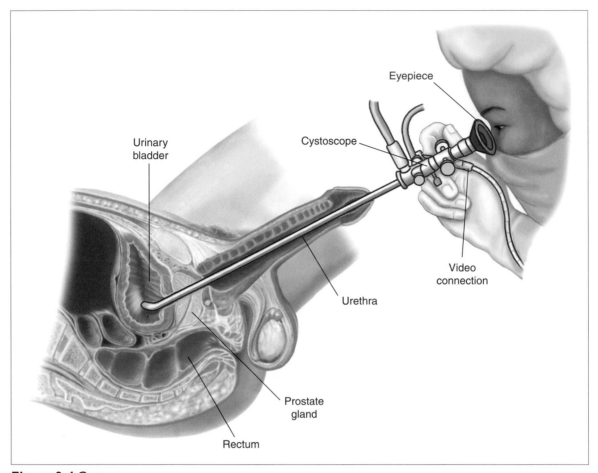

Figure 8-4 Cystoscopy.

lithotripsy
LĬTH-ō-trĭp-sē
  lith/o: stone, calculus
  -tripsy: crushing
	Method of removing stones by crushing them into smaller pieces so that they can be expelled in the urine

extracorporeal shock-wave lithotripsy (ESWL)
ĕks-tră-kor-POR-ē-ăl SHŎK-wāv
  extra: outside
  corpor: body
    -eal: pertaining to
  lith/o: stone, calculus
  -tripsy: crushing
	Use of powerful sound wave vibrations to break up stones in the kidney (See Figure 8-5.)

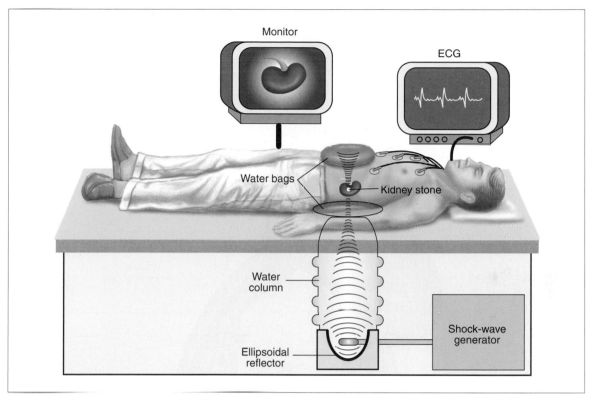

Figure 8-5 Extracorporeal shock-wave lithotripsy.

nephrolithotomy něf-rō-lĭth-ŎT-ō-mē *nephr/o:* kidney *lith/o:* stone, calculus *-tomy:* incision	Surgical procedure that involves a small incision in the skin and insertion of an endoscope into the kidney to remove a renal calculus
renal transplantation RĒ-năl trăns-plăn-TĀ-shŭn *ren:* kidney *-al:* pertaining to	Organ transplant of a kidney in a patient with end-stage renal disease; also called *kidney transplantation* (See Figure 8-6.)
ureteral stent ū-RĒ-těr-ăl *ureter:* ureter *-al:* pertaining to	Insertion of a thin tube into the ureter to prevent or treat obstruction of urine flow from the kidney (See Figure 8-7.)

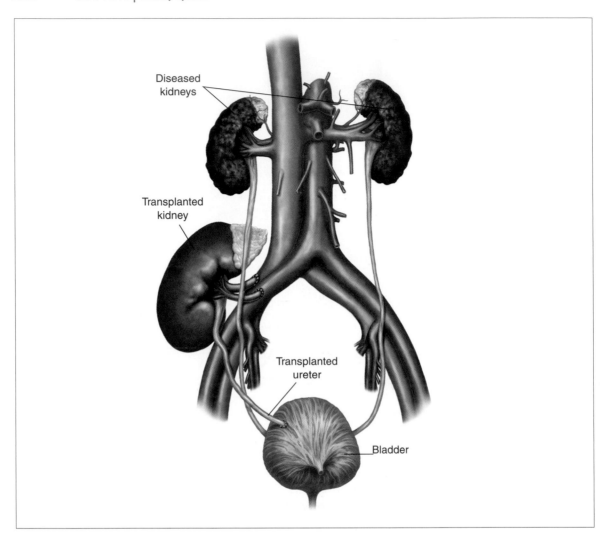

Figure 8-6 Renal transplantation in which the donor kidney is typically placed inferior to the normal anatomical location, and the patient's kidneys are usually left in place.

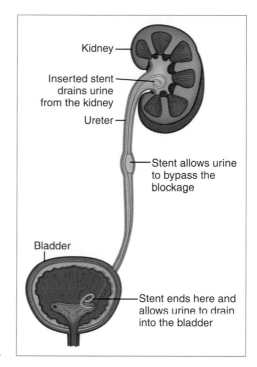

Figure 8-7 Ureteral stent placement.

Pharmacology

antibiotics ăn-tĭ-bī-ŎT-ĭks	Treat bacterial infections of the urinary tract by acting on the bacterial membrane or one of its metabolic processes
antispasmodics ăn-tē-spăz-MŎD-ĭks	Decrease spasms in the urethra and bladder (caused by UTIs and catheterization) by relaxing the smooth muscles lining their walls, allowing normal emptying of the bladder
diuretics dī-ū-RĔT-ĭks	Block reabsorption of sodium by the kidneys, increasing the amount of salt and water excreted in the urine (causes reduction of fluid retained in the body and prevents edema)

Pronunciation Help	Long Sound	ā in rāte	ē in rēbirth	ī in īsle	ō in ōver	ū in ūnite
	Short Sound	ă in ălone	ĕ in ĕver	ĭ in ĭt	ŏ in nŏt	ŭ in cŭt

A Closer Look

Take a closer look at the following urological conditions and procedures to enhance your understanding of the medical terminology associated with them.

Hydronephrosis

Hydronephrosis is an excessive accumulation of urine in the renal pelvis as a result of obstruction of a ureter. Because urine is blocked from flowing into the bladder, it flows backward **(refluxes)** into the renal pelvis and calyces. This reflux causes hydronephrosis and results in abnormal dilation of the renal pelvis and the calyces of one or both kidneys. The main cause of urinary tract obstruction leading to hydronephrosis is a stone or **stricture.** Other causes include tumor growth, thickening of the bladder wall, and **prostatomegaly.**

The illustration that follows depicts urinary obstruction in the proximal part of the ureter caused by a stone **(calculus),** a condition called **hydroureter.** The illustration also shows the enlarged right kidney, which is caused by pressure from urine reflux, a condition called **hydronephrosis.**

Although a partial obstruction and hydronephrosis may not produce symptoms initially, the pressure built up behind the area of obstruction eventually results in symptoms of renal dysfunction.

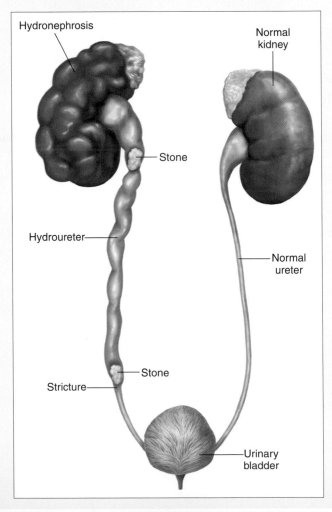

Hydronephrosis

A Closer Look—cont'd

Dialysis

Dialysis is the process of removing waste products from the blood when the kidneys are unable to do so. There are two types of dialysis: hemodialysis and peritoneal dialysis.

Hemodialysis involves passing the blood through an artificial kidney for filtering out impurities. The illustration that follows shows the process of hemodialysis.

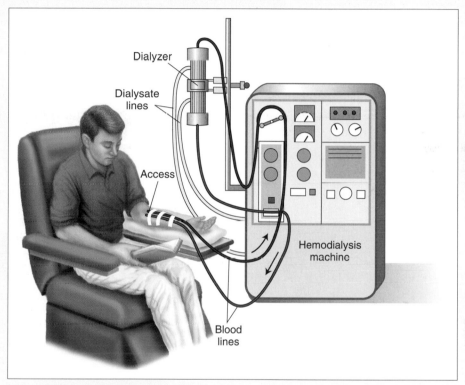

Hemodialysis

(Continued)

A Closer Look—cont'd

Peritoneal dialysis involves introducing fluid into the abdomen through a catheter. Dialysate fluid flows through the catheter and remains in the abdominal cavity for several hours. During that time, the fluid pulls body wastes from the blood into the abdominal cavity. The fluid is then removed from the abdomen via a catheter. The illustration that follows shows the introduction of dialysis fluid into the peritoneal cavity (A) and draining the fluid with waste products from the peritoneal cavity (B).

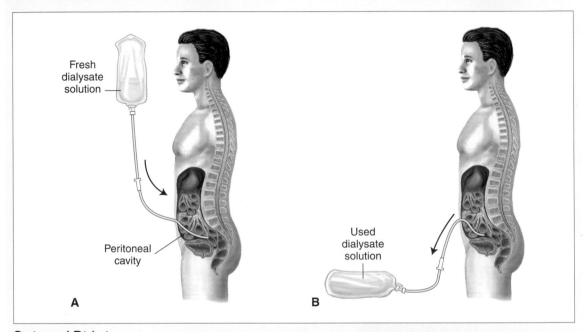

Peritoneal Dialysis

Medical Vocabulary Recall

Match the medical terms below with the definitions in the numbered list.

azoturia	dialysis	enuresis	renal hypertension	uremia
BUN	diuresis	hydronephrosis	retrograde pyelography	VCUG
catheterization	dysuria	interstitial nephritis	UA	Wilms tumor

1. _____ refers to physical, chemical, and microscopic examination of urine.

2. _____ is a malignant neoplasm in the kidney that occurs in young children.

3. _____ is an increase in nitrogenous compounds in urine.

4. _____ means painful or difficult urination, which is a symptom of numerous conditions.

5. _____ means increased formation and secretion of urine.

6. _____ is a radiologic technique in which a contrast medium is introduced through a cystoscope to provide detailed visualization of the urinary collecting system.

7. _____ accumulation of urine in the kidney as a result of an obstruction in a ureter.

8. _____ is associated with pathological changes in the renal interstitial tissue, which may be primary or due to a toxic agent.

9. _____ is a test that measures the amount of urea excreted by kidneys into the blood.

10. _____ means urinary incontinence, including bed-wetting.

11. _____ refers to insertion of a hollow, flexible tube into a body cavity or organ to instill a substance or remove fluid.

12. _____ is radiography of the bladder and urethra after introduction of a contrast medium and during the process of urination.

13. _____ refers to an elevated level of urea and other nitrogenous waste products in blood.

14. _____ refers to high blood pressure that results from kidney disease.

15. _____ is the mechanical filtering process used to cleanse blood of high concentrations of metabolic waste products.

 Competency Verification: Check your answers in Appendix B, Answer Key, on page 379. Review material that you did not answer correctly.

Correct Answers: _____ × **6.67 =** _____ %

Pronunciation and Spelling

Use the following list to practice correct pronunciation and spelling of medical terms. First practice the pronunciation aloud. Then write the correct spelling of the term. The first word is completed for you.

Pronunciation	Spelling
1. ăz-ō-TĒ-mē-ă	*azotemia*
2. kăth-ĕ-tĕr-ĭ-ZĀ-shŭn	
3. sĭs-TŎS-kō-pē	
4. sĭs-tō-ū-RĒ-thrō-skōp	
5. glō-mĕr-ū-lō-nĕ-FRĪ-tĭs	
6. ĭn-KŎN-tĭ-nĕns	
7. LĬTH-ō-trĭp-sē	
8. nĕf-rō-lĭth-ŎT-ō-mē	
9. nĕf-rŏp-TŌ-sĭs	
10. nĕf-rō-sklĕ-RŌ-sĭs	
11. ŏl-ĭg-Ū-rē-ă	
12. pŏl-ē-Ū-rē-ă	
13. prō-tēn-Ū-rē-ă	
14. PĪ-ĕ-lō-plăs-tē	
15. pī-ō-nĕf-RŌ-sĭs	
16. RĔT-rō-grād pī-ĕ-LŎG-ră-fē	
17. ū-rē-tĕr-ĔK-tă-sĭs	
18. ū-rē-tĕr-ō-stĕ-NŌ-sĭs	
19. ū-RĒ-thrō-sēl	
20. ū-RŎL-ō-jĭst	

✓ **Competency Verification:** Check your answers in Appendix B, Answer Key, on page 379. Review material that you did not answer correctly.

Correct Answers: _____ × 5 = _____ %

ABBREVIATIONS

The following table introduces abbreviations associated with the urinary system.

Abbreviation	Meaning	Abbreviation	Meaning
BUN	blood urea nitrogen	PKD	polycystic kidney disease
C&S	culture and sensitivity	RP	retrograde pyelography
CKD	chronic kidney disease	pH	symbol for degree of acidity or alkalinity
CRF	chronic renal failure	TURP	transurethral resection of the prostate
cysto	cystoscopy	UA	urinalysis
ESRD	end-stage renal disease	US	ultrasound, ultrasonography
ESWL	extracorporeal shock-wave lithotripsy	UTI	urinary tract infection
IVP	intravenous pyelography	VCUG	voiding cystourethrography
KUB	kidneys, ureters, bladder	WBC, wbc	white blood cell

CHART NOTES

Chart notes make up part of the medical record and are used in various types of health care facilities. The chart notes that follow were dictated by the patient's physician and reflect common clinical events using medical terminology to document the patient's care. Studying and completing the terminology and chart note analysis sections below will help you learn and understand terms associated with the medical specialty of urology.

Terminology

The following terms are linked to chart notes in the medical specialty of urology and nephrology. Practice pronouncing each term aloud, and then use a medical dictionary such as *Taber's Cyclopedic Medical Dictionary; Appendix A: Glossary of Medical Word Elements,* or other resources to define each term.

Term	Meaning
cholecystec-tomy kō-lē-sĭs- TĔK-tō-mē	
choledocholi-thiasis kō-lĕd-ō-kō-lĭ-THĪ-ă-sĭs	
choledo-cholithotomy kō-lĕd-ō-kō-lĭth-ŎT- ō-mē	
cholelithiasis kō-lē-lĭ-THĪ-ă-sĭs	
cystoscopy sĭs-TŎS-kō-pē	
hematuria hĕm-ă-TŪ-rē-ă	
incontinence ĭn-KŎNT-ĭn-ĕns	
nocturia nŏk-TŪ-rē-ă	
polyuria pŏl-ē-Ū-rē-ă	

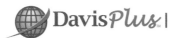**DavisPlus** | Visit *Medical Terminology Express* at *DavisPlus* Online Resource Center. Use it to practice pronunciations and reinforce the meanings of the terms in this chart note.

Cystitis

Read the chart note that follows aloud. Underline any term you have trouble pronouncing and any terms that you cannot define. If needed, refer to the Terminology section on page 209 for correct pronunciations and meanings of terms.

This 50-year-old white woman has been complaining of diffuse pelvic pain with urinary bladder spasm since cystoscopy 10 days ago, at which time marked cystitis was noted. She reports nocturia three to four times each night, urinary frequency, urgency, and epigastric discomfort. The patient has a history of polyuria, hematuria, and urinary incontinence. There is a history of numerous stones, large and small, in the gallbladder. In 19xx, she was admitted to the hospital with cholecystitis, chronic and acute; cholelithiasis; and choledocholithiasis. Subsequently, cholecystectomy, choledocholithotomy, and incidental appendectomy were performed.

Impression: Urinary incontinence caused by cystitis and is temporary in nature.

Chart Note Analysis

From the preceding chart note, select the medical word that means

1. inflammation of the bladder: _____

2. urination at night: _____

3. blood in the urine: _____

4. visual examination of the bladder: _____

5. region above the stomach: _____

6. frequent urge to urinate: _____

7. excision of the appendix: _____

8. abnormal condition of gallstones: _____

9. inflammation of the gallbladder: _____

10. abnormal condition of stones in the bile duct: _____

11. excessive urination: _____

12. uncontrolled loss of urine from the bladder: _____

13. incision into the bile duct to remove stones: _____

14. excision of the gallbladder: _____

15. organ that stores bile: _____

Competency Verification: Check your answers in Appendix B, Answer Key, on page 379. Review material that you did not answer correctly.

Correct Answers: _____ × **6.67** = _____ %

Demonstrate What You Know!

To evaluate your understanding of how medical terms you have studied in this and previous chapters are used in a clinical environment, complete the numbered sentences by selecting an appropriate term from the words below.

anuria	edema	intravenous	nephromegaly	pyuria
continence	hematuria	lithotomy	pus	urinary
diuretic	hernia	nephrologist	pyelopathy	urologist

1. A person with nephrosis exhibits swelling, or _____, around the ankles, feet, and eyes.

2. To stimulate the flow of urine, a patient would be prescribed a _____.

3. A diagnosis of hydronephrosis would indicate an obstruction in the _____ tract.

4. Any disease of the renal pelvis is known as _____.

5. Medication administered into a vein is said to be given by an _____ method.

6. _____ is evident in a urine sample that contains red blood cells.

7. A patient with cystitis usually shows pus in the urine. This condition is called _____.

8. A person who is not forming urine has a condition called _____.

9. A physician who treats disorders of the urinary tract is a _____.

10. When a person has the ability to control his or her bladder, it is known as urinary _____.

11. A diseased kidney can lead to _____, also called *enlarged kidney.*

12. The rupture or protrusion of an organ through a wall of a body cavity is called a _____.

13. In pyonephrosis, there is an accumulation of _____ in the kidneys.

14. An incision to remove a calculus is a surgical procedure known as _____.

15. A physician who manages kidney transplants and dialysis therapies is a _____.

✓ **Competency Verification:** Check your answers in Appendix B, Answer Key, on page 379. Review material that you did not answer correctly.

Correct Answers: _____ × **6.67** = _____ %

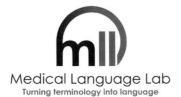

Medical Language Lab
Turning terminology into language

If you are not satisfied with your retention level of the urinary chapter, visit *DavisPlus* Student Online Resource Center and the Medical Language Lab to complete the website activities linked to this chapter.

Reproductive System

Objectives

Upon completion of this chapter, you will be able to:

- Describe types of medical treatment provided by gynecologists, obstetricians, and urologists.
- Name the primary structures of the female and male reproductive systems and discuss their functions.
- Identify combining forms, suffixes, and prefixes associated with the female and male reproductive systems.
- Recognize, pronounce, build, and spell medical terms and abbreviations associated with the female and male reproductive systems.
- Demonstrate your knowledge of this chapter by successfully completing the activities in this chapter.

VOCABULARY PREVIEW

Term	Meaning
fertilization FĔR-tĭ-lĭ-zā-shŭn	Union of the male and female gametes to form a zygote, leading to the development of a new individual
gamete GĂM-ēt	Reproductive cell (spermatozoon in the male and ovum in the female)
infertility ĭn-fĕr-TĬL-ĭ-tē	Persistent inability to conceive a child
neonate NĒ-ō-nāt	Infant from birth to 28 days of age
ova Ō-văh	Female reproductive cells (plural of *ovum*)
postpartum pōst-PĂR-tĕm *post-:* after, behind *-partum:* childbirth; labor	Occurring after childbirth

Pronunciation Help	Long Sound	ā in rāte	ē in rēbirth	ī in īsle	ō in ōver	ū in ūnite
	Short Sound	ă in ălone	ĕ in ĕver	ĭ in ĭt	ŏ in nŏt	ŭ in cŭt

MEDICAL SPECIALTIES OF GYNECOLOGY AND OBSTETRICS AND UROLOGY

Gynecology and Obstetrics

Gynecology is the medical specialty concerned with diagnosis and treatment of female reproductive disorders, including conditions affecting the breasts. The **gynecologist** is a physician who specializes in gynecology. Unlike most medical specialties, gynecology includes both the surgical and the nonsurgical expertise of the physician. Because obstetrics is studied in conjunction with gynecology, the physician's medical practice commonly includes both areas of expertise. This branch of medicine is called **obstetrics and gynecology (OB-GYN).** The obstetrician and gynecologist possess knowledge of endocrinology because hormones play an important role in the functions of the female reproductive system, especially the process of secondary sex characteristics, menstruation, pregnancy, and menopause. **Infertility**, birth control, and hormone imbalance all are part of the treatment provided by an OB-GYN physician.

Obstetrics is the branch of medicine concerned with pregnancy and childbirth, including the study of the physiological and pathological functions of the female reproductive tract. It also involves the care of the mother and fetus throughout pregnancy, childbirth, and the immediate **postpartum** period. An **obstetrician** is a physician who specializes in obstetrics. The branch of medicine that concentrates on the care of the **neonate** and in the diagnosis and treatment of disorders of neonates is known as **neonatology.** When an infant is born, physicians called **neonatologists** specialize in providing medical care to the infant.

Urology

Urology is the branch of medicine specializing in treating disorders of the male reproductive system. The **urologist** is a specialist who diagnoses and manages male reproductive dysfunctions. The urologist uses diagnostic tests, medical and surgical procedures, and drugs to treat diseases, sexual dysfunctions, and infertility in male patients. The urologist also diagnoses and treats diseases that affect the urinary system of men and women.

REPRODUCTIVE SYSTEMS QUICK STUDY

Although anatomical structures of the female and male reproductive systems differ, both have a common purpose. They are specialized to produce and unite **gametes** and transport them to sites of **fertilization**. Reproductive systems of both sexes are designed specifically to perpetuate the species and pass genetic material from generation to generation. In addition, both sexes produce hormones, which are vital in development and maintenance of sexual characteristics and regulation of reproductive physiology. In women, the reproductive system includes the ovaries, fallopian tubes, uterus, vagina, clitoris, and vulva. In men, the reproductive system includes the testes, epididymis, vas deferens, seminal vesicles, ejaculatory duct, prostate, and penis.

Female Reproductive System

The female reproductive system is composed of **internal organs of reproduction** and **external genitalia.** The internal organs are the ovaries, fallopian tubes (oviducts, uterine tubes), uterus, and vagina. External organs are known collectively as the **vulva** or **genitalia.** Included in the vulva are the mons pubis, labia majora, labia minora, clitoris, and Bartholin glands. The combined organs of the female reproductive system are designed to produce and transport **ova** and discharge ova from the body if fertilization does not occur. The female reproductive system also nourishes and provides a place for the developing fetus throughout pregnancy if fertilization occurs. The ovaries of the female reproductive system also produce the female sex hormones estrogen and progesterone, which are responsible for development of secondary sex characteristics, including breast development and regulation of the menstrual cycle.

Male Reproductive System

The primary sex organs of the male reproductive system are called **gonads,** specifically the **testes** (singular, **testis**). Gonads produce gametes (sperm) and secrete sex hormones. The remaining accessory reproductive organs are structures that are essential in caring for and transporting sperm. These organs and structures are designed to accomplish the man's reproductive role of producing and delivering sperm to the woman's reproductive tract, where fertilization can occur.

These structures can be divided into three categories:

1. sperm-transporting ducts, which include the epididymis, ductus deferens, ejaculatory duct, and urethra
2. accessory glands, which include the seminal vesicles, prostate gland, and bulbourethral glands
3. copulatory organ, the penis, which contains erectile tissue

ALERT: An extensive self-paced anatomy and physiology multimedia review is included in *TermPlus,* a powerful, interactive CD-ROM program that can be purchased separately from F.A. Davis Company.

MEDICAL WORD BUILDING

Constructing medical words using word elements (combining forms, suffixes, and prefixes) related to the female and male reproductive systems will enhance your understanding of those terms and reinforce your ability to use terms correctly.

Combining Forms

Begin your study of female and male reproductive terminology by reviewing the organs and their associated combining forms (CFs), which are illustrated in the figure *Female Reproductive System* below and the figure *Male Reproductive System* that follows.

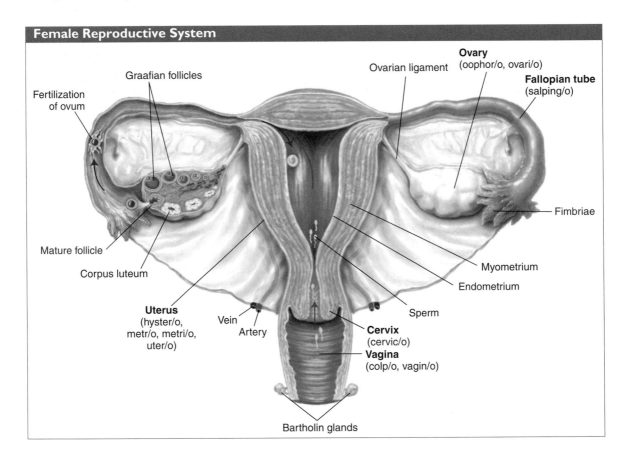

Female Reproductive System

Male Reproductive System

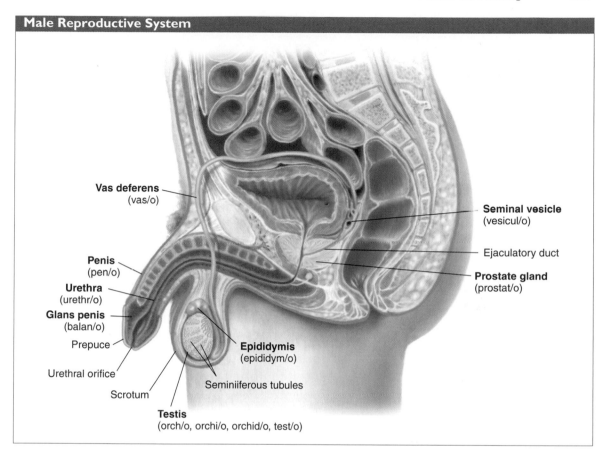

Vas deferens
(vas/o)

Seminal vesicle
(vesicul/o)

Ejaculatory duct

Penis
(pen/o)

Prostate gland
(prostat/o)

Urethra
(urethr/o)

Glans penis
(balan/o)

Prepuce

Epididymis
(epididym/o)

Urethral orifice

Seminiiferous tubules

Scrotum

Testis
(orch/o, orchi/o, orchid/o, test/o)

In the table that follows, CFs are listed alphabetically, and other word parts are defined as needed. Review the medical word and study the elements that make up the term. Then complete the meaning of the medical words in the right-hand column. The first one is completed for you. You may also refer to *Appendix A: Glossary of Medical Word Elements* to complete this exercise.

Combining Form	Meaning	Medical Word	Meaning
Female Reproductive System			
amni/o	amnion (amniotic sac)	**amni/o**/centesis (ăm-nē-ō-sĕn-TĒ-sĭs) *-centesis:* surgical puncture Get a closer look at amniocentesis on page 238.	*surgical puncture of the amniotic sac (to remove fluid for laboratory analysis)*
cervic/o	neck; cervix uteri (neck of uterus)	**cervic**/itis (sĕr-vĭ-SĪ-tĭs) *-itis:* inflammation	
colp/o	vagina	**colp/o**/scopy (kŏl-PŎS-kō-pē) *-scopy:* visual examination	
vagin/o	vagina	**vagin/o**/cele (VĂJ-ĭn-ō-sēl) *-cele:* hernia, swelling	
galact/o	milk	**galact/o**/rrhea (gă-lăk-tō-RĒ-ă) *-rrhea:* discharge, flow	
lact/o		**lact/o**/gen (LĂK-tō-jĕn) *-gen:* forming, producing; origin	
gynec/o	woman, female	**gynec/o**/logist (gī-nĕ-KŎL-ō-jĭst) *-logist:* specialist in study of	
hyster/o	uterus (womb)	**hyster**/ectomy (hĭs-tĕr-ĔK-tō-mē) *-ectomy:* excision, removal	
uter/o		**uter/o**/vagin/al (ū-tĕr-ō-VĂJ-ĭ-năl) *vagin:* vagina *-al:* pertaining to	

Combining Form	Meaning	Medical Word	Meaning
Female Reproductive System			
mamm/o	breast	**mamm/o**/gram (MĂM-ō-grăm) *-gram:* record, writing	
mast/o		**mast/o**/pexy (MĂS-tō-pĕks-ē) *-pexy:* fixation (of an organ)	
men/o	menses, menstruation	**men/o**/rrhagia (mĕn-ō-RĀ-jē-ă) *-rrhagia:* bursting forth (of)	
metr/o	uterus (womb); measure	endo/**metr**/itis (ĕn-dō-mē-TRĪ-tĭs) *endo-:* in, within *-itis:* inflammation	
nat/o	birth	pre/**nat**/al (prē-NĀ-tl) *pre-:* before, in front of *-al:* pertaining to	
oophor/o	ovary	**oophor**/oma (ō-ŏf-ōr-Ōmă) *-oma:* tumor	
ovari/o		**ovari/o**/tomy (ō-vā-rē-ŎT-ō-mē) *-tomy:* incision	
perine/o	perineum	**perine/o**/rrhaphy (pĕr-ĭ-nē-OR-ă-fē) *-rrhaphy:* suture	
salping/o	tube (usually fallopian or eustachian [auditory] tubes)	**salping**/ectomy (săl-pĭn-JĔK-tō-mē) *-ectomy:* excision, removal	
vulv/o	vulva	**vulv/o**/pathy (vŭl-VŎP-ă-thē) *-pathy:* disease	
episi/o		**episi/o**/tomy (ĕ-pĭs-ē-ŎT-ō-mē) *-tomy:* incision	

Combining Form	Meaning	Medical Word	Meaning
Male Reproductive System			
andr/o	male	**andr/o**/gen (ĂN-drō-jĕn) *-gen:* forming, producing; origin	
balan/o	glans penis	**balan**/itis (băl-ă-NĪ-tĭs) *-itis:* inflammation	
gonad/o	gonads, sex glands	**gonad/o**/tropin (gŏn-ă-dō-TRŌ-pĭn) *-tropin:* stimulate	

olig/o	scanty	**olig/o**/sperm/ia
		(ŏl-ĭ-gō-SPĔR-mē-ă)
		sperm: spermatozoa,
		   sperm cells
		   -ia: condition	

orch/o	testis (plural, testes)	crypt/**orch**/ism (krĭpt-OR-kĭzm) *crypt:* hidden *-ism:* condition	
orchi/o		**orchi/o**/pexy (OR-kē-ō-pĕk-sē) *-pexy:* fixation (of an organ)	
orchid/o		**orchid**/ectomy (or-kĭ-DĔK-tō-mē) *-ectomy:* excision, removal	
test/o		**test**/algia (tĕs-TĂL-jē-ă) *-algia:* pain	
prostat/o	prostate gland	**prostat**/itis (prŏs-tă-TĪ-tĭs) *-itis:* inflammation	

Combining Form	Meaning	Medical Word	Meaning
Male Reproductive System			
spermat/o	spermatozoa, sperm cells	**spermat/o**/cide (SPĔR-mă-tō-sīd) *-cide:* killing	
sperm/i*		**sperm/i**/cide (SPĔR-mĭ-sīd) *-cide:* killing	
sperm/o		a/**sperm**/ia (ă-SPĔR-mē-ă) *a-:* without, not *-ia:* condition	
varic/o	dilated vein	**varic/o**/cele (VĂR-ĭ-kō-sēl) *-cele:* hernia, swelling	
vas/o	vessel; vas deferens; duct	**vas**/ectomy (văs-ĔK-tō-mē) *-ectomy:* excision, removal Get a closer look at vasectomy on page 239.	
vesicul/o	seminal vesicle	**vesicul**/itis (vĕ-sĭk-ū-LĪ-tĭs) *-itis:* inflammation	

*Using the combining vowel i instead of o is an exception to the rule.

Suffixes and Prefixes

In the table that follows, suffixes and prefixes are listed alphabetically, and other word parts are defined as needed. Review the medical word and study the elements that make up the term. Then complete the meaning of the medical words in the right-hand column. You may also refer to *Appendix A: Glossary of Medical Word Elements* to complete this exercise.

Word Element	Meaning	Medical Word	Meaning
Suffixes			
-arche	beginning	men/**arche** (mĕn-ĂR-kē) *men:* menses, menstruation	
-cyesis	pregnancy	pseudo/**cyesis** (soo-dō-sī-Ē-sĭs) *pseudo-:* false	
-gravida	pregnant woman	primi/**gravida** (prī-mĭ-GRĂV-ĭ-dă) *primi-:* first	
-para	to bear (offspring)	multi/**para** (mŭl-TĬP-ă-ră) *multi-:* many, much	
-salpinx	tube (usually fallopian or eustachian [auditory] tubes)	hemat/o/**salpinx** (hĕm-ă-tō-SĂL-pinks) *hemat/o:* blood	
-tocia	childbirth, labor	dys/**tocia** (dĭs-TŌ-sē-ă) *dys-:* bad; painful; difficult	
Prefix			
retro-	backward, behind	**retro**/version (rĕt-rō-VĔR-shŭn) *-version:* turning	

 Competency Verification: Check your answers in Appendix B, Answer Key, pages 380–381. If you are not satisfied with your level of comprehension, review the terms in the table and retake the review.

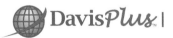 Visit the *Medical Terminology Express* online resource center at *DavisPlus* for an audio exercise of the terms in this table. Other activities are also available to reinforce content.

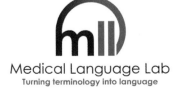
Medical Language Lab
Turning terminology into language

Visit the Medical Language Lab at *medicallanguagelab.com* to enhance your study and reinforce this chapter's word elements with the flash-card activity. We recommend you complete the flash-card activity before continuing with the next section.

Medical Terminology Word Building

In this section, combine the word parts you have learned to construct medical terms related to the male and female reproductive systems.

Use *gynec/o* (woman, female) to build words that mean:

1. disease (specific to) women _____

2. physician who specializes in diseases of the female _____

Use *cervic/o* (neck; cervix uteri) to build words that mean:

3. inflammation of cervix uteri and vagina _____

4. excision of cervix uteri _____

Use *colp/o* (vagina) to build words that mean:

5. instrument used to examine the vagina _____

6. visual examination of the vagina _____

Use *hyster/o* (uterus) to build words that mean:

7. rupture of the uterus _____

8. disease of the uterus _____

Use *metr/o* (uterus) to build words that mean:

9. hemorrhage from the uterus _____

10. inflammation of the uterus _____

Use *salping/o* (tube [usually fallopian or eustachian tube]) to build words that mean:

11. herniation of the fallopian tube _____

12. inflammation of the fallopian tube _____

13. fixation of a fallopian tube _____

Use *prostat/o* (prostate gland) to build words that mean:

14. enlargement of the prostate gland _____

15. pain in the prostate gland _____

Use *orchid/o* or *orchi/o* (testes) to build words that mean:

16. disease of testes _____

17. pain in testes _____

Use *balan/o* (glans penis) to build words that mean:

18. discharge from the glans penis _____

19. inflammation of the glans penis _____

20. surgical repair of the glans penis _____

 Competency Verification: Check your answers in Appendix B, Answer Key, on page 382. Review material that you did not answer correctly.

Correct Answers: _____ × **5** = _____ %

MEDICAL VOCABULARY

The following tables consist of selected terms that pertain to diseases and conditions of the female and male reproductive systems. Terms related to diagnostic, medical, and surgical procedures are included as well as pharmacological agents used to treat diseases. Recognizing and learning these terms will help you understand the connection between diseases and their treatments. Word analyses for selected terms are also provided.

Diseases and Conditions

Female Reproductive System

candidiasis kăn-dĭ-DĪ-ă-sĭs	Vaginal fungal infection caused by *Candida albicans* and characterized by a curdy or cheeselike discharge and extreme itching
cervicitis sĕr-vĭ-SĪ-tĭs *cervic:* neck; cervix uteri (neck of uterus) *-itis:* inflammation	Inflammation of the uterine cervix, which is usually the result of infection or a sexually transmitted infection
ectopic pregnancy ĕk-TŎP-ĭk	Implantation of the fertilized ovum outside of the uterine cavity, most commonly in the oviducts (tubal pregnancy) (See Figure 9-1.)

endometriosis
ĕn-dō-mē-trē-Ō-sĭs
endo-: in, within
metri: uterus (womb)
 -osis: abnormal condition;
    increase (used
    primarily
    with blood cells)
	Presence of endometrial tissue outside (ectopic) the uterine cavity, such as the pelvis or abdomen (See Figure 9-2.)

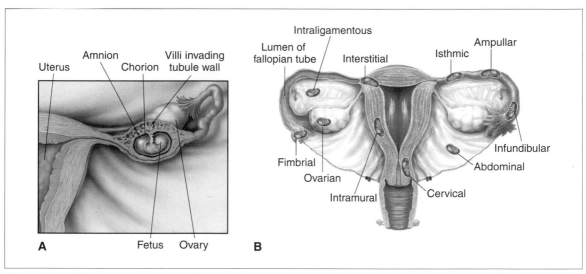

Figure 9-1 (A) Tubal pregnancy. (B) Other sites of ectopic pregnancy.

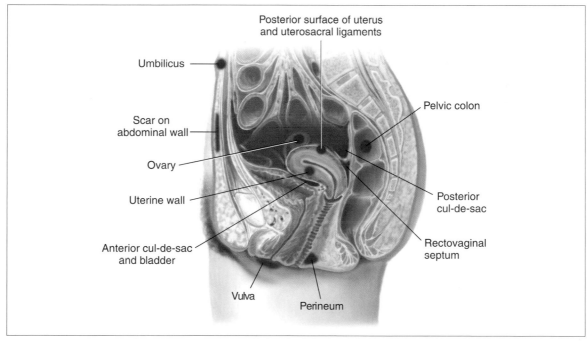

Figure 9-2 Endometriosis.

fibroid FĪ-broyd *fibr:* fiber, fibrous tissue *-oid:* resembling	Benign neoplasm in the uterus that is composed largely of fibrous tissue; also called *leiomyoma*
fistula FĬS-tū-lă	Abnormal tunnel connecting two body cavities, such as the rectum and the vagina, or a body cavity to the skin, such as the rectum to the outside of the body, caused by an injury, infection, or inflammation
vesicovaginal vĕs-ĭ-kō-VĂJ-ĭ-năl *vesic/o:* bladder *vagin:* vagina *-al:* pertaining to	Abnormal duct between the bladder and vagina that results in severe urine loss from the vagina (See Figure 9-3.)
gestational hypertension jĕs-TĀ-shŭn-ăl hī-pĕr-TĔN-shŭn	Potentially life-threatening condition of high blood pressure; usually develops after the 20th week of pregnancy and is characterized by edema and proteinuria
preeclampsia prē-ē-KLĂMP-sē-ă	Nonconvulsive form of gestational hypertension that, if left untreated, may progress to eclampsia
eclampsia ē-KLĂMP-sē-ă	Convulsive form of gestational hypertension that is a medical emergency and life-threatening to the mother, baby, or both
sterility stĕr-ĬL-ĭ-tē	Inability of a woman to become pregnant or for a man to impregnate a woman
toxic shock syndrome (TSS) TŎK-sĭk SHŎK *tox:* poison *-ic:* pertaining to	Rare, sometimes fatal, staphylococcal infection that generally occurs in menstruating women, most of whom use vaginal tampons

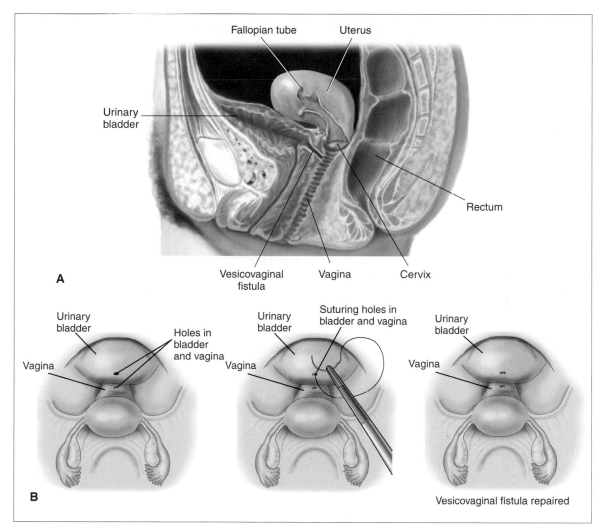

Figure 9-3 Vesicovaginal fistula. (A) Lateral view of the female reproductive system with vesico-vaginal fistula. (B) Frontal view of the urinary bladder and vagina with vesicovaginal fistula repair.

Male Reproductive System

anorchism ăn-ŎR-kĭzm *an:* without, not *orch:* testis (plural, *testes*) *-ism:* condition	Congenital absence of one or both testes; also called *anorchia*

balanitis băl-ă-NĪ-tĭs *balan:* glans penis *-itis:* inflammation	Inflammation of the skin covering the glans penis caused by irritation and invasion of microorganisms and commonly associated with inadequate hygiene of the prepuce and phimosis
benign prostatic hyperplasia (BPH) bē-NĪN prŏs-TĂT-ĭk hī-pĕr-PLĀ-zē-ă	Gradual enlargement of the prostate gland that normally occurs as a man ages and is common in men older than age 60 (See Figure 9-4.)

cryptorchidism
krĭpt-OR-kĭd-ĭzm
  crypt: hidden
orchid: testis (plural, *testes*)
  -ism: condition
	Failure of one or both testicles to descend into the scrotum

epispadias ĕp-ĭ-SPĀ-dē-ăs *epi-:* above, upon *-spadias:* slit, fissure	Congenital defect in which the urethra opens on the upper side of the penis near the glans penis instead of the tip

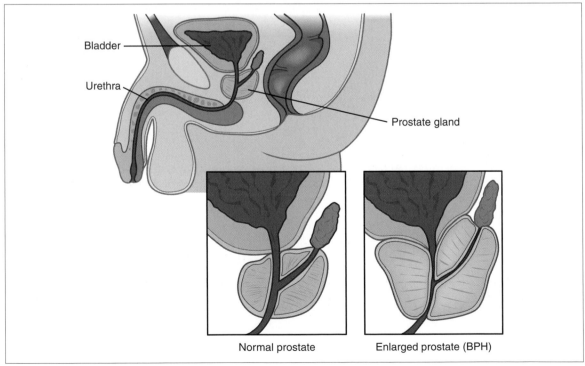

Figure 9-4 Benign prostatic hyperplasia.

hypospadias
hī-pō-SPĀ-dē-ăs
  hyp/o: under, below,
      deficient
-spadias: slit, fissure
	Congenital defect in which the male urethra opens on the undersurface of the penis instead of the tip

impotence ĬM-pō-tĕns	Inability of a man to achieve or maintain a penile erection; also called *erectile dysfunction*

phimosis
fĭ-MŌ-sĭs
phim: muzzle
-osis: abnormal condition;
    increase (used
    primarily with
    blood cells)
	Stenosis or narrowing of the preputial orifice so that the foreskin cannot be pushed back over the glans penis

sexually transmitted infections (STIs)	Any disease affecting the male or female reproductive system that is acquired as a result of sexual intercourse or other intimate contact with an infected individual; also called *venereal disease*
chlamydia klă-MĬD-ē-ă	One of the most damaging STIs caused by the bacterium *Chlamydia trachomatis*, causing cervicitis in women and urethritis in men

genital warts
  JĔN-ĭ-tăl WORTZ
  genit: genitalia
    -al: pertaining to
	Wart(s) in the genitalia caused by human papillomavirus (HPV) and possibly associated with cervical cancer in women

gonorrhea
  gŏn-ō-RĒ-ă
  gon/o: seed (ovum or
      spermatozoon)
  -rrhea: discharge, flow
	Contagious STI caused by the bacterium *Neisseria gonorrhoeae* and most commonly affecting the genitourinary tract and occasionally the pharynx or rectum

herpes genitalis HĔR-pēz jĕn-ĭ-TĂL-ĭs	Infection with herpes simplex virus type 2 of the male or female genital and anorectal skin and mucosa that may be transmitted through the placenta to the fetus during delivery
syphilis SĬF-ĭ-lĭs	Infectious, chronic STI characterized by a skin lesion (chancre) typically on the genitals, rectum, or mouth, which may cause long-term complications, including death if left untreated
trichomoniasis trĭk-ō-mō-NĪ-ă-sĭs	Protozoal infestation of the vagina, urethra, or prostate and the most common STI affecting men and women, although symptoms are more common in women

Diagnostic Procedures

Female Reproductive System

colposcopy kŏl-PŎS-kō-pē *colp/o:* vagina *-scopy:* visual examination	Examination of the vagina and cervix with an optical magnifying instrument (colposcope) (See Figure 9-5.)
hysterosalpingography hĭs-tĕr-ō-săl-pĭn-GŎG-ră-fē *hyster/o:* uterus (womb) *salping/o:* tube (usually fallopian or eustachian [auditory] tube) *-graphy:* process of recording	Radiography of the uterus and oviducts after injection of a contrast medium
laparoscopy lăp-ăr-ŎS-kō-pē *lapar/o:* abdomen *-scopy:* visual examination	Visual examination of the abdominal cavity with a laparoscope through one or more small incisions in the abdominal wall, usually at the umbilicus (See Figure 9-6.)
mammography măm-ŎG-ră-fē *mamm/o:* breast *-graphy:* process of recording	Radiography of the breasts used to diagnose benign and malignant tumors
Papanicolaou (Pap) test pă-pă-NĬ-kō-lŏw	Microscopic analysis of a small tissue sample obtained from the cervix and vagina using a swab to detect carcinoma

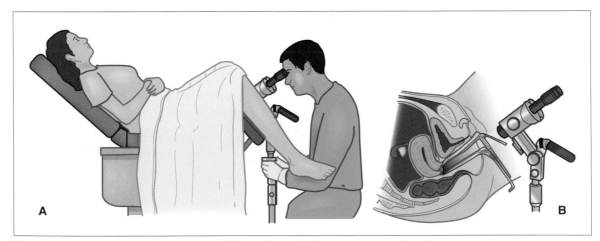

Figure 9-5 Colposcopy. (A) A woman lies in dorsal lithotomy position for this examination. (B) Colposcope.

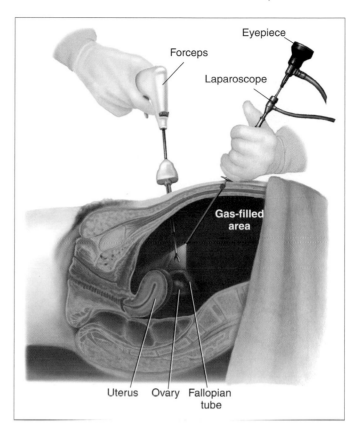

Figure 9-6 Laparoscopy.

Male Reproductive System

digital rectal examination (DRE) DĬJ-ĭ-tăl RĔK-tăl *rect:* rectum *-al:* pertaining to	Examination of the prostate gland by finger palpation through the anal canal and the rectum (See Figure 9-7.)
prostate-specific antigen (PSA) test PRŎS-tāt ĂN-tĭ-jĕn	Blood test used to screen for prostate cancer in which elevated levels of PSA are associated with prostate enlargement and cancer

transrectal ultrasound (TRUS) and biopsy of the prostate
trans: across, through
 rect: rectum
  -al: pertaining to
   bi-: two
-opsy: view of
	An ultrasound probe is inserted into the rectum to obtain an image of the prostate gland and collect multiple needle biopsy specimens of the prostate gland tissues where abnormalities are detected (See Figure 9-8.)

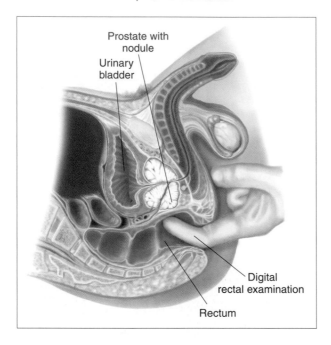

Figure 9-7 Digital rectal examination.

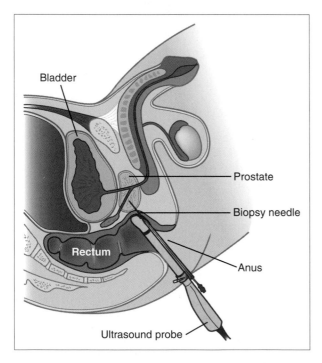

Figure 9-8 Transrectal ultrasound and biopsy of the prostate.

Medical and Surgical Procedures

Female Reproductive System

cerclage sĕr-KLĂZH	Obstetric procedure in which a nonabsorbable suture is used for holding the cervix closed to prevent spontaneous abortion in a woman who has an incompetent cervix
dilation and curettage (D&C) DĬ-lā-shŭn, kū-rĕ-TĂZH	Surgical procedure that widens the cervical canal of the uterus (dilation) so that the endometrium of the uterus can be scraped (curettage) to stop prolonged or heavy uterine bleeding, diagnose uterine abnormalities, and obtain tissue for microscopic examination (See Figure 9-9.)

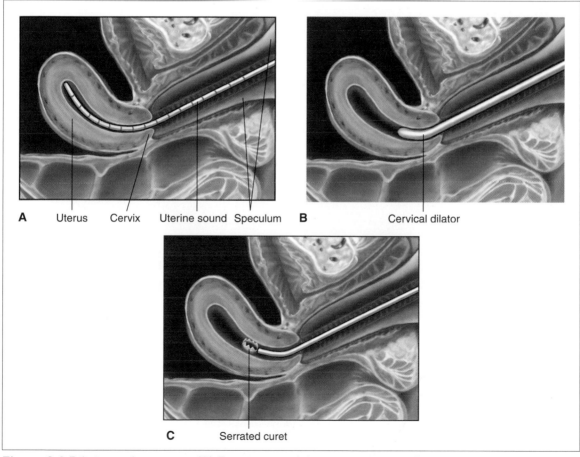

A   Uterus   Cervix   Uterine sound   Speculum   B   Cervical dilator

C   Serrated curet

Figure 9-9 Dilation and curettage. (A) Examination of the uterine cavity with a uterine sound. (B) Dilation of the cervix using dilators of increasing size to allow insertion of a curet. (C) Curettage (scraping) of the uterine lining with a serrated uterine curet to collect tissue samples for diagnostic purposes.

hysterosalpingo-oophorectomy hĭs-tĕr-ō-săl-pĭng-gō-ō-ŏ-for-ĔK-tō-mē *hyster/o:* uterus (womb) *salping/o:* tube (usually fallopian or eustachian [auditory] tube) *oophor:* ovary *-ectomy:* excision	Surgical removal of the uterus, a fallopian tube, and an ovary
lumpectomy lŭm-PĔK-tō-mē	Excision of a small primary breast tumor ("lump") and some of the normal tissue that surrounds it (See Figure 9-10.)

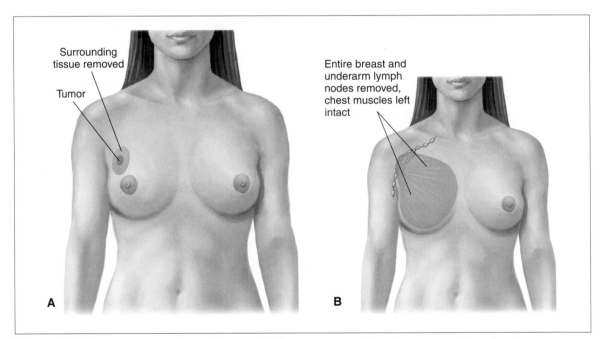

Figure 9-10 Lumpectomy and mastectomy. (A) Lumpectomy with primary tumor in red and surrounding tissue removed in pink. (B) Modified radical mastectomy.

mastectomy măs-TĔK-tō-mē *mast:* breast *-ectomy:* excision, removal	Complete or partial excision of one or both breasts, most commonly performed to remove a malignant tumor
modified radical	Mastectomy that involves excision of an entire breast, including lymph nodes in the underarm (axillary dissection) (See Figure 9-10.)
radical	Mastectomy that involves excision of an entire breast, all underarm lymph nodes, and chest wall muscles under the breast
total	Mastectomy that involves excision of an entire breast, nipple, areola, and the involved overlying skin; also called *simple mastectomy*
reconstructive breast surgery	Reconstruction of a breast that has been removed because of cancer or other disease; commonly possible immediately after mastectomy so the patient awakens from anesthesia with a breast mound already in place
tissue (skin) expansion	Common breast reconstruction technique in which a balloon expander is inserted beneath the skin and chest muscle, saline solution is gradually injected to increase size, and the expander is replaced with a more permanent implant (See Figure 9-11.)
transverse rectus abdominis muscle (TRAM) flap	Surgical creation of a skin flap (using skin and fat from the lower half of the abdomen), which is passed under the skin to the breast area, shaped into a natural-looking breast, and sutured into place (See Figure 9-12.)

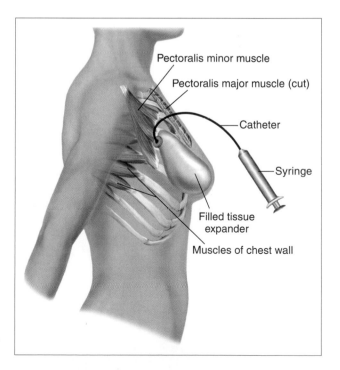

Figure 9-11 Tissue expander for breast reconstruction.

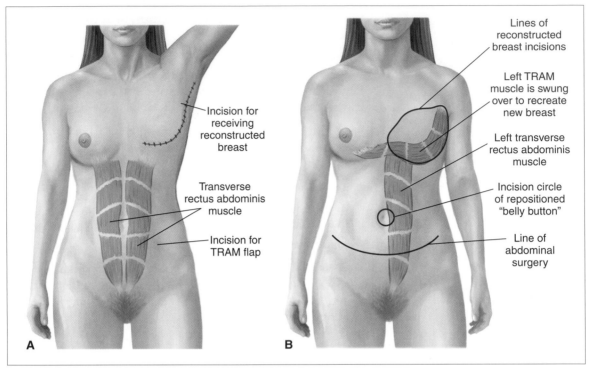

Figure 9-12 Transverse rectus abdominis muscle (TRAM) flap. (A) After mastectomy. (B) Process of TRAM reconstruction.

tubal ligation TŪ-băl lī-GĀ-shŭn	Sterilization procedure that involves blocking both fallopian tubes by cutting or burning them and tying them off

Male Reproductive System

circumcision sĕr-kŭm-SĬ-zhŭn	Surgical removal of the foreskin or prepuce of the penis; usually performed on a male infant
transurethral resection of the prostate (TURP) trăns-ū-RĒ-thrăl PRŎS-tāt	Surgical procedure to relieve obstruction caused by benign prostatic hyperplasia (excessive overgrowth of normal tissue) by insertion of a resectoscope into the penis and through the urethra to "chip away" at prostatic tissue and flush out chips using an irrigating solution (See Figure 9-13.)

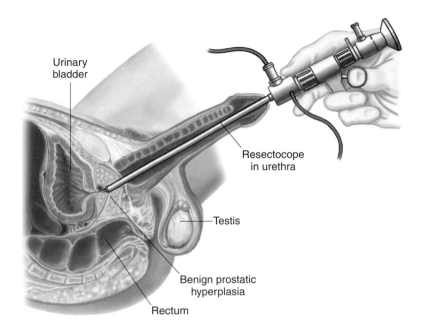

Urinary
bladder

Resectocope
in urethra

Testis

Benign prostatic
hyperplasia

Rectum

Figure 9-13 Transurethral
resection of the prostate
(TURP).

Pharmacology

Female Reproductive System

antifungals ăn-tĭ-FŬN-gălz	Treat vaginal fungal infection, such as candidiasis
estrogens ĔS-trō-jĕnz	Treat symptoms of menopause (hot flashes, vaginal dryness) through hormone replacement therapy (HRT)
hormone replacement therapy (HRT)	Synthetic hormone used to correct a deficiency of estrogen, progesterone, testosterone, or testosterone hormone; relieve symptoms of menopause; and prevent osteoporosis in women
oral contraceptives (OCPs) kŏn-tră-SĔP-tĭvz	Prevent ovulation to avoid pregnancy; also known as *birth control pills*

Male Reproductive System

gonadotropins gŏn-ă-dō-TRŌ-pĭns	Hormonal preparation used to increase sperm count in cases of infertility
spermicides SPĔR-mĭ-sīdz	Method of birth control; destroy sperm by creating a highly acidic environment in the uterus

Pronunciation Help	Long Sound	ā in rāte	ē in rēbirth	ī in īsle	ō in ōver	ū in ūnite
	Short Sound	ă in ălone	ĕ in ĕver	ĭ in ĭt	ŏ in nŏt	ŭ in cŭt

A Closer Look

Take a closer look at the following female and male reproductive procedures to enhance your understanding of the medical terminology associated with them.

Amniocentesis

Amniocentesis, also referred to as **amniotic fluid test,** is an obstetric procedure. It is used in prenatal diagnosis of abnormalities and fetal infections. It involves a surgical puncture of the amniotic sac to remove amniotic fluid, which contains fetal cells. After the amniotic fluid is extracted, the fetal cells are separated from the sample. The cells are grown in a culture medium and then fixed and stained. Under a microscope, fetal DNA is examined for genetic abnormalities. The most common abnormalities detected are **Down syndrome, Edward syndrome (trisomy 18),** and **Turner syndrome (monosomy X).**

Amniocentesis is a routine procedure; however, possible complications include infection of the amniotic sac from the needle and failure of the puncture to heal properly, which can result in leakage or infection. Serious complications can result in miscarriage. Otherwise, the puncture heals, and the amniotic sac replenishes the liquid over the next 24 to 48 hours. The illustration that follows shows how amniocentesis is performed.

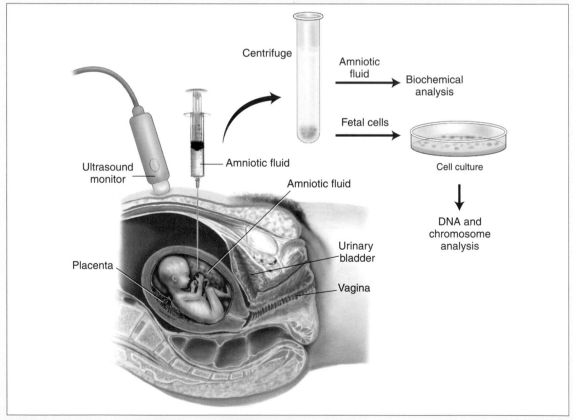

Amniocentesis

A Closer Look—cont'd

Vasectomy and Its Reversal

During a **vasectomy,** the urologist makes an incision through the scrotal sac with the patient under local anesthesia. The urologist cuts the vas deferens from each testicle, removes a small segment, and ties and binds off **(ligates)** the ends with sutures.

This procedure impedes sperm from entering the seminal stream **(ejaculate)** and thereby prevents fertilization from occurring. Nevertheless, the testicles continue to produce sperm, which is reabsorbed by the body. Vasectomy is a surgical procedure for male sterilization and/or a permanent method of birth control, but advances in **microsurgery** have made it possible for vasectomy reversal. A urologist performs vasectomy reversal, also called **vasovasostomy,** if a man wants to regain his fertility. Vasovasostomy is more complicated than a vasectomy and is typically an outpatient procedure with the patient under spinal or general anesthesia. Vasovasostomy has the greatest chance of success within the first 3 years after vasectomy. The illustration that follows shows the vasectomy procedure and its reversal.

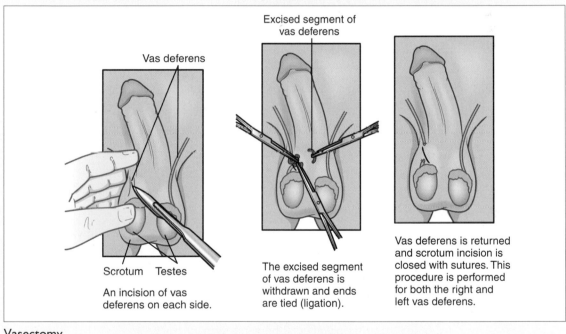

Vas deferens

Excised segment of
vas deferens

Scrotum   Testes

An incision of vas
deferens on each side.

The excised segment
of vas deferens is
withdrawn and ends
are tied (ligation).

Vas deferens is returned
and scrotum incision is
closed with sutures. This
procedure is performed
for both the right and
left vas deferens.

Vasectomy

Medical Vocabulary Recall

Match the medical terms below with the definitions in the numbered list.

anorchism	cryptorchidism	impotence	PSA
candidiasis	D&C	lumpectomy	sterility
cerclage	endometriosis	mammography	syphilis
chlamydia	fistula	phimosis	trichomoniasis
circumcision	gonorrhea	preeclampsia	TSS

1. _____ refers to failure of the testicles to descend into the scrotum.

2. _____ blood test to screen for prostate cancer.

3. _____ refers to a woman's inability to become pregnant or a man's inability to impregnate a woman.

4. _____ refers to congenital absence of one or both testes.

5. _____ is a vaginal fungal infection caused by *Candida albicans* and marked by a curdy discharge and extreme itching.

6. _____ is caused by infection with the bacterium *Chlamydia trachomatis* and occurs in both sexes.

7. _____ is surgical removal of the foreskin or prepuce of the penis.

8. _____ is an obstetric procedure to prevent spontaneous abortion in a woman who has an incompetent cervix.

9. _____ is excision of a small primary breast tumor and some of the normal surrounding tissue.

10. _____ is a condition in which endometrial tissue is found in various abnormal sites throughout the pelvis or in the abdominal wall.

11. _____ refers to x-ray of the breast; used to diagnose benign and malignant tumors.

12. _____ is an STI caused by the bacterium *Neisseria gonorrhoeae* that most commonly affects the genitourinary tract

13. _____ is an STI characterized initially by a skin lesion (chancre).

14. _____ is a rare, sometimes fatal staphylococcal infection that occurs in menstruating women who use vaginal tampons.

15. _____ is a protozoal infestation of the vagina, urethra, or prostate.

16. _____ refers to widening of the uterine cervix so that the surface lining of the uterus can be scraped.

17. _____ means stenosis of the preputial orifice so that the foreskin does not retract over the glans penis.

18. _____ refers to the inability of a man to achieve a penile erection.

19. _____ is a nonconvulsive form of gestational hypertension.

20. _____ is an abnormal passageway between two body cavities.

✓ **Competency Verification:** Check your answers in Appendix B, Answer Key, on page 382. Review material that you did not answer correctly.

Correct Answers: _____ × 10 = _____ %

Pronunciation and Spelling

Use the following list to practice correct pronunciation and spelling of medical terms. Practice the pronunciation aloud and then write the correct spelling of the term. The first word is completed for you.

Pronunciation	Spelling
1. sĕr-KLĂZH	*cerclage*
2. sĕr-vĭ-SĪ-tĭs	
3. klă-MĬD-ē-ă	
4. sĕr-kŭm-SĪ-zhŭn	
5. ĕp-ĭ-SPĀ-dē-ăs	
6. gŏn-ă-dō-TRŌ-pĭn	
7. gī-nĕ-KŎL-ō-jĭst	
8. hĭs-tĕr-ō-săl-pĭng-gō-ō-ŏ-for-ĔK-tō-mē	
9. măm-ŎG-ră-fē	
10. ō-ŏf-ō-RŌmă	
11. ŌR-kē-ō-pĕk-sē	
12. pă-pă-NĪ-kō-lŏw	
13. pĕr-ĭ-nē-OR-ă-fē	
14. fĭ-MŌ-sĭs	
15. prŏs-tă-TĪ-tĭs	
16. soo-dō-sī-Ē-sĭs	

(Continued)

Pronunciation	Spelling
17. SPĔR-mĭ-sīd	
18. SĬF-ĭ-lĭs	
19. trĭk-ō-mō-NĪ-ă-sĭs	
20. VĂR-ĭ-kō-sĕl	

 Competency Verification: Check your answers in Appendix B, Answer Key, on page 382. Review material that you did not answer correctly.

Correct Answers: _____ × 10 = _____ %

ABBREVIATIONS

The following table introduces abbreviations associated with the female and male reproductive systems.

Abbreviation	Meaning	Abbreviation	Meaning
Female Reproductive System			
CS, C-section	cesarean section	Pap	Papanicolaou (test)
D&C	dilation and curettage	para 1, 2, 3	unipara, bipara, tripara (number of viable births)
HRT	hormone replacement therapy	PID	pelvic inflammatory disease
IVF	in vitro fertilization	TAH	total abdominal hysterectomy
LMP	last menstrual period	TRAM	transverse rectus abdominis muscle
US	ultrasound, ultrasonography	TSS	toxic shock syndrome
OB-GYN	obstetrics and gynecology	TVH	total vaginal hysterectomy
Male Reproductive System			
BPH	benign prostatic hyperplasia, benign prostatic hypertrophy	PSA	prostate-specific antigen
DRE	digital rectal examination	TURP	transurethral resection of the prostate
Sexually Transmitted Infections			
GC	gonorrhea	STI	sexually transmitted infection
HPV	human papillomavirus	VD	venereal disease

CHART NOTES

Chart notes make up part of the medical record and are used in various types of health care facilities. The chart notes that follow were dictated by the patient's physician and reflect common clinical events using medical terminology to document the patient's care. Studying and completing the terminology and chart note analysis sections below can help you learn and understand terms associated with the medical specialty of obstetrics-gynecology.

Terminology

The following terms are linked to chart notes in the medical specialty of obstetrics-gynecology. Practice pronouncing each term aloud and then use a medical dictionary such as *Taber's Cyclopedic Medical Dictionary; Appendix A: Glossary of Medical Words Elements,* or other resources to define each term.

Term	Meaning
axilla ăk-SĬL-ă	
D&C	
gravida 4 GRĂV-ĭ-dă	
laparoscopy lăp-ăr-ŎS-kō-pē	
lesion LĒ-zhŭn	
menstrual MĔN-stroo-ăl	
metastases mĕ-TĂS-tă-sēz	
neoplastic nē-ō-PLĂS-tĭk	
para 4 PĂR-ă	
post- menopausal pōst-mĕn-ō-PAW-zăl	

(Continued)

Term	Meaning
Premarin PRĔM-ă-rĭn	
preulcerating prē-ŬL-sĕr-āt-ĭng	

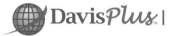 **Davis*Plus*** | Visit *Medical Terminology Express* at *DavisPlus* Online Resource Center. Use it to practice pronunciations and reinforce the meanings of the terms in this chart note.

Postmenopausal Bleeding

Read the chart note that follows aloud. Underline any term you have trouble pronouncing and any terms that you cannot define. If needed, refer to the Terminology section on page 243 for correct pronunciations and meanings of terms.

A 52-year-old gravida 4, para 4 woman had her last menstrual period at age 48. She was in our office last month for an evaluation because of postmenopausal bleeding. She has been taking Premarin and has had vaginal bleeding. Patient is currently admitted for gynecological laparoscopy and diagnostic D&C to rule out the possibility of a neoplastic process.

Last year this patient was admitted to the hospital for a simple mastectomy. Patient had a large preulcerating lesion of the left breast with metastases to the axilla, liver, and bone. Further medical evaluation will be performed next week.

Chart Note Analysis

From the preceding chart note, select the medical word that means

1. movement of cancer cells from one part of the body to another part: _____

2. occurring after menopause: _____

3. an injury or wound that alters tissue: _____

4. pertaining to new tissue formation: _____

5. trade name for estrogen pills: _____

6. removal of a breast: _____

7. pertaining to menstruation: _____

8. visual examination of the abdomen: _____

9. four pregnancies: _____

10. four live births: _____

Competency Verification: Check your answers in Appendix B, Answer Key, page 382. Review material that you did not answer correctly.

Correct Answers: _____ × 10 = _____ %

Demonstrate What You Know!

To evaluate your understanding of how medical terms you have studied in this and previous chapters are used in a clinical environment, complete the numbered sentences by selecting an appropriate term from the words below.

aspermia	dystocia	galactorrhea	obstetrics	sperm
colpocystocele	fallopian tube	hysterectomy	ovaries	spermicide
cryptorchidism	fertilization	infertility	prostatitis	urologists

1. The _____ produce estrogen and progesterone.

2. Discharge or flow of milk is known as _____.

3. _____ is the surgical procedure to remove the uterus.

4. _____ is the branch of medicine concerned with pregnancy and childbirth.

5. After giving birth, some women develop a condition in which the bladder herniates into the vaginal wall. This condition is known as _____.

6. When a woman has difficulty achieving pregnancy, she is experiencing a condition known as

   _____.

7. Hematosalpinx is a collection of blood in the _____.

8. _____ is a condition of a woman who is experiencing painful childbirth.

9. When an ovum and a sperm unite, the outcome is called _____, or *pregnancy*.

10. When testicles are retained in the abdomen, it is a condition called _____.

11. _____ is an effective agent that destroys spermatozoa.

12. _____ treat male reproductive disorders, such as sexual dysfunction and infertility.

13. A man who has an inflammation of the prostate is experiencing _____.

14. A man who is unable to form sperm has a condition called _____.

15. The male gonads produce _____ and secrete sex hormones.

✓ **Competency Verification:** Check your answers in Appendix B, Answer Key, on page 382. Review material that you did not answer correctly.

Correct Answers: _____ × **6.67** = _____ %

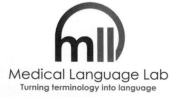

Medical Language Lab
Turning terminology into language

If you are not satisfied with your retention level of the reproductive chapter, visit *DavisPlus* Student Online Resource Center and the Medical Language Lab to complete the website activities linked to this chapter.

Endocrine System

Objectives

Upon completion of this chapter, you will be able to:

- Describe types of medical treatment provided by endocrinologists.
- Name the primary structures of the endocrine system.
- Discuss the primary function of the endocrine system.
- Identify combining forms, suffixes, and prefixes associated with the endocrine system.
- Recognize, pronounce, build, and spell medical terms and abbreviations associated with the endocrine system.
- Demonstrate your knowledge by successfully completing the activities in this chapter.

VOCABULARY PREVIEW

Term	Meaning
homeostasis hō-mē-ō-STĀ-sĭs *home/o-:* same, alike *-stasis:* standing still	Ability of the body to maintain a state of equilibrium within its internal environment, regardless of changing conditions in the outside environment
hormone HOR-mōn	Chemical substance produced by specialized cells of the body that works slowly and affects many different processes, including growth and development, sexual function, mood, and metabolism
metabolism mĕ-TĂB-ō-lĭzm	Sum of all chemical and physical processes occurring within living cells

Pronunciation Help	Long Sound	ā in rāte	ē in rēbirth	ī in īsle	ō in ōver	ū in ūnite
	Short Sound	ă in ălone	ĕ in ĕver	ĭ in ĭt	ŏ in nŏt	ŭ in cŭt

MEDICAL SPECIALTY OF ENDOCRINOLOGY

Endocrinology is the branch of medicine concerned with diagnosis and treatment of **hormone** imbalances and diseases that affect the endocrine glands. Endocrine disorders include:

- diabetes
- thyroid diseases
- metabolic disorders
- overproduction or underproduction of hormones
- menopause
- osteoporosis
- hypertension
- cholesterol (lipid) disorders
- infertility
- lack of growth (short stature)
- cancers of the endocrine glands

Endocrinologists also conduct basic research to learn the ways glands work and clinical research to learn the best methods to treat patients with a hormone imbalance. Through research, endocrinologists develop new drugs and treatments for hormone problems.

ENDOCRINE SYSTEM QUICK STUDY

The endocrine system consists of a network of ductless glands with a rich blood supply that enables the hormones (chemical substances) they produce to enter the bloodstream. These hormones regulate various body functions and keep the internal environment of the body in **homeostasis**. The endocrine system is instrumental in regulating mood, body growth and development, tissue function, and **metabolism**. Sexual functions and reproductive processes are also influenced by the secretions of hormones.

ALERT: An extensive anatomy and physiology review is included in *TermPlus,* a powerful, interactive CD-ROM program that can be purchased separately from F.A. Davis Company.

MEDICAL WORD BUILDING

Constructing medical words using word elements related to the endocrine system will enhance your understanding of those terms and reinforce your ability to use terms correctly.

Combining Forms

Begin your study of endocrine terminology by reviewing their associated combining forms (CFs), which are illustrated in the figure *Endocrine System* that follows.

Endocrine System

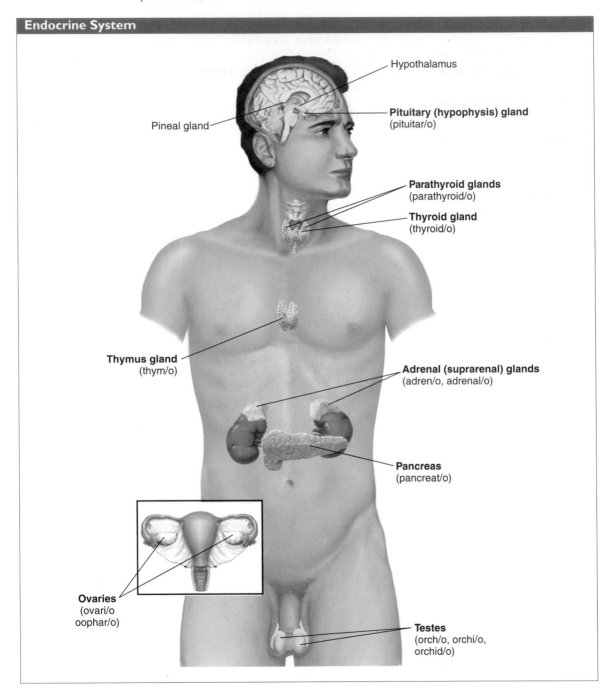

Hypothalamus

Pituitary (hypophysis) gland
(pituitar/o)

Pineal gland

Parathyroid glands
(parathyroid/o)

Thyroid gland
(thyroid/o)

Thymus gland
(thym/o)

Adrenal (suprarenal) glands
(adren/o, adrenal/o)

Pancreas
(pancreat/o)

Ovaries
(ovari/o
oophar/o)

Testes
(orch/o, orchi/o,
orchid/o)

In the table that follows, CFs are listed alphabetically, and other word parts are defined as needed. Review the medical word and study the elements that make up the term. Then complete the meaning of the medical words in the right-hand column. The first one is completed for you. You may also refer to *Appendix A: Glossary of Medical Word Elements* to complete this exercise.

Combining Form	Meaning	Medical Word	Meaning
aden/o	gland	**aden**/oma (ăd-ĕ-NŌ-mă) *-oma:* tumor	*tumor composed of glandular tissue*
adrenal/o	adrenal glands	**adrenal**/ectomy (ăd-rē-năl-ĔK-tō-mē) *-ectomy:* excision, removal	excision of adrenal glands
adren/o	adrenal glands	**adren**/al (ăd-RĒ-năl) *-al:* pertaining to	Pertaining to adrenal glands
calc/o	calcium	hypo/**calc**/emia (hī-pō-kăl-SĒ-mē-ă) *hypo-:* under, below, deficient *-emia:* blood condition	calcium deficient blood condition
gluc/o	sugar, sweetness	**gluc/o**/genesis (gloo-kō-JĔN-ĕ-sĭs) *-genesis:* forming, producing; origin	production of sugar
glyc/o	sugar, sweetness	hyper/**glyc**/emia (hī-pĕr-glī-SĒ-mē-ă) *hyper-:* excessive, above normal *-emia:* blood condition	elevated blood glucose
pancreat/o	pancreas	**pancreat**/itis (păn-krē-ă-TĪ-tĭs) *-itis:* inflammation	inflammation of pancreas
parathyroid/o	parathyroid glands	**parathyroid**/ectomy (păr-ă-thī-royd-ĔK-tō-mē) *-ectomy:* excision, removal	excision of parathyroid glands

(Continued)

Combining Form	Meaning	Medical Word	Meaning
pituitar/o	pituitary gland	hypo/**pituitar**/ism (hī-pō-pǐ-TŪ-ǐ-tǎ-rǐzm) *hypo-:* under, below, deficient *-ism:* condition	deficient pituitary gland condition
thym/o	thymus gland	**thym**/oma (thī-MŌ-mǎ) *-oma:* tumor	thymus gland tumor
thyr/o	thyroid gland	**thyr/o**/megaly (thī-rō-MĔG-ǎ-lē) *-megaly:* enlargement 🔍 Get a closer look at thyroid disorders on page 258.	enlargement of thyroid gland
thyroid/o	thyroid gland	**thyroid**/ectomy (thī-royd-ĔK-tō-mē) *-ectomy:* excision, removal	excision of thyroid
toxic/o	poison	**toxic/o**/logist (tŏks-ǐ-KŌL-ō-jǐst) *-logist:* specialist in the study of	specialist in the study of poison

Suffixes and Prefixes

In the table that follows, suffixes and prefixes are listed alphabetically, and other word parts are defined as needed. Review the medical word and study the elements that make up the term. Then complete the meaning of the medical words in the right-hand column. You may also refer to *Appendix A: Glossary of Medical Word Elements* to complete this exercise.

Word Element	Meaning	Medical Word	Meaning
Suffixes			
-crine	to secrete	endo/**crine** (ĔN-dō-krǐn) *endo:* in, within	to secrete within
-ism	condition	hirsut/**ism** (HŬR-sūt-ǐzm) *hirsut:* hairy	hairy condition
-toxic	poison	thyr/o/**toxic** (thī-rō-TŎKS-ǐk) *thyr/o:* thyroid gland	thyroid gland poison

Word Element	Meaning	Medical Word	Meaning
Prefixes			
hyper-	excessive, above normal	**hyper**/thyroid/ism (hī-pĕr-THĪ-royd-ĭzm) *thyroid:* thyroid gland *-ism:* condition Get a closer look at thyroid disorders on page 258.	*excessive thyroid gland condition*
poly-	many, much	**poly**/dipsia (pŏl-ē-DĬP-sē-ă) *-dipsia:* thirst	*much thirst*

✓ **Competency Verification:** Check your answers in Appendix B, Answer Key, pages 382–383. If you are not satisfied with your level of comprehension, review the terms in the table and retake the review.

DavisPlus | Visit the *Medical Terminology Express* online resource center at *DavisPlus* for an audio exercise of the terms in this table. Other activities are also available to reinforce content.

mll Medical Language Lab
Turning terminology into language

Visit the Medical Language Lab at *medicallanguagelab.com* to enhance your study and reinforce this chapter's word elements with the flash-card activity. We recommend you complete the flash-card activity before continuing with the next section.

Medical Terminology Word Building

In this section, combine the word parts you have learned to construct medical terms related to the endocrine system.

Use *glyclo* (sugar) to build words that mean:

1. blood condition of excessive glucose _hyperglycemia_
2. blood condition of glucose deficiency _hypoglycemia_
3. forming, producing, or origin of glycogen _glycogenesis_

Use *pancreat/o* (pancreas) to build words that mean:

4. inflammation of the pancreas _pancreatitis_
5. destruction of the pancreas _pancreatolysis_
6. disease of the pancreas _pancreatopathy_

Use **thyr/o** or **thyroid/o** (thyroid gland) to build words that mean:

7. inflammation of the thyroid gland _thyroiditis_

8. enlargement of the thyroid _thyromegaly_

Build surgical words that mean:

9. excision of a parathyroid gland _parathyroidectomy_

10. removal of the adrenal gland _adrenalectomy_

 Competency Verification: Check your answers in Appendix B, Answer Key, on page xxx. Review material that you did not answer correctly.

Correct Answers: _____ × 10 = _____ %

MEDICAL VOCABULARY

The following tables list additional terms related to the endocrine system. Recognizing and learning these terms will help you understand the connection between common signs, symptoms, and diseases and their diagnoses. Medical and surgical procedures are included as well as pharmacological agents used to treat diseases.

Diseases and Conditions

Addison disease Ă-dĭ-sŭn	Hypofunctioning of the adrenal cortex that results in generalized malaise, weakness, muscle atrophy, severe loss of fluids and electrolytes, low blood pressure, hypoglycemia, and hyperpigmentation of the skin
Cushing syndrome KOOSH-ĭng	Cluster of symptoms caused by excessive amounts of cortisol (glucocorticoid) or adrenocorticotropic hormone (ACTH) circulating in the blood; may be due to the use of oral corticosteroid medication or by tumors that produce cortisol or ACTH (See Figure 10-1.)
diabetes mellitus (DM) dī-ă-BĒ-tēz MĚ-lĭ-tŭs	Group of metabolic diseases characterized by high glucose levels that result from defects in insulin secretion, action, or both and that occur in two primary forms: type 1 and type 2
type 1 diabetes	Abrupt onset of DM, usually in childhood, caused by destruction of beta islet cells of the pancreas with complete deficiency of insulin secretion
type 2 diabetes	Gradual onset of DM, usually appearing in middle age and caused by a deficiency in production of insulin or a resistance to the action of insulin by the cells of the body

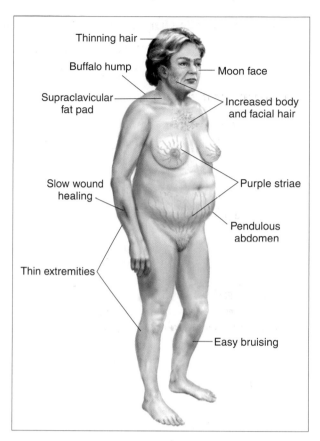

Thinning hair

Buffalo hump

Moon face

Supraclavicular fat pad

Increased body and facial hair

Slow wound healing

Purple striae

Pendulous abdomen

Thin extremities

Easy bruising

Figure 10-1 Physical manifestations of Cushing syndrome.

insulinoma ĭn-sū-lĭn-Ō-mā *insulin:* insulin *-oma:* tumor	Tumor of the islets of Langerhans in the pancreas
pancreatitis păn-krē-ă-TĪ-tĭs *pancreat:* pancreas *-itis:* inflammation	Inflammation of the pancreas that occurs when pancreatic enzymes that digest food are activated in the pancreas instead of the duodenum and attack pancreatic tissue, causing damage to the gland; most commonly caused by alcoholism and biliary tract disease
panhypopituitarism păn-hī-pō-pĭ-TŪ-ĭ-tăr-ĭzm *pan-:* all *hyp/o:* under, below, deficient *pituitar:* pituitary gland *-ism:* condition	Total pituitary impairment that brings about a progressive and general loss of hormone activity
pheochromocytoma fē-ō-krō-mō-sī-TŌ-mă	Rare adrenal gland tumor that causes excessive release of epinephrine (adrenaline) and norepinephrine (hormones that regulate heart rate and blood pressure) and induces severe blood pressure elevation

Diagnostic Procedures

fasting blood glucose (FBG) GLOO-kōs	Test that measures glucose levels in the blood after the patient has fasted (not eaten) for at least 8 hours; used to diagnose pancreatic disorders, such as diabetes and hypoglycemia; also called *fasting blood sugar (FBS)*
glucose tolerance test (GTT) GLOO-kōs	Test in which a patient fasts for 8 to 12 hours and then ingests glucose, and blood samples are taken to determine how quickly the glucose is cleared from the blood; used to diagnose diabetes with higher accuracy than other blood glucose tests; also called *oral glucose tolerance test (OGTT)*
radioactive iodine uptake test (RAIU)	Imaging procedure that measures levels of radioactivity in the thyroid after oral or intravenous administration of radioactive iodine; used to determine thyroid function by monitoring the ability of the thyroid to take up (uptake) iodine from the blood.
thyroid function test (TFT)	Blood test that measures thyroid hormone levels to detect an increase or decrease in thyroid function
total calcium	Blood test that measures calcium to detect parathyroid and bone disorders

Medical and Surgical Procedures

lobectomy lō-BĔK-tō-mē *lob:* lobe *-ectomy:* excision, removal	Removal of one lobe in treatment of endocrine diseases such as hyperthyroidism
thymectomy thī-MĔK-tō-mē *thym:* thymus gland *-ectomy:* excision, removal	Excision of the thymus gland in cases of myasthenia gravis or a tumor
transsphenoidal hypophysectomy trăns-sfē-NOY-dăl hī-pō-fĭ-SĔK-tō-mē	Minimally invasive endoscopic surgery that removes pituitary tumors through the nasal cavity via the sphenoid sinus (transsphenoidal) without affecting brain (See Figure 10-2.)

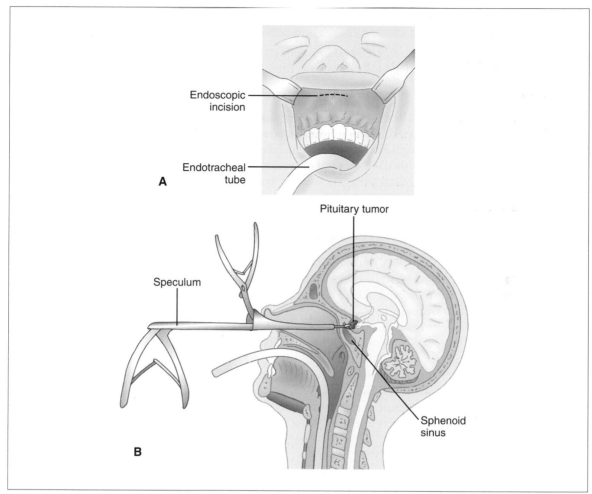

Figure 10-2 Transsphenoidal hypophysectomy. (A) Incision beneath the upper lip to enter the nasal cavity and gain access to the pituitary gland. (B) Insertion of a speculum and special forceps to remove the pituitary tumor.

Pharmacology

hormone replacement therapy (HRT)	Synthetic hormone used to correct a deficiency of estrogen, progesterone, testosterone, or testosterone hormone; relieve symptoms of menopause; and prevent osteoporosis in women
insulins ĬN-sŭ-lĭns	Replace insulin in patients with type 1 diabetes or severe type 2 diabetes
oral antidiabetics ăn-tĭ-dī-ă-BĔT-ĭks	Treat type 2 diabetes by stimulating the pancreas to produce more insulin or lower glucose levels in the blood

Pronunciation Help	Long Sound	ā in rāte	ē in rēbirth	ī in īsle	ō in ōver	ū in ūnite
	Short Sound	ă in ălone	ĕ in ĕver	ĭ in ĭt	ŏ in nŏt	ŭ in cŭt

A Closer Look

Take a closer look at the thyroid and pituitary gland disorders to enhance your understanding of the medical terminology associated with them.

Thyroid Disorders

Disorders of the thyroid include thyroid hormone deficiency **(hypothyroidism)** or overproduction **(hyperthyroidism)** and gland inflammation and enlargement **(thyromegaly).** These disorders are common and may develop at any age. They may be the result of a developmental problem, injury, disease, or dietary deficiency. With treatment, most of these conditions have a good prognosis. However, if untreated, they progress to medical emergencies or irreversible disabilities.

One form of hypothyroidism, called **cretinism,** develops in infants. If not treated, this disorder leads to mental retardation, impaired growth, low body temperatures, and abnormal bone formation. These symptoms usually do not appear at birth because the infant has received thyroid hormones from the mother's blood during fetal development.

When hypothyroidism develops during adulthood, it is called **myxedema.** Myxedema is characterized by **edema,** low blood levels of thyroid hormones, weight gain, cold intolerance, fatigue, depression, muscle or joint pain, and sluggishness. Recovery may be complete if thyroid hormone is administered soon after symptoms appear.

Hyperthyroidism results from excessive secretion of thyroid hormones, which results in a metabolic imbalance. The most common form of hyperthyroidism is **Graves disease.** Graves disease is an autoimmune disease that increases production of thyroid hormones, enlarges the thyroid gland **(goiter),** and causes multiple system changes. Graves disease is characterized by an elevated metabolic rate, abnormal weight loss, excessive perspiration, muscle weakness, and emotional instability. Also, the eyes are likely to protrude **(exophthalmos)** because of edematous swelling in the tissues behind them. The figures that follow show exophthalmos caused by Graves disease and enlargement of the thyroid gland in goiter.

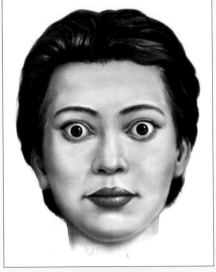

Exophthalmos caused by Graves disease.

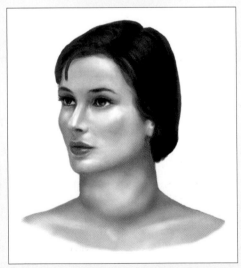

Enlargement of the thyroid gland in goiter.

A Closer Look—cont'd

Pituitary Gland Disorders

Growth hormone (GH) is synthesized and secreted by the anterior pituitary gland and is responsible for normal growth of bones, cartilage, and soft tissue. Several disorders of the anterior pituitary gland involve GH. A deficiency or absence of GH **(hyposecretion)** during childhood slows bone growth and results in underdevelopment of the body **(hypopituitarism),** a disorder known as **pituitary dwarfism.** The individual is extremely short (final height of only 3 to 4 feet) but has normal body proportions. Pituitary dwarfism may be linked to other defects and a varying degree of mental retardation. Treatment of dwarfism includes administration of GH during childhood, before skeletal growth is completed. The illustration that follows shows the physical manifestations of pituitary dwarfism.

Excessive secretion of GH **(hypersecretion)** during childhood causes an abnormal increase in the length of long bones and results in a disorder known as **giantism.** The individual grows to be very tall (may attain 8 feet), but body proportions are about normal. Although many basketball players are very tall, they are not considered giants. These individuals are tall as a result of their genetic makeup and healthy nutrition.

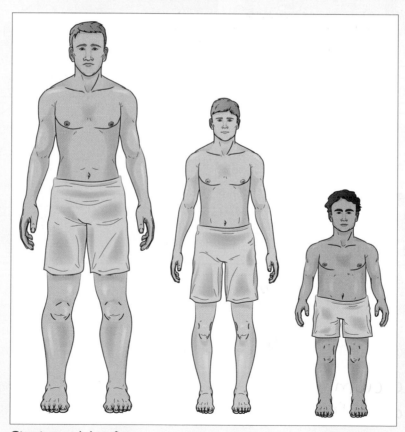

Giantism and dwarfism.

(Continued)

A Closer Look—cont'd

When hypersecretion of GH occurs after puberty, an overgrowth of the bones of the face, hands, and feet results in a disorder known as **acromegaly.** This condition is often seen in persons 30 to 40 years old after they experience years of excessive GH. The individual may experience joint pain resulting from osteoarthritis and a host of other clinical features in the body systems. As with gigantism, a pituitary tumor or adenoma often is the cause of acromegaly. It affects women and men with equal frequency. Treatment of acromegaly requires surgical removal of the tumor or tumor destruction by radiation. The figure that follows shows a patient with acromegaly as a result of hypersecretion of GH that occurred after puberty.

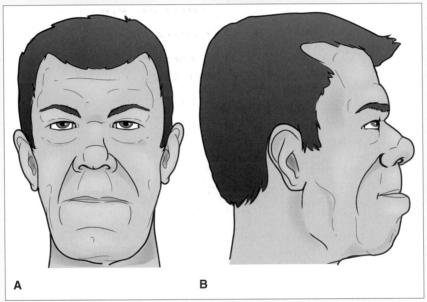

Acromegaly in frontal view (A) and lateral view (B).

Medical Vocabulary Recall

Match the medical terms below with the definitions in the numbered list.

Addison disease	exophthalmos	insulinoma	panhypopituitarism	total calcium
cretinism	FGB	myxedema	pheochromocytoma	type 1 diabetes
Cushing syndrome	HRT	pancreatitis	TFT	type 2 diabetes

1. _total calcium_ is a blood test to detect bone and parathyroid abnormalities.
2. _type 1 diabetes_ is a disease caused by failure of the pancreas to produce insulin.

3. __Cretinism__ is a congenital condition characterized by severe hypothyroidism commonly associated with other endocrine disorders.

4. __exophthalmos__ is abnormal protrusion of eyeball possibly caused by thyrotoxicosis.

5. __insulinoma__ is a tumor of the pancreas.

6. __myxedema__ is hypothyroidism that develops during adulthood.

7. __TFT__ measures thyroid hormone levels in the blood.

8. __Cushing Syndrome__ is caused by excessive amounts of cortisol or ACTH circulating in the blood.

9. __panhypopituitarism__ brings about a progressive and general loss of hormone activity.

10. __HRT__ is used to correct hormone deficiencies.

11. __Addison disease__ is caused by a deficiency of cortical hormones as a result of hypofunctioning of the adrenal cortex.

12. __FBG__ measures blood glucose levels after fasting at least 8 hours.

13. __pheochromocytoma__ is a rare adrenal gland tumor that induces severe blood pressure elevation.

14. __pancreatitis__ is most commonly caused by alcoholism and biliary tract disease.

15. __type 2 diabetes__ usually appears in middle age and is caused by a deficiency of insulin production

Competency Verification: Check your answers in Appendix B, Answer Key, on page 383. Review material that you did not answer correctly.

Correct Answers: _____ × 10 = _____ %

Pronunciation and Spelling

Use the following list to practice correct pronunciation and spelling of medical terms. Practice the pronunciation aloud and then write the correct spelling of the term. The first word is completed for you.

Pronunciation	Spelling
1. ăd-ĕ-Nō-mă	*adenoma*
2. ăd-rē-năl-ĔK-tō-mē	adrenalectomy
3. dī-ă-BĒ-tēz	diabetes

(Continued)

Pronunciation	Spelling
4. ĕks-ŏf-THĂL-mŏs	exophthalmos
5. GLOO-kōs	glucose
6. hī-pō-kăl-SĒ-mē-ă	hypocalcemia
7. hī-pĕr-glī-SĒ-mē-ă	hyperglycemia
8. ĭn-sū-lĭn-Ō-mă	insulinoma
9. MĚ-lĭ-tŭs	melitus
10. mĭks-ĕ-DĒ-mă	myxedema
11. păn-krē-ă-TĪ-tĭs	pancreatitis
12. pĕr-ĬF-ĕr-ăl	peripheral
13. pĭ-TŪ-ĭ-tă-rĭzm	pituitarism
14. pŏl-ē-DĬP-sē-ă	polydipsia
15. tŏks-ĭ-KŎL-ō-jĭst	toxicologist

 Competency Verification: Check your answers in Appendix B, Answer Key, page 384. Review material that you did not answer correctly.

Correct Answers: _____ × **6.67** = _____ %

ABBREVIATIONS

The table below introduces abbreviations associated with the endocrine system.

Abbreviation	Meaning	Abbreviation	Meaning
ADH	antidiuretic hormone	GTT	glucose tolerance test
BS	blood sugar	HRT	hormone replacement therapy
DM	diabetes mellitus	IV	intravenously
FBG	fasting blood glucose	RAIU	radioactive iodine uptake
FBS	fasting blood sugar	TFT	thyroid function test
GH	growth hormone	TSH	thyroid-stimulating hormone

CHART NOTES

Chart notes comprise part of the medical record and are used in various types of health care facilities. The chart notes that follow were dictated by the patient's physician and reflect common clinical events using medical terminology to document the patient's care. Studying and completing the terminology and chart notes sections below will help you learn and understand terms associated with the medical specialty of cardiology.

Terminology

The following terms are linked to chart notes in the specialty of endocrinology. Practice pronouncing each term aloud and then use a medical dictionary such as *Taber's Cyclopedic Medical Dictionary; Appendix A: Glossary of Medical Word Elements,* or other resources to define each term.

Term	Meaning
aerobic ĕr-Ō-bĭk	
anaerobic ĂN-ĕr-ō-bĭk	
calcaneal kăl-KĀ-nē-ăl	
erythema ĕr-ĭ-THĒ-mă	
malleolus măl-Ē-ŏ-lŭs	
peripheral diabetic neuropathy pĕr-ĬF-ĕr-ăl dī-ă-BĔT-ĭk nū-RŎP-ă-thē	
trophic TRŌF-ĭk	
type I diabetes mellitus dī-ă-BĒ-tēz MĔ-lĭ-tŭs	

(Continued)

Term	Meaning
ulceration ŬL-sĕr-ā-shŭn	
vascular VĂS-kŭ-lăr	

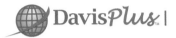 **DavisPlus** | Visit *Medical Terminology Express* at *DavisPlus* Online Resource Center. Use it to practice pronunciations and reinforce the meanings of the terms in this chart note.

Infected Foot

Read the chart note below aloud. Underline any term you have trouble pronouncing or cannot define. If needed, refer to the Terminology section on page 263 for correct pronunciations and meanings of terms.

SUBJECTIVE: The patient is a 59-year-old man with long-term type 1 diabetes mellitus never well controlled. He complains of a hot, swollen left heel and came in through the emergency department.

OBJECTIVE: Physical examination revealed trophic changes in the feet bilaterally with amputation of the right great toe. There is a significant ulceration with early infection in the right heel. In the left heel, there is erythema to the level of the upper malleolus bilaterally, and there is marked erythema at the entire calcaneal bed. There is an open foul ulceration of the heel. There are no palpable pulses in either foot, no reflexes, and no sensation to deep palpation.

ASSESSMENT: Nonsalvageable anaerobic/aerobic infection of the left heel in the context of peripheral diabetic neuropathy and poor circulation.

PLAN:
1. Vascular consultation for amputation.
2. Infectious disease consultation for appropriate antibiotic coverage.

Chart Note Analysis

From the preceding chart note, select the medical word that means

1. redness of skin: _erythema_

2. agent used to treat infection: _antibiotic_

3. composed of blood vessels: _vascular_

4. pertaining to the heel: calcaneal

5. nonhealing lesion on the surface of the skin or mucous membrane: ulceration

6. nerve damage to extremities from diabetes: peripheral diabetic neuropathy

7. bony prominence on both sides of the ankle joint: malleolus

8. pertaining to development or nourishment: trophic

9. insulin-dependent diabetes: type 1 diabetes mellitus

10. without oxygen: anaerobic

DavisPlus | Visit *Medical Terminology Express* at *DavisPlus* Online Resource Center. Use it to practice pronunciations and reinforce the meanings of the terms in this chart note.

Competency Verification: Check your answers in Appendix B, Answer Key, on page 384. Review material that you did not answer correctly.

Correct Answers: _____ × 10 = _____ %

Demonstrate What You Know!

To evaluate your understanding of how medical terms you have studied in this and previous chapters are used in a clinical environment, complete the numbered sentences by selecting an appropriate term from the words below.

aerobic	Graves	hyperglycemia	insulin	thymoma
FBG	homeostasis	hypersecretion	pancreas	toxicologist
GTT	hormones	hypocalcemia	RAIU	ulceration

1. If a patient has an abnormally low level of blood calcium, this condition is diagnosed as hypocalcemia

2. The term used to describe excessive secretion of a hormone by a gland is hypersecretion

3. Treatment for type 1 diabetes includes insulin injections to maintain a normal level of glucose in the blood.

4. aerobic is a condition that requires oxygen for respiration.

5. A(n) ulceration is an open lesion on the surface of the skin or mucous membrane.

6. hormones are chemical substances produced by specialized cells of the body that travel in the bloodstream to tissues and organs.

7. RAIU is a test in which radioactive iodine is administered to determine thyroid function.

8. Graves disease is characterized by an enlarged thyroid gland and exophthalmos (bulging eyes).

9. **GTT** _____ measures blood glucose levels at specified intervals (usually over a period of 3 hours) after administration of glucose.

10. **homeostasis** _____ is relative equilibrium in the internal environment of the body.

11. A specialist who studies poisons and their effects on the human body is called a(n) **toxicologist**

12. The gland responsible for production of insulin is the **pancreas** _____.

13. Results of a blood test show a greater than normal amount of glucose in the blood. This condition is charted as **hyperglycemia** _____.

14. **FBG** _____ measures the level of circulating glucose in the blood after a 12-hour fast.

15. A tumor of the thymus gland is indicated in the chart as a(n) **thymoma** _____.

✓ **Competency Verification:** Check your answers in Appendix B, Answer Key, on page 384. Review material that you did not answer correctly.

Correct Answers: _____ × **6.67 =** _____ %

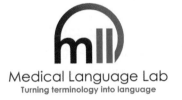

Medical Language Lab
Turning terminology into language

If you are not satisfied with your retention level of the endocrine chapter, visit *DavisPlus* Student Online Resource Center and the Medical Language Lab to complete the website activities linked to this chapter.

Nervous System

OBJECTIVES

Upon completion of this chapter, you will be able to:

- Describe types of medical treatment provided by neurologists.
- Name the primary structures of the nervous system and discuss their functions.
- Identify combining forms, suffixes, and prefixes associated with the nervous system.
- Recognize, pronounce, build, and spell medical terms and abbreviations associated with the nervous system.
- Demonstrate your knowledge of this chapter by successfully completing the activities.

VOCABULARY PREVIEW

Term	Meaning
cognition kŏg-NĬSH-ŭn	Process of thought—including reasoning, judgment, and perception
nerve impulse	Electrical signal transmitted along the nerve fiber in response to a stimulus
neurotransmitters nū-rō-TRĂNS-mĭt-ĕrz	Chemicals in the brain that transmit messages between nerve cells (neurons)
peripheral pĕr-ĬF-ĕr-ăl	Pertaining to the outside, surface, or surrounding area of an organ or structure or occurring away from its center
traumatic traw-MĂT-ĭk	Caused by or pertaining to an injury
vascular VĂS-kū-lăr *vascul:* vessel (usually blood or lymph) *-ar:* pertaining to	Pertaining to or composed of blood vessels

Pronunciation Help	Long Sound	ā in rāte	ē in rēbirth	ī in īsle	ō in ōver	ū in ūnite
	Short Sound	ă in ălone	ĕ in ĕver	ĭ in ĭt	ŏ in nŏt	ŭ in cŭt

MEDICAL SPECIALTY OF NEUROLOGY

Neurology is the branch of medicine concerned with diagnosis and treatment of diseases of the nervous system, which include the brain, spinal cord, and **peripheral** nerves. The nervous system controls voluntary and involuntary movements as well as some organ and gland functioning. It also controls all the processes of **cognition**, such as thinking, feeling, and remembering. The **neurologist** detects, diagnoses, and treats symptoms and disorders that indicate an impairment of any of these functions. These disorders can include, but are not limited to, **vascular** problems that affect the brain, infections or inflammations of the brain or the spinal cord tissue, nervous tissue tumors, degenerative neuromuscular disorders, and **traumatic** brain or spinal cord injury. The branch of surgery involving the nervous system, including the brain and spinal cord, is called **neurosurgery.** The physician who specializes in neurosurgery is a **neurosurgeon.**

NERVOUS SYSTEM QUICK STUDY

The nervous system controls all critical body activities and reactions and is one of the most complicated systems of the body. In contrast to the endocrine system, which slowly discharges hormones into the bloodstream, the nervous system is designed to act instantaneously by transmitting electrical impulses to specific body locations. The nervous system coordinates voluntary (conscious) activities, such as walking, talking, and eating. It also controls involuntary (unconscious) functions, such as reflexes to pain, body changes related to stress, and processes related to thought and emotions.

The nervous system consists of two main divisions: the **central nervous system (CNS)** and the **peripheral nervous system (PNS).** The **CNS** consists of the brain and spinal cord and is the control center of the body. The **PNS** consists of the peripheral nerves, which include the cranial nerves (emerging from the base of the skull) and the spinal nerves (emerging from the spinal cord). The PNS connects the CNS to remote body parts to relay and receive messages, and its autonomic nerves regulate involuntary functions of the internal organs. (See *Nervous System: Brain and Spinal Cord,* page 270.)

Despite the complex organization of the nervous system, it consists of only two principal types of cells, **neurons** and **neuroglia.** Neurons are the basic structural and functional units of the nervous system. They are grouped into bundles of nerves or nerve tracts that carry electrical messages throughout the body, while **neurotransmitters** assist in transmitting messages between neurons. Neurons perform functions such as perception of sensory stimuli, learning, memory, and control of muscles and glands. Neuroglia do not carry messages; they perform the functions of support and protection. Many neuroglial, or glial, cells form a supporting network by twining around nerve cells or lining certain structures in the brain and spinal cord. Others bind nervous tissue to supporting structures and attach the neurons to their blood vessels. Certain small glial cells are phagocytic. In other words, they protect the CNS from disease by engulfing invading microbes and clearing away debris. Neuroglia are of clinical interest because they are a common source of tumors (gliomas) of the nervous system.

ALERT: An extensive anatomy and physiology review is included in *TermPlus,* a powerful, interactive CD-ROM program that can be purchased separately from F.A. Davis Company.

MEDICAL WORD BUILDING

Constructing medical words using word elements (combining forms, suffixes, and prefixes) related to the nervous system will enhance your understanding of those terms and reinforce your ability to use terms correctly.

Combining Forms

Begin your study of nervous system terminology by reviewing the organs and their associated combining forms (CFs), which are illustrated in the figure *Nervous System: Brain and Spinal Cord* that follows.

Nervous System: Brain and Spinal Cord

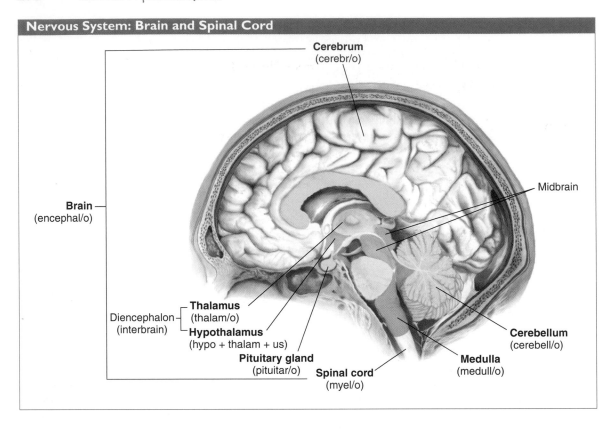

In the table that follows, CFs are listed alphabetically, and other word parts are defined as needed. Review the medical word and study the elements that make up the term. Then complete the meaning of the medical words in the right-hand column. The first one is completed for you. You may also refer to *Appendix A: Glossary of Medical Word Elements* to complete this exercise.

Combining Form	Meaning	Medical Word	Meaning
cerebr/o	cerebrum	cerebr/o/spin/al (sĕr-ĕ-brō-SPĪ-năl) *spin:* spine *-al:* pertaining to	*Pertaining to the brain and spine or spinal cord*
encephal/o	brain	encephal/itis (ĕn-sĕf-ă-LĪ-tĭs) *-itis:* inflammation	*inflammation of brain*
gli/o	glue; neuroglial tissue	gli/oma (glī-Ō-mă) *-oma:* tumor	*tumor glue*

Combining Form	Meaning	Medical Word	Meaning
mening/o	meninges (membranes covering brain and spinal cord)	mening/o/cele (měn-ĬN-gō-sēl) *-cele:* hernia, swelling	*hernia of meninges*
meningi/o		meningi/oma (měn-ĭn-jē-Ō-mă) *-oma:* tumor	*tumor of meninges*
myel/o	bone marrow; spinal cord	myel/algia (mī-ĕl-ĂL-jē-ă) *-algia:* pain	*bone marrow pain*
neur/o	nerve	neur/o/lysis (nū-RŎL-ĭs-ĭs) *-lysis:* separation; destruction; loosening	*destruction of pain*

Suffixes and Prefixes

In the table that follows, suffixes and prefixes are listed alphabetically, and other word parts are defined as needed. Review the medical word and study the elements that make up the term. Then complete the meaning of the medical words in the right-hand column. You may also refer to *Appendix A: Glossary of Medical Word Elements* to complete this exercise.

Word Element	Meaning	Medical Word	Meaning
Suffixes			
-lepsy	seizure	epi/**lepsy** (ĔP-ĭ-lĕp-sē) *epi-:* above, upon	*above seizure*
-phasia	speech	a/**phasia** (ă-FĀ-zē-ă) *a-:* without, not	*without speech*
Prefixes			
dys-	bad, painful, difficult	dys/phasia (dĭs-FĀ-zē-ă) *-phasia:* speech	*painful speech*
hemi-	one half	hemi/paresis (hĕm-ē-păr-Ē-sĭs) *-paresis:* partial paralysis	*partial paralysis of one half*

(Continued)

Word Element	Meaning	Medical Word	Meaning
Prefixes			
para-	near; beside; beyond	**para**/plegia (păr-ă-PLĒ-jē-ă) *-plegia:* paralysis	*near paralysis*
quadri-	four	**quadri**/plegia (kwŏd-rĭ-PLĒ-jē-ă) *-plegia:* paralysis Get a closer look at quadriplegia, see page 281.	*4 paralysis*

Competency Verification: Check your answers in Appendix B, Answer Key, pages 381–385. If you are not satisfied with your level of comprehension, review the terms in the table and retake the review.

DavisPlus | Visit the *Medical Terminology Express* online resource center at *DavisPlus* for an audio exercise of the terms in this table. Other activities are also available to reinforce content.

Medical Language Lab
Turning terminology into language

Visit the Medical Language Lab at *medicallanguagelab.com* to enhance your study and reinforce this chapter's word elements with the flash-card activity. We recommend you complete the flash-card activity before continuing with the next section.

Medical Terminology Word Building

In this section, combine the word parts you have learned to construct medical terms related to the nervous system.

Use *neur/o* (nerve) to build words that mean:

1. tumor composed of nervous (tissue) _neuroma_

2. separation or destruction of a nerve _neurolysis_

Use *encephal/o* (brain) to build words that mean:

3. inflammation of the brain _encephalitis_

4. tumor composed of brain (tissue) _encephaloma_

5. herniation or protrusion of brain (tissue) _encephalocele_

Use *myel/o* (bone marrow; spinal cord) to build words that mean:

6. pain in the spinal cord __Myelalgia__

7. herniation of the spinal cord __Myelocele__

Use *cerebr/o* (cerebrum) to build a word that means:

8. pertaining to the cerebrum and spinal cord __Cerebrospinal__

Use the suffix *-phasia* to build words that mean:

9. without or lacking speech __aphasia__

10. difficult speech __dysphasia__

✓ **Competency Verification:** Check your answers in Appendix B, Answer Key, on page 385. Review material that you did not answer correctly.

Correct Answers: _____ × 10 = _____ %

MEDICAL VOCABULARY

The following tables consist of selected terms that pertain to diseases and conditions of the nervous system. Terms related to diagnostic, medical, and surgical procedures are included as well as pharmacological agents used to treat diseases. Recognizing and learning these terms will help you understand the connection between diseases and their treatments. Word analyses for selected terms are also provided.

Diseases and Conditions

amyotrophic lateral sclerosis (ALS) ă-mī-ō-TRŌ-fĭk, sklĕ-RŌ-sĭs	Degenerative disorder that manifests in adulthood with symptoms of difficulty in swallowing and talking, dyspnea, muscle weakness, and paralysis; also called *Lou Gehrig disease* (named after the baseball player who became afflicted with ALS)
dementia dĭ-MĔN-shē-ă	Progressive, irreversible deterioration of mental function marked by memory impairment and, commonly, deficits in reasoning, judgment, abstract thought, comprehension, learning, task execution, and use of language
Alzheimer disease ĂLTS-hī-mĕr	Chronic, organic brain syndrome characterized by death of neurons in the cerebral cortex and their replacement by microscopic "plaques," which results in dementia that progresses to complete loss of mental, emotional, and physical functioning and personality changes
epilepsy ĔP-ĭ-lĕp-sē	Disorder that results from the generation of electrical signals inside the brain, causing recurring seizures in which some people simply stare blankly for a few seconds during a seizure, whereas others have extreme convulsions

Huntington chorea HŬN-tĭng-tŭn kō-RĒ-ă	Inherited, degenerative disease of the CNS with symptoms developing in middle age as nerve cells in the brain waste away, resulting in uncontrolled bizarre movements, emotional disturbances, and mental deterioration
hydrocephalus hī-drō-SĔF-ă-lŭs *hydro:* water *cephal:* head *-us:* condition, structure	Excessive accumulation of cerebrospinal fluid (CSF) within the ventricles of the brain that is most common in neonates, but can also occur in adults as a result of injury or disease; if left untreated, causes an enlarged head and cognitive decline

multiple sclerosis (MS)
MŬL-tĭ-pl sklĕ-RŌ-sĭs
scler: hardening; sclera
  (white of eye)
-osis: abnormal condition;
  increase (used primarily
  with blood cells)
	Progressive degenerative disease of the CNS characterized by inflammation, hardening, and loss of myelin throughout the spinal cord and brain, which produces weakness and other muscular symptoms

neuroblastoma
nū-rō-blăs-TŌ-mă
neur/o: nerve
  blast: embryonic cell
  -oma: tumor
	Malignant tumor composed mainly of cells resembling neuroblasts that occurs most commonly in infants and children

neurosis
nū-RŌ-sĭs
neur/o: nerve
  -osis: abnormal condition;
    increase (used
    primarily with
    blood cells)
	Nonpsychotic mental illness that triggers feelings of distress and anxiety and impairs normal behavior

palsy PAWL-zē	Partial or complete loss of motor function; also called *paralysis*
Bell	Facial paralysis on one side of the face as a result of inflammation of a facial nerve
cerebral sĕ-RĒ-brăl *cerebr:* cerebrum *-al:* pertaining to	Bilateral, symmetrical, nonprogressive motor dysfunction and partial paralysis, which is usually caused by damage to the cerebrum during gestation or birth trauma but can also be hereditary

paralysis pă-RĂL-ĭ-sĭs *para-:* near, beside; beyond *-lysis:* separation; destruction; loosening	Loss of muscle function, loss of sensation, or both as a result of spinal cord injury Get a closer look at spinal cord injuries on pages 280 and 281.
Parkinson disease	Progressive neurological disorder caused by a neurotransmitter deficiency (dopamine) that affects the portion of the brain responsible for controlling movement and results in hand tremors; uncontrollable head nodding; shuffling gait; and difficulty talking, swallowing, or completing simple tasks
poliomyelitis pō-lē-ō-mī-ĕl-Ī-tĭs *poli/o:* gray; gray matter (of brain or spinal cord) *myel:* bone marrow; spinal cord *-itis:* inflammation	Inflammation of the gray matter of the spinal cord caused by a virus, commonly resulting in spinal and muscle deformity and paralysis
psychosis sī-KŌ-sĭs *psych/o:* mind *-osis:* abnormal condition; increase (used primarily with blood cells)	Mental disorder marked by loss of contact with reality; often with delusions and hallucinations
sciatica sī-ĂT-ĭ-kă	Severe pain in the leg along the course of the sciatic nerve, which travels from the hip to the foot (See Figure 11-1.)
shingles SHĬNG-lz	Chronic viral disease in which painful blisters appear on the skin along the course of a peripheral nerve that is caused by inflammation secondary to *herpes zoster* virus, the same virus that causes chickenpox; also called *herpes zoster* (See Figure 11-2.)
spina bifida SPĪ-nă BĬF-ĭ-dă	Congenital neural tube defect characterized by incomplete closure of the spinal canal through which the spinal cord and meninges may or may not protrude (See Figure 11-3.)
spina bifida occulta SPĪ-nă BĬF-ĭ-dă ŏ-KŬL-tă	Most common and least severe form of spina bifida without protrusion of the spinal cord or meninges
spina bifida cystica SPĪ-nă BĬF-ĭ-dă SĬS-tĭk-ă	More severe type of spina bifida that involves protrusion of the meninges (meningocele), spinal cord (myelocele), or both (meningomyelocele)

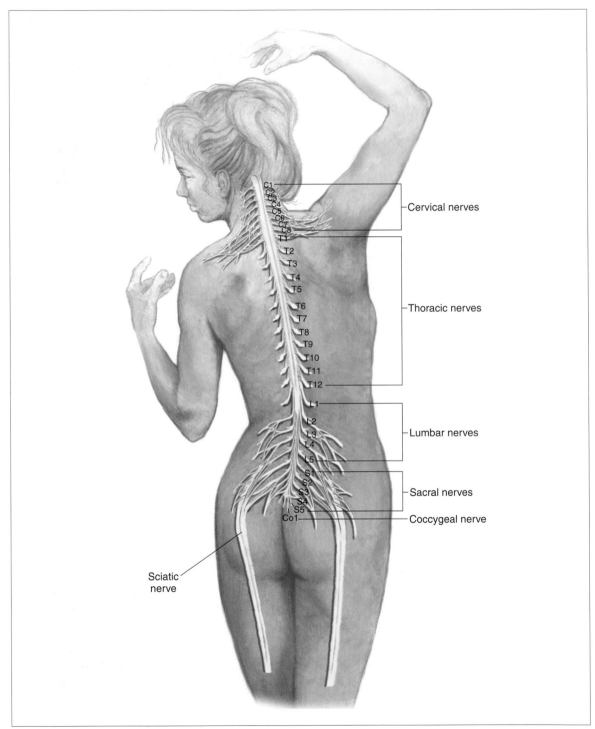

Figure 11-1 Spinal nerves.

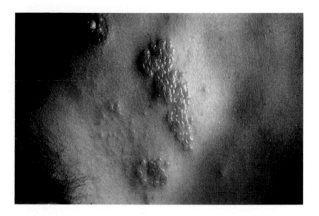

Figure 11-2 Shingles (herpes zoster).

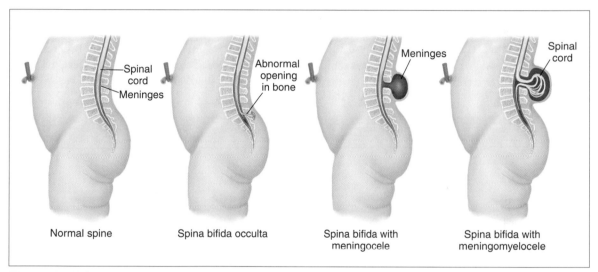

Figure 11-3 Spina bifida.

stroke STRŌK	Inadequate supply of blood and oxygen to the brain due to a clot or rup- tured blood vessel (hemorrhage), which allows brain tissue to die and becomes a medical emergency; also called *cerebrovascular accident* (CVA)
transient ischemic attack (TIA) TRĂN-zhĕnt ĭs-KĒ-mĭk *ischem:* to hold back, block *-ic:* pertaining to	Interruption in blood supply to the brain that does not cause permanent brain damage but may be an indication of a higher risk of a more serious and debilitating condition (stroke); also called *ministroke*

Diagnostic Procedures

cerebrospinal fluid (CSF) analysis sĕr-ĕ-brō-SPĪ-năl *cerebr/o:* cerebrum *spin:* spine *-al:* pertaining to	Laboratory test that examines a sample of CSF obtained from a lumbar puncture, which is analyzed for the presence of blood, bacteria, and malignant cells as well as for the amount of protein and glucose present
electroencephalography (EEG) ē-lĕk-trō-ĕn-sĕf-ă-LŎG-ră-fē *electr/o:* electricity *encephal/o:* brain *-graphy:* process of recording	Electrodes are placed on the scalp to record electrical activity within the brain; used to evaluate seizure and sleep disorders and periods of unconsciousness, monitor brain surgeries, and determine whether a person is in a coma or brain dead
lumbar puncture (LP) LŬM-băr *lumb:* loins (lower back) *-ar:* pertaining to	Insertion of a needle into the subarachnoid space of the spinal column to withdraw a sample of CSF used for biochemical, microbiological, and cytological laboratory analysis; also called *spinal tap* or *spinal puncture* (See Figure 11-4.)

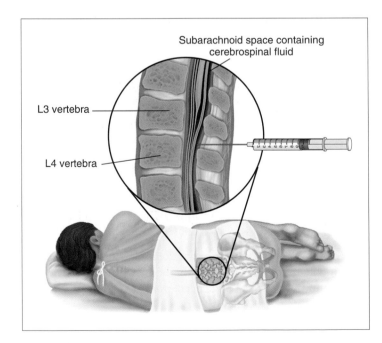

Figure 11-4 Lumbar puncture.

Medical and Surgical Procedures

craniotomy krā-nē-ŎT-ō-mē *crani/o:* cranium (skull) *-tomy:* incision	Surgical procedure that creates an opening in the skull to gain access to the brain during neurosurgical procedures
thalamotomy thăl-ă-MŎT-ō-mē *thalam/o:* thalamus *-tomy:* incision	Partial destruction of the thalamus to treat psychosis or intractable pain
trephination trĕf-ĭn-Ā-shŭn	Excision of a circular disk of bone using a specialized saw called a trephine to reveal brain tissue during neurosurgery, or to relieve intracranial pressure (ICP)

Pharmacology

anesthetics ăn-ĕs-THĔT-ĭks	Produce partial or complete loss of sensation with or without loss of consciousness
general	Produce complete loss of feeling with loss of consciousness
local	Produce loss of feeling and affect a local area only
anticonvulsants ăn-tĭ-kŏn-VŬL-sănts	Prevent or control seizures
antiparkinsonian agents ăn-tĭ-păr-kĭn-SŌN-ē-ăn	Reduce signs and symptoms associated with Parkinson disease
antipsychotics ăn-tĭ-sī-KŎT-ĭks	Alter neurotransmitters in the brain to alleviate symptoms of delusions and hallucinations
thrombolytics thrŏm-bō-LĬT-ĭks	Dissolve blood clots in a process known as *thrombolysis*

Pronunciation Help	Long Sound	ā in rāte	ē in rēbirth	ī in īsle	ō in ōver	ū in ūnite
	Short Sound	ă in ălone	ĕ in ĕver	ĭ in ĭt	ŏ in nŏt	ŭ in cŭt

A Closer Look

Take a closer look at the following nervous system disorders to enhance your understanding of the medical terminology associated with them.

Trigeminal Neuralgia

Trigeminal neuralgia (TN) is a neuropathic pain syndrome that involves the facial area stimulated by the trigeminal nerve **(cranial nerve V)**. This syndrome results in flashes of pain radiating along the course of the nerve and is the most common cause of facial pain. TN often produces unilateral, abrupt, brief but severe pain, which becomes more frequent over time; successive occurrences can lead to incapacitation. The pain may arise spontaneously but is often associated with particular triggers, such as sensory stimulus to the face. The trigeminal nerve branches stimulate areas of the face, including the forehead, nose, cheek, gums, and jaw. Irritation or chronic compression of the nerve is suspected to initiate symptoms.

Most cases of TN are believed to be caused by blood vessels pressing on the root of the trigeminal nerve; this causes the nerve to transmit pain signals, which are experienced as the stabbing pains of TN. Pressure on the trigeminal nerve may also be caused by trauma, a tumor, multiple sclerosis, or herpes zoster. TN is seen more often in women and usually begins around age 50 to 60 years. Most patients respond well to pharmacological therapy; patients who do not may require surgical intervention to relieve the pain. However, nerve function of the affected nerve may be compromised as a result. Gamma Knife radiosurgery is also an option. The Gamma Knife creates a lesion on the nerve to block the pain signals. The following illustration depicts the facial areas of pain caused by stimulation by the branches of the trigeminal nerve in patients who experience TN.

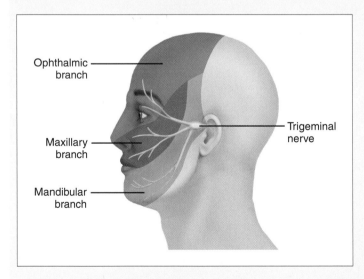

Trigeminal nerve (fifth cranial nerve) and branches.

Spinal Cord Injuries

Vertebral fractures and dislocations are severe injuries to the spinal cord that result in impairment of spinal cord function below the level of the injury. Spinal cord injuries are commonly the result of **trauma** caused by motor vehicle accidents, falls, diving in shallow water, or accidents associated with contact sports. Such trauma may cause varying degrees of paralysis. These injuries are seen most commonly in adolescent boys and young adults. The loss of motor function may be confined to the lower extremities

A Closer Look—cont'd

(paraplegia) or may be present in all four extremities **(quadriplegia),** accompanied by increased muscular tension and hyperactive reflexes **(spastic)** or by loss of reflexes and tone **(flaccid).**

  Paraplegia is paralysis of the lower portion of the body and both legs. It results in loss of sensory and motor control below the level of injury. **Quadriplegia** is paralysis of all four extremities and, usually, the trunk. It generally results in loss of motor and sensory function below the level of injury. Paralysis includes the trunk, legs, and pelvic organs with partial or total paralysis in the upper extremities. The higher the trauma, the more debilitating the motor and sensory impairments will be. The following illustration shows spinal cord injuries and their extent of paralysis.

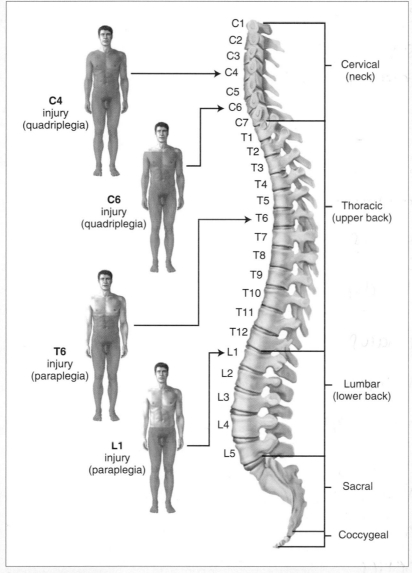

Spinal cord injuries.

Medical Vocabulary Recall

Match the medical terms below with the definitions in the numbered list.

Alzheimer disease	Bell palsy	hydrocephalus	Parkinson disease	spina bifida
anesthetics	craniotomy	LP	poliomyelitis	stroke
anticonvulsants	dementia	neuroblastoma	sciatica	thalamotomy
antiparkinsonian	epilepsy	paralysis	shingles	TIA

1. _Bell palsy_ is facial paralysis caused by inflammation of a facial nerve.

2. _Stroke_ refers to brain tissue damage caused by formation of a clot or a ruptured blood vessel; also called _CVA_.

3. _epilepsy_ is a CNS disorder characterized by recurrent seizures.

4. _thalamotomy_ is a partial destruction of the thalamus to treat psychosis or intractable pain.

5. _LP_ involves insertion of a needle into the subarachnoid space to withdraw a sample of CSF for laboratory analysis.

6. _TIA_ is a temporary interruption of blood supply to the brain without permanent brain damage.

7. _Parkinson disease_ is a progressive degenerative neurological disorder that causes tremors, uncontrollable head nodding, and a shuffling gait.

8. _poliomyelitis_ refers to inflammation of the gray matter caused by a virus.

9. _Sciatica_ refers to severe pain in the leg along the course of the sciatic nerve.

10. _Spina bifida_ is a congenital defect characterized by incomplete closure of the spinal canal through which the spinal cord and meninges may or may not protrude.

11. _hydrocephalus_ is a cranial enlargement caused by accumulation of fluid within the ventricles of the brain.

12. _neuroblastoma_ is a malignant tumor, composed principally of cells resembling neuroblasts, that occurs mainly in infants and children.

13. _Alzheimer disease_ results in memory loss, mental deterioration, and decline in social skills and physical functioning.

14. _anticonvulsants_ are used to prevent or control seizure activity.

15. _dementia_ is a general term that refers to cognitive deficit, including memory impairment.

16. _Shingles_ refers to eruption of acute, inflammatory, herpetic vesicles on the trunk of the body along a peripheral nerve.

17. _anesthetics_ produce partial or complete loss of sensation without loss of consciousness.

18. <u>antiparkinsonian</u> agents reduce symptoms, such as tremors, in Parkinson disease.

19. <u>craniotomy</u> is the creation of an opening in the skull to gain access to the brain during neurosurgical procedures.

20. <u>paralysis</u> is a loss of muscle function, sensation, or both resulting from spinal cord injury.

 Competency Verification: Check your answers in Appendix B, Answer Key, on page 385. Review material that you did not answer correctly.

Correct Answers: _____ × **5** = _____ %

Pronunciation and Spelling

Use the following list to practice correct pronunciation and spelling of medical terms. First practice the pronunciation aloud. Then write the correct spelling of the term. The first word is completed for you.

Pronunciation	Spelling
1. ĂLTS-hī-m ĕr	*Alzheimer*
2. sĕr-ĕ-brō-VĂS-kū-lăr	cerebrovascular
3. krā-nē-ŎT-ō-mē	craniotomy
4. ĔP-ĭ-l ĕp-sē	epilepsy
5. LŬM-băr	lumbar
6. PAWL-zē	palsy
7. pō-lē-ō-mī-ĕl-Ī-tĭs	poliomyelitis
8. pă-RĂL-ĭ-sĭs	paralysis
9. păr-ă-PLĒ-jē-ă	paraplegia
10. nū-rō-blăs-TŌ-mă	neuroblastoma
11. kwŏd-rĭ-PLĒ-jē-ă	quadriplegia
12. SPĪ-nă BĬF-ĭ-dă ŏ-KŬL-tă	spina bifida occulta
13. sī-ĂT-ĭ-kă	sciatica
14. SĒ-zhūr	seizure
15. SHĬNG-lz	shingles

 Competency Verification: Check your answers in Appendix B, Answer Key, on page 385. Review material that you did not answer correctly.

Correct Answers: _____ × **6.67** = _____ %

ABBREVIATIONS

The table that follows introduces abbreviations associated with the nervous system.

Abbreviation	Meaning	Abbreviation	Meaning
ALS	amyotrophic lateral sclerosis	LP	lumbar puncture
C1, C2, and so on	first cervical vertebra, second cervical vertebra, and so on	MS	mitral stenosis; musculoskeletal; multiple sclerosis; mental status; magnesium sulfate
CNS	central nervous system	PNS	peripheral nervous system
CSF	cerebrospinal fluid	S1, S2, and so on	first sacral vertebra, second sacral vertebra, and so on
CVA	cerebrovascular accident; costovertebral angle	T1, T2, and so on	first thoracic vertebra, second thoracic vertebra, and so on
CVD	cerebrovascular disease	TIA	transient ischemic attack
EEG	electroencephalogram; electroencephalography	TN	trigeminal neuralgia
L1, L2, and so on	first lumbar vertebra, second lumbar vertebra, and so on		

CHART NOTES

Chart notes make up part of the medical record and are used in various types of health care facilities. The chart notes that follow were dictated by the patient's physician and reflect common clinical events using medical terminology to document the patient's care. Studying and completing the terminology and chart notes sections that follow will help you learn and understand terms associated with the medical specialty of neurology.

Terminology

The following terms are linked to chart notes in the medical specialty of neurology. Practice pronouncing each term aloud and then use a medical dictionary such as *Taber's Cyclopedic Medical Dictionary; Appendix A: Glossary of Medical Word Elements,* or other resources to define each term.

Term	Meaning
adenocarcinoma ăd-ĕ-nō-kăr-sĭn-Ō-mă	
anorexia ăn-ō-RĔK-sē-ă	
aphasia ă-FĀ-zē-ă	
biliary BĬL-ē-ār-ē	
cholecystojejunostomy kō-lē-sĭs-tō- jĕ-jū-NŎS-tō-mē	
deglutition dē-gloo-TĬSH-ŭn	
diplopia dĭp-LŌ-pē-ă	
jaundice JAWN-dĭs	
jejunojejunostomy jĕ-jū-nō-jĕ-jū-NŎS-tō-mē	
metastasis mĕ-TĂS-tă-sis	
pruritus proo-RĪ-tŭs	
stroke STRŌK	
vertigo VĔR-tĭ-gō	

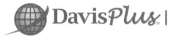 **DavisPlus** | Visit *Medical Terminology Express* at *DavisPlus* Online Resource Center. Use it to practice pronunciations and reinforce the meanings of the terms in this medical report.

Stroke

Read the chart note that follows aloud. Underline any term you have trouble pronouncing and any terms that you cannot define. If needed, refer to the Terminology section on page 284 for correct pronunciations and meanings of terms.

Patient is a moderately obese white woman who was admitted to Riverside Hospital because of a sudden episode of stroke. She recalls an episode of vertigo 3 days ago. Patient is being nursed at home by her daughter because of terminal adenocarcinoma of the head of the pancreas with metastasis to the liver, which was diagnosed in December. Patient fell to the floor with paralysis of the right arm and right leg and aphasia. She has not noticed any difficulty with deglutition. Apparently with the onset of the stroke, she also experienced diplopia. She denies any difficulty with her cardio-vascular system in the past. Patient was in the hospital 5 years ago be-cause of generalized biliary-type disease with jaundice, pruritus, weight loss, and anorexia. Subsequently, she was seen in consultation, and chole-cystojejunostomy and jejunojejunostomy were performed.

Diagnosis:
1. Stroke, probably secondary to metastatic lesion of the brain or cere-brovascular disease.
2. Evidence of the previously described deterioration secondary to carci-noma of the pancreas with metastases to the liver.

Chart Note Analysis

From the preceding chart note, select the medical word that means

1. loss of appetite: _anorexia_
2. the act of swallowing: _deglutition_
3. double vision: _diplopia_
4. condition of yellowness of the skin and the mucous membranes: _jaundice_
5. a sensation of moving around in space: _vertigo_
6. a loss of sensation and voluntary movement: _paralysis_
7. a malignant tumor of a glandular organ: _adenocarcinoma_
8. creation of an opening between the gallbladder and the jejunum: _Cholecytojejunostomy_

9. pertaining to bile: _biliary_

10. spread of cancer (to the liver): _metastasis_

11. inability to communicate through speech: _aphasia_

12. itchy skin sensation that prompts a person to rub or scratch: _pruritus_

> **Competency Verification:** Check your answers in Appendix B, Answer Key, on page 385. Review material that you did not answer correctly.
>
> **Correct Answers:** _____ × 8.4 = _____ %

Demonstrate What You Know!

To evaluate your understanding of how medical terms you have studied in this and previous chapters are used in a clinical environment, complete the numbered sentences by selecting an appropriate term from the words below.

aphasia	homeostasis	paresis
CNS	meningitis	PNS
cognition	meningomyelocele	quadriplegia
diplopia	myelalgia	TIAs
flaccid	neurosurgeon	vertigo

1. Baby John is born with herniation of the meninges and spinal cord, a condition which the nurse charts as _meningomyelocele_.

2. Paralysis of four limbs is charted as _quadriplegia_.

3. CSF analysis indicates a patient has an infection of the meninges called _meningins_.

4. Partial paralysis is charted as _paresis_.

5. _cognition_ refers to the ability to think and reason.

6. The brain and spinal cord are divisions of the _CNS_.

7. A patient complains of strange sensations of moving around in space. This condition is diagnosed as _vertigo_.

8. The peripheral nerves are part of the _PNS_.

9. The term used to describe pain in the spinal cord is _myelagia_.

10. A relative equilibrium in the internal environment of the body is called _homeostasis_.

11. The aging process results in a loss of reflexes and body tone, a condition called _flacid_.

12. The physician who specializes in neurosurgery is a _neurosurgeon_.

13. A patient has a history of ministrokes, or __T I A S_____, that preceded her stroke.

14. __aphasia_____ is an absence of language function that may be the result of an injury to the cerebral cortex.

15. With the onset of stroke, a patient experiences double vision, or __diplopia_____.

✓ **Competency Verification:** Check your answers in Appendix B, Answer Key, on page 385. Review material that you did not answer correctly.

Correct Answers: _____ × **6.67** = _____ %

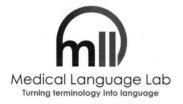

Medical Language Lab
Turning terminology into language

If you are not satisfied with your retention level of the nervous system chapter, visit *DavisPlus* Student Online Resource Center and the Medical Language Lab to complete the website activities linked to this chapter.

Musculoskeletal System

OBJECTIVES

Upon completion of this chapter, you will be able to:

- Describe types of medical treatment provided by orthopedists and chiropractors.
- Name the primary structures of the musculoskeletal system and discuss their functions.
- Identify combining forms, suffixes, and prefixes associated with the musculoskeletal system.
- Recognize, pronounce, build, and spell medical terms and abbreviations associated with the musculoskeletal system.
- Demonstrate your knowledge of this chapter by successfully completing the activities in this chapter.

VOCABULARY PREVIEW

Term	Meaning
arthritis ăr-THRĪ-tĭs *arthr:* joint *-itis:* inflammation	Inflammation of a joint, usually accompanied by pain, swelling, and stiffness
arthroplasty ĂR-thrō-plăs-tē *arthr:* joint *-plasty:* surgical repair	Surgery to reshape, reconstruct, or replace a diseased or damaged joint
articulate ăr-TĬK-ū-lāt	Site of contact between two bones; also called a *joint*
contraction kŏn-TRĂK-shŭn	Shortening or tightening of a muscle
musculoskeletal mŭs-kū-lō-SKĔL-ĕ-tăl *muscul/o:* muscle *skelet:* skeleton *-al:* pertaining to	Pertaining to muscles and the skeleton
radiography rā-dē-ŎG-ră-fē *radi/o:* radiation, x-ray; radius (lower arm bone on thumb side) *-graphy:* process of recording	Production of captured shadow images on photographic film through the action of ionizing radiation passing through the body from an external source
synovial fluid sĭn-Ō-vē-ăl	Lubricating fluid secreted by the synovial membrane in the joint

Pronunciation Help	Long Sound Short Sound	ā in rāte ă in ălone	ē in rēbirth ĕ in ĕver	ī in īsle ĭ in ĭt	ō in ōver ŏ in nŏt	ū in ūnite ŭ in cŭt

MEDICAL SPECIALTIES OF ORTHOPEDICS AND CHIROPRACTIC MEDICINE

The **musculoskeletal** system is associated with the medical specialties of orthopedics and chiropractic medicine.

Orthopedics

Orthopedics is the branch of medicine concerned with prevention, diagnosis, care, and treatment of musculoskeletal disorders. These disorders include injury to or disease of the body's bones, joints, ligaments, muscles, and tendons. **Orthopedists** employ medical, physical, and surgical methods, such as hip **arthroplasty**, to restore function that is lost as a result of injury or disease to the musculoskeletal system. They also coordinate their treatments with other health care providers, such as physical therapists, occupational therapists, and sports medicine physicians. In addition to the orthopedist who treats bone and joint diseases, the **rheumatologist** (also a medical doctor) specializes in treatment of **arthritis** and other diseases of joints, muscles, and bones.

Chiropractic Medicine

Another health care provider who treats musculoskeletal disorders is the **chiropractor.** In contrast to orthopedists, chiropractors are not physicians. They do not employ drugs or surgery, the primary basis of treatment used by medical physicians. **Chiropractic medicine** is a system of therapy based on the theory that disease is caused by pressure on nerves. Chiropractors do employ **radiography** to diagnose pathological disorders and determine the most effective type of treatment. In most instances, chiropractic treatment involves physical manipulation of the spinal column.

MUSCULOSKELETAL SYSTEM QUICK STUDY

The musculoskeletal system includes muscles, bones, joints, and related structures, such as the tendons and connective tissue. These structures function to support and move body parts and organs.

Muscles perform four primary functions: producing body movements, stabilizing body positions, storing and moving substances within the body, and generating heat. Through **contraction**, muscles help maintain body posture. Less apparent involuntary motions provided by muscles include the passage and elimination of food through the digestive system, propulsion of blood through the arteries, and contraction of the bladder to eliminate urine.

The main function of bones is to form a skeleton that supports and protects the body. It also serves as a storage area for mineral salts, especially calcium and phosphorus. Joints are the places where two bones **articulate**. **Synovial fluid** lubricates the joints to minimize friction upon motion. Because bones cannot move without the help of muscles, contraction must be provided by muscular tissue. (See *Anterior View of the Skeleton*, page 292.)

ALERT: An extensive anatomy and physiology multimedia review is included in *TermPlus*, a powerful, interactive CD-ROM program that can be purchased separately from F.A. Davis Company.

MEDICAL WORD BUILDING

Constructing medical words using word elements (combining forms, suffixes, and prefixes) related to the musculoskeletal system will enhance your understanding of those terms and reinforce your ability to use terms correctly.

Combining Forms

Begin your study of musculoskeletal terminology by reviewing the structures of the musculoskeletal system and their associated combining forms (CFs), which are illustrated in the figure *Anterior View of the Skeleton* that follows.

Anterior View of the Skeleton

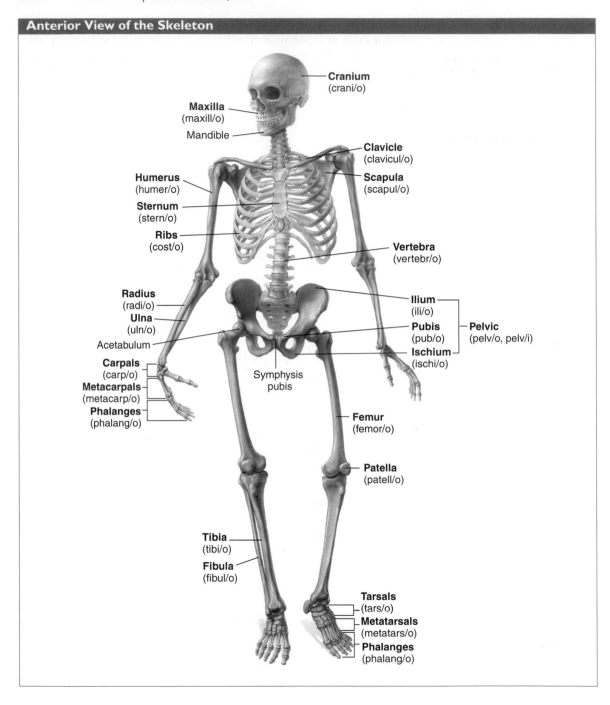

Cranium
(crani/o)

Maxilla
(maxill/o)

Mandible

Clavicle
(clavicul/o)

Humerus
(humer/o)

Scapula
(scapul/o)

Sternum
(stern/o)

Ribs
(cost/o)

Vertebra
(vertebr/o)

Radius
(radi/o)

Ilium
(ili/o)

Ulna
(uln/o)

Pubis
(pub/o)

Pelvic
(pelv/o, pelv/i)

Acetabulum

Ischium
(ischi/o)

Carpals
(carp/o)

Metacarpals
(metacarp/o)

Symphysis
pubis

Phalanges
(phalang/o)

Femur
(femor/o)

Patella
(patell/o)

Tibia
(tibi/o)

Fibula
(fibul/o)

Tarsals
(tars/o)

Metatarsals
(metatars/o)

Phalanges
(phalang/o)

In the table that follows, CFs are listed alphabetically, and other word parts are defined as needed. Review the medical word and study the elements that make up the term. Then complete the meaning of the medical words in the right-hand column. The first one is completed for you. You may also refer to *Appendix A: Glossary of Medical Word Elements* to complete this exercise.

Combining Form	Meaning	Medical Word	Meaning
Muscles and Related Structures			
fasci/o	band, fascia (fibrous membrane supporting and separating muscles)	fasci/o/plasty (FĂSH-ē-ō-plăs-tē) *-plasty*: surgical repair	*surgical repair of fascia*
fibr/o	fiber, fibrous tissue	fibr/oma (fī-BRŌ-mă) *-oma*: tumor	tumor fiber
leiomy/o	smooth muscle (visceral)	leiomy/oma (lī-ō-mī-Ō-mă) *-oma*: tumor	smooth muscle tumor
lumb/o	loins (lower back)	lumb/o/cost/al (lŭm-bō-KŎS-tăl) *cost*: ribs *-al*: pertaining to	pertaining to low back
muscul/o	muscle	muscul/ar (MŬS-kū-lăr) *-ar*: pertaining to	pertaining to muscle
my/o		my/o/rrhexis (mī-or-ĔK-sĭs) *-rrhexis*: rupture	muscle rupture
ten/o	tendon	ten/o/tomy (tĕn-ŎT-ō-mē) *-tomy*: incision	tendon incision
tend/o		tend/o/plasty (TĔN-dō-plăs-tē) *-plasty*: surgical repair	tendon surgical repair
tendin/o		tendin/itis (tĕn-dĭn-Ī-tĭs) *-itis*: inflammation	tendon inflammation

(Continued)

Combining Form	Meaning	Medical Word	Meaning
Bones of the Upper Extremities			
carp/o	carpus (wrist bones)	**carp/o**/ptosis (kăr-pŏp-TŌ-sĭs) *-ptosis:* prolapse, downward displacement	*carpus prolapse*
cervic/o	neck; cervix uteri (neck of uterus)	**cervic**/al (SĔR-vĭ-kăl) *-al:* pertaining to	*pertaining to neck*
cost/o	ribs	sub/**cost**/al (sŭb-KŎS-tăl) *sub-:* under, below *-al:* pertaining to	*pertaining to under ribs*
crani/o	cranium (skull)	**crani/o**/tomy (krā-nē-ŎT-ō-mē) *-tomy:* incision	*cranium incision*
humer/o	humerus (upper arm bone)	**humer**/al (HŪ-mĕr-ăl) *-al:* pertaining to	*pertaining to humerus*
metacarp/o	metacarpus (hand bones)	**metacarp**/ectomy (mĕt-ă-kăr-PĔK-tō-mē) *-ectomy:* excision, removal	*removal of metacarpus*
phalang/o	phalanges (bones of fingers and toes)	**phalang**/itis (făl-ăn-JĪ-tĭs) *-itis:* inflammation	*inflammation of phalanges*
spondyl/o*	vertebra (backbone)	**spondyl**/itis (spŏn-dĭl-Ī-tĭs) *-itis:* inflammation	*inflammation of vertebra*
vertebr/o*		**vertebr**/al (VĔR-tĕ-brăl) *-al:* pertaining to	*pertaining to vertebra*
stern/o	sternum (breastbone)	**stern/o**/cost/al (stĕr-nō-KŎS-tăl) *cost:* ribs *-al:* pertaining to	*pertaining to sternum*

*The CF spondyl/o is used to form words about the condition of the structure; the CF vertebr/o is used to form words that describe the structure.

Combining Form	Meaning	Medical Word	Meaning
Bones of the Lower Extremities			
calcane/o	calcaneum (heel bone)	calcane/o/dynia (kăl-kăn-ē-ō-DĬN-ē-ă) -*dynia:* pain	*calcaneal pain*
femor/o	femur (thigh bone)	femor/al (FĔM-or-ăl) -*al:* pertaining to	*pertaining to femur*
fibul/o	fibula (smaller, outer bone of lower leg)	fibul/ar (FĬB-ū-lăr) -*ar:* pertaining to	*pertaining to fibula*
patell/o	patella (kneecap)	patell/ectomy (păt-ē-LĔK-tō-mē) -*ectomy:* excision, removal	*removal of patella*
pelv/i**	pelvis	pelv/i/metry (pĕl-VĬM-ĕ-trē) -*metry:* act of measuring	*act of measuring pelvis*
pelv/o		pelv/is (PĔL-vĭs) -*is:* noun ending	*pelvis*
radi/o	radiation, x-ray; radius (lower arm bone, thumb side)	radi/o/graph (RĀ-dē-ō-grăf) -*graph:* instrument for recording	*instrument for recording radiation*
tibi/o	tibia (larger bone of lower leg)	tibi/al (TĬB-ē-ăl) -*al:* pertaining to	*pertaining to tibia*
Other Related Structures			
ankyl/o	stiffness; bent, crooked	ankyl/osis (ăng-kĭ-LŌ-sĭs) -*osis:* abnormal condition; increase (used primarily with blood cells)	*abnormal crooked condition*
arthr/o	joint	arthr/o/desis (ăr-thrō-DĒ-sĭs) -*desis:* binding, fixation (of a bone or joint)	*joint binding*

**The i in pelv/i/metry is an exception to the rule of using the connecting vowel o.*

(Continued)

Combining Form	Meaning	Medical Word	Meaning
Other Related Structures			
chondr/o	cartilage	cost/o/**chondr**/itis (kŏs-tō-kŏn-DRĪ-tĭs) *cost/o:* ribs *–itis:* inflammation	*inflammation of rib cartilage*
lamin/o	lamina (part of vertebral arch)	**lamin**/ectomy (lăm-ĭ-NĔK-tŏ-mē) *–ectomy:* excision, removal	*removal of lamina*
myel/o	bone marrow; spinal cord	**myel**/o/cele (MĪ-ĕ-lō-sēl) *–cele:* hernia, swelling	*Swelling of bone marrow*
orth/o	straight	**orth**/o/ped/ics (or-thō-PĒ-dĭks) *ped:* foot; child *–ics:* pertaining to	*pertaining to straight foot*
oste/o	bone	**oste**/o/porosis (ŏs-tē-ō-por-Ō-sĭs) *–porosis:* porous	*porous bone*

Suffixes and Prefixes

In the table that follows, suffixes and prefixes are listed alphabetically, and other word parts are defined as needed. Review the medical word and study the elements that make up the term. Then complete the meaning of the medical words in the right-hand column. You may also refer to *Appendix A: Glossary of Medical Word Elements* to complete this exercise.

Word Element	Meaning	Medical Word	Meaning
Suffixes			
-clasia	to break; surgical fracture	arthr/o/**clasia** (ăr-thrō-KLĀ-zē-ă) *arthr/o:* joint	*joint break*
-clast	to break	oste/o/**clast** (ŎS-tē-ō-klăst) *oste/o:* bone	*bone break*
-plegia	paralysis	hemi/**plegia** (hĕm-ē-PLĒ-jē-ă) *hemi–:* half	*half paralysis*

Word Element	Meaning	Medical Word	Meaning
Suffixes			
-sarcoma	malignant tumor of connective tissue	**my/o/sarcoma** (mī-ō-sar-KŌ-mă) *my/o:* muscle	malignant muscle tumor
Prefixes			
dia-	through, across	**dia/physis** (dī-ĂF-ĭ-sĭs) *-physis:* growth	growth across
peri-	around	**peri/oste/um** (pĕr-ē-ŎS-tē-ŭm) *oste:* bone *um:* structure, thing	around bone structure

 Competency Verification: Check your answers in Appendix B, Answer Key, pages 386–388. If you are not satisfied with your level of comprehension, review the terms in the table and retake the review.

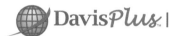 Visit the *Medical Terminology Express* online resource center at *DavisPlus* for an audio exercise of the terms in this table. Other activities are also available to reinforce content.

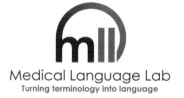

Medical Language Lab
Turning terminology into language

Visit the Medical Language Lab at *medicallanguagelab.com* to enhance your study and reinforce this chapter's word elements with the flash-card activity. We recommend you complete the flash-card activity before continuing with the next section.

Medical Terminology Word Building

In this section, combine the word parts you have learned to construct medical terms related to the musculoskeletal system.

Use **oste/o** (bone) to build words that mean:

1. bone cells _opthalmoplegia_
2. pain in bones _ophthalmology_
3. disease of bones and joints _pupilloscopy_
4. beginning or formation of bones _keratometer_

Use **cervic/o** (neck) to build words that mean:

5. pertaining to the neck _Scleritis_

6. pertaining to the neck and arm _Scleromalacia_

7. pertaining to the neck and face _iridoplegia_

Use **myel/o** (bone marrow; spinal cord) to build words that mean:

8. tumor of bone marrow _iridoplegia_

9. sarcoma of bone marrow (cells) _iridocele_

10. radiography of the spinal cord _retinopathy_

11. abnormal softening of the spinal cord _retinitis_

Use **stern/o** (sternum) to build words that mean:

12. pertaining to above the sternum _blepharoplegia_

13. resembling the breastbone _blepharoptosis_

Use **arthr/o** (joint) or **chondr/o** (cartilage) to build words that mean:

14. embryonic cell that forms cartilage _blepharoplasty_

15. inflammation of a joint _otopyorrhea_

16. inflammation of bones and joints _audiometer_

Use **pelv/i** (pelvis) to build a word that means:

17. instrument for measuring the pelvis _myringotome_

Use **my/o** (muscle) to build words that mean:

18. twitching of a muscle _myringoplasty_

19. any disease of muscle _salpingitis_

20. rupture of a muscle _salpingopharyngeal_

> **Competency Verification:** Check your answers in Appendix B, Answer Key, on page 388. Review material that you did not answer correctly.
>
> **Correct Answers:** _____ × 5 = _____ %

MEDICAL VOCABULARY

The following tables consist of selected terms that pertain to diseases and conditions of the musculoskeletal system. Terms related to diagnostic, medical, and surgical procedures are included as well as pharmacological agents used to treat diseases. Recognizing and learning these terms will help you understand the connection between diseases and their treatments. Word analyses for selected terms are also provided.

Diseases and Conditions

Muscles

muscular dystrophy (MD) MŬS-kū-lăr DĬS-trō-fē *muscul:* muscle 　*-ar:* pertaining to 　*dys-:* bad; painful; difficult 　*-trophy:* development, 　　nourishment	Group of hereditary diseases characterized by progressive degeneration of the muscles, leading to increasing weakness and debilitation, including Duchenne dystrophy (most common form)
myasthenia gravis (MG) mī-ăs-THĒ-nē-ă GRĂV-ĭs	Autoimmune neuromuscular disorder characterized by progressive fatigue and severe muscle weakness, particularly evident with facial muscles and ptosis of the eyelids
rotator cuff injury	Injury to the capsule of the shoulder joint, which is reinforced by muscles and tendons; also called *musculotendinous rotator cuff injury*
sprain	Trauma to a joint that causes injury to the surrounding ligament, accompanied by pain and disability, such as an eversion sprain that occurs when the foot is twisted outward
strain	Trauma to a muscle from overuse or excessive forcible stretch
tendinitis těn-dĭn-Ī-tĭs	Inflammation of a tendon, usually caused by injury or overuse; also called *tendonitis*
torticollis tōr-tĭ-KŎL-ĭs	Spasmodic contraction of the neck muscles, causing stiffness and twisting of the neck; also called *wryneck*

Bones and Joints

arthritis ăr-THRĪ-tĭs *arthr:* joint 　*-itis:* inflammation	Inflammation of a joint usually accompanied by pain, swelling, and, commonly, changes in structure
gouty GOWT-ē	Arthritis caused by excessive uric acid in the body; also called *gout*
osteoarthritis ŏs-tē-ō-ăr-THRĪ-tĭs *oste/o:* bone *arthr:* joint 　*-itis:* inflammation	Progressive, degenerative joint disease characterized by bone spurs (osteophytes) and destruction of articular cartilage

rheumatoid arthritis (RA) ROO-mă-toyd ăr-THRĪ-tĭs	Chronic, systemic inflammatory disease affecting the synovial membranes of multiple joints, eventually resulting in crippling deformities and immobility Get a closer look at rheumatoid arthritis on page 309.
bunion BŬN-yŭn	Deformity characterized by lateral deviation of the great toe as it turns in toward the second toe (angulation) with an abnormal enlargement of the joint at the base of the great toe (See Figure 12-1.)
carpal tunnel syndrome (CTS) KĂR-păl TŬN-ĕl SĬN-drōm	Pain or numbness resulting from compression of the median nerve within the carpal tunnel (wrist canal through which the flexor tendons and median nerve pass)
contracture kŏn-TRĂK-chŭr	Fibrosis of connective tissue in the skin, fascia, muscle, or joint capsule that prevents normal mobility of the related tissue or joint
crepitation krĕp-ĭ-TĀ-shŭn	Grating sound made by movement of bone ends rubbing together, indicating a fracture or joint destruction
Ewing sarcoma Ū-ĭng săr-KŌ-mă	Malignant tumor that develops from bone marrow, usually in long bones or the pelvis, and most commonly affecting adolescent boys
fracture (Fx) FRĂK-chŭr	Any break in a bone Get a closer look at bone fractures on pages 307 and 308.

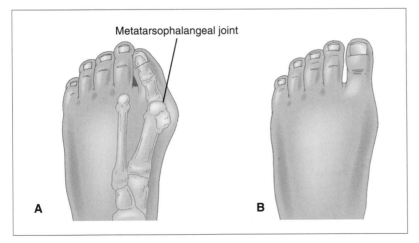

Metatarsophalangeal joint

A

B

Figure 12-1 (A, B) Bunion.

ganglion cyst GĂNG-lē- ŏn s ĭst	Noncancerous, jelly-like fluid–filled lumps that most commonly develop along the tendons or joints of the wrists or hands, but may also appear in the feet (See Figure 12-2.)
herniated disk HĔR-nē-āt-ĕd	Herniation or rupture of the nucleus pulposus (center gelatinous material within an intervertebral disk) between two vertebrae; also called *prolapsed disk* (See Figure 12-3.)
osteomyelitis ŏs-tē-ō-mī-ĕ-LĪ-tĭs	Infection that encompasses all bone (osseous) components, including the bone marrow (See Figure 12-4.)

osteoporosis
ŏs-tē-ō-pōr-Ō-sĭs
   oste/o: bone
  -porosis: porous
	Decrease in bone density with an increase in porosity, causing bones to become brittle and increasing the risk of fractures

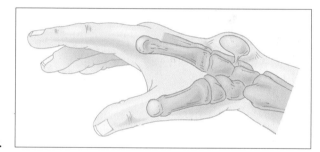

Figure 12-2 Ganglion cyst of the wrist.

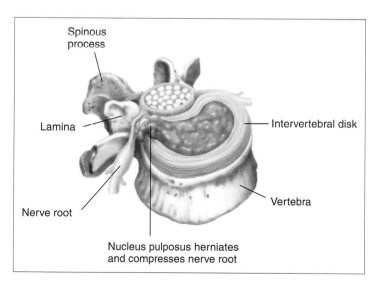

Figure 12-3 Herniated disk.

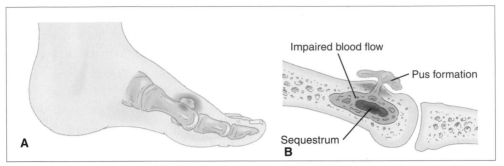

Figure 12-4 Osteomyelitis. (A) Bone infection in the toe. (B) Blocked blood flow in the area of infection with sequestrum (bone death) and pus formation at infection site.

Paget disease PĂ-jĕt	Abnormal bone destruction and regrowth of either one or several bones at numerous sites that results in deformity; most commonly occurs in the pelvis, skull, spine, and legs; also called *osteitis deformans*
rickets RĬK-ĕts	Form of osteomalacia in children caused by vitamin D deficiency; also called *rachitis*
sequestrum sē-KWĔS-trŭm	Fragment of a necrosed bone that has become separated from surrounding tissue
talipes equinovarus TĂL-ĭ-pēz ē-kwī-nō-VĀR-ŭs	Congenital deformity in which the great toe is angled laterally toward the other toes; also called *clubfoot* (See Figure 12-5.)

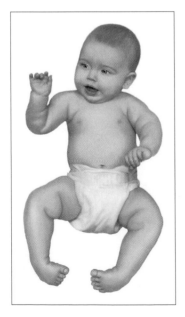

Figure 12-5 Talipes equinovarus.

Spine

spinal curvatures SPĪ-năl	Abnormal deviation of the spine from its normal position that results in a misalignment or exaggeration in certain areas, as occurs in kyphosis, lordosis, and scoliosis

kyphosis
kī-FŌ-sĭs
kyph: humpback
-osis: abnormal condition;
    increase (used
    primarily with
    blood cells)
	Increased curvature of the thoracic region of the vertebral column, leading to a humpback posture; also called *hunchback* (See Figure 12-6.)

lordosis
lŏr-DŌ-sĭs
lord: curve, swayback
-osis: abnormal condition;
    increase (used
    primarily with blood
    cells)
	Forward curvature of the lumbar region of the vertebral column, leading to a swayback posture (See Figure 12-6.)

scoliosis
skō-lē-Ō-sĭs
scoli: crooked, bent
-osis: abnormal condition;
    increase (used
    primarily with
    blood cells)
	Abnormal sideward curvature of the spine to the left or right that eventually causes back pain, disk disease, or arthritis (See Figure 12-6.)

spondylitis spŏn-dĭl-Ī-tĭs	Inflammation of one or more vertebrae

ankylosing spondylitis
ăng-kĭ-LŌS-ĭng spŏn-dĭl-Ī-tĭs
spondyl: vertebra
        (backbone)
   -itis: inflammation
	Chronic inflammatory disease of unknown origin that first affects the spine and is characterized by fusion and loss of mobility of two or more vertebrae; also called *rheumatoid spondylitis*

spondylolisthesis spŏn-dĭ-lō-lĭs-THĒ-sĭs *spondyl/o:* vertebra (backbone) *-listhesis:* slipping	Partial forward dislocation of one vertebra over the one below it, most commonly the fifth lumbar vertebra over the first sacral vertebra; also called *spinal cord compression*
subluxation sŭb-lŭk-SĀ-shŭn	Partial or incomplete dislocation of a bone from its normal location within a joint, causing loss of function of the joint; also called *partial dislocation*

Figure 12-6 Spinal curvatures.

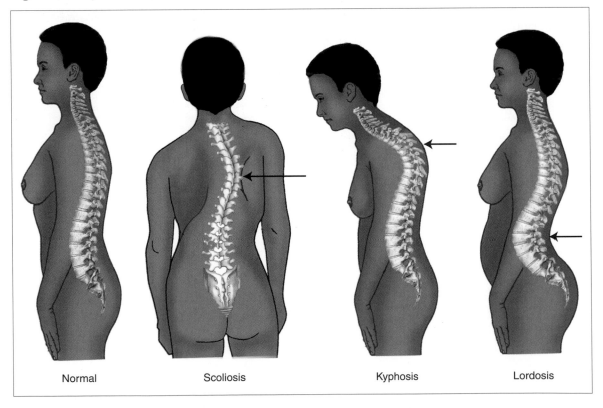

| Normal | Scoliosis | Kyphosis | Lordosis |

Diagnostic Procedures

arthrocentesis ăr-thrō-sĕn-TĒ-sĭs *arthr/o:* joint *-centesis:* surgical puncture	Puncture of a joint space with a needle to obtain samples of synovial fluid for diagnostic purposes, instill medications, or remove accumulated fluid from joints to relieve pain
arthroscopy ăr-THRŎS-kō-pē *arthr/o:* joint *-scopy:* visual examination	Visual examination of the interior of a joint and its structures using a thin, flexible, fiberoptic scope called an *arthroscope,* which contains a miniature camera and projects images on a monitor to guide instruments during procedures (See Figure 12-7.)

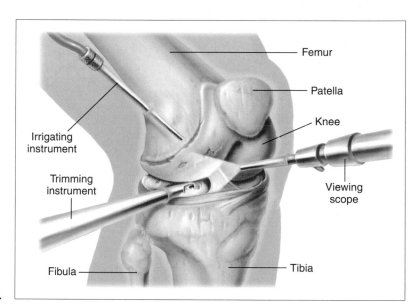

Figure 12-7 Arthroscopy.

Medical and Surgical Procedures

arthroplasty ĂR-thrō-plăs-tē *arthr/o:* joint *-plasty:* surgical repair	Surgical reconstruction or replacement of a painful, degenerated joint to restore mobility in rheumatoid arthritis or osteoarthritis or to correct a congenital deformity
total hip arthroplasty	Replacement of the femoral head and acetabulum with prostheses that are fastened into the bone; also called *total hip replacement* (THR) (See Figure 12-8.)
sequestrectomy sē-kwĕs-TRĔK-tō-mē *sequestr:* separation *-ectomy:* excision, removal	Excision of a sequestrum (segment of necrosed bone)

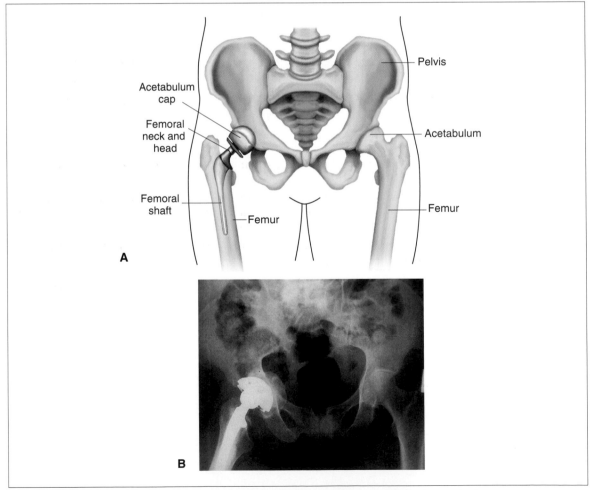

Figure 12-8 Total hip replacement. (A) Right total hip replacement. (B) Radiograph showing total hip replacement of arthritic hip.

Pharmacology

bone reabsorption inhibitors	Reduce the reabsorption of bones in treatment of weak and fragile bones as seen in osteoporosis and Paget disease
gold salts	Treat rheumatoid arthritis by inhibiting activity within the immune system and preventing further disease progression
muscle relaxants	Relieve muscle spasms, pain, and stiffness
nonsteroidal anti-inflammatory drugs (NSAIDs) nŏn-STĔR-oyd-ăl ăn-tē-ĭn-FLĂM-ă-tō-rē	Relieve mild to moderate pain and reduce inflammation in treatment of musculoskeletal conditions, such as sprains and strains, and inflammatory disorders, including rheumatoid arthritis, osteoarthritis, bursitis, gout, and tendinitis

Pronunciation Help	Long Sound	ā in rāte	ē in rēbirth	ī in īsle	ō in ōver	ū in ūnite
	Short Sound	ă in ălone	ĕ in ĕver	ĭ in ĭt	ŏ in nŏt	ŭ in cŭt

A Closer Look

Take a closer look at the following musculoskeletal conditions to enhance your understanding of the medical terminology associated with them.

Bone Fractures

A **fracture** is a break or crack in a bone. Fractures occur when bones are broken as a result of an injury, an accident, or a disease process. They are classified according to the way in which the bone breaks and whether or not the skin is pierced with a bony fragment. A fracture that is caused by a disease process, such as **osteoporosis** or bone cancer, is known as a **pathologic fracture.** The illustration that follows identifies and describes some common types of fractures. Specific methods of treatment for fractures depend on the type of fracture sustained, its location, and any related injuries. X-rays help confirm and determine the severity of the fracture.

(Continued)

A Closer Look—cont'd

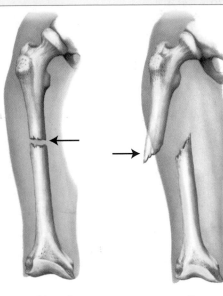

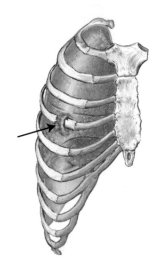

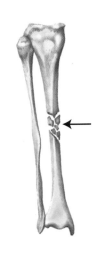

Closed
Bone is broken but
no open wound in skin

Open
Bone breaks
through skin

Complicated
Extensive soft tissue
injury such as a
broken rib piercing the lung above

Comminuted
Bone is crushed
into several pieces

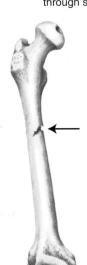

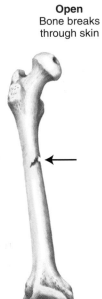

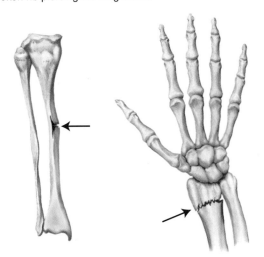

Impacted
Broken ends of a bone
are forced into one another

Incomplete
Line of fracture
does not include
the whole bone

Greenstick
Bone is broken only
on one side, commonly occurs
most in children because
growing bones are soft

Colles fracture
Distal radius is
broken by falling
onto an outstretched
hand

Types of Fractures.

A Closer Look—cont'd

Rheumatoid Arthritis

Rheumatoid arthritis (RA) is a chronic, systemic inflammatory disease that primarily attacks peripheral joints and surrounding muscles, tendons, ligaments, and blood vessels. Spontaneous remissions and unpredictable exacerbations mark the course of this potentially crippling disease. RA is an **autoimmune disease** in which a reaction against one's own joint tissues, especially synovial fluid, occurs. As RA develops, there is congestion and edema of the synovial membrane and joint, causing formation of a thick layer of granulation tissue. This tissue invades cartilage, destroying the joint and bone. Eventually, a fibrous immobility of joints **(ankylosis)** occurs, causing immobility and visible deformities, as seen in the illustration that follows. The disease is three times more common in women than men. RA usually requires lifelong treatment, and surgery is occasionally required. The prognosis worsens with the development of nodules, **vasculitis,** and the presence of **rheumatoid factor** (substance detected in blood test of patients with rheumatoid arthritis).

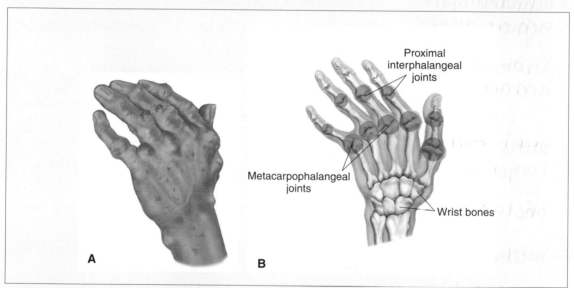

Rheumatoid arthritis with deformity of the left hand (A) and the joints affected (B).

Treatment consists of physical therapy, heat applications, and drugs such as aspirin, nonsteroidal anti-inflammatory drugs (NSAIDs), and **corticosteroids** to reduce pain and inflammation. Other therapeutic drugs include disease-modifying antirheumatic drugs (DMARDs).

Medical Vocabulary Recall

Match the medical terms below with the definitions in the numbered list.

arthroplasty	gout	myasthenia gravis	sequestrum
contracture	herniated disk	osteoporosis	sprain
crepitation	kyphosis	Paget disease	strain
CTS	lordosis	RA	tendinitis
Ewing sarcoma	muscular dystrophy	scoliosis	torticollis

1. _tinnitus_ means a decrease in bone density and an increase in porosity, causing the risk of fractures.

2. _otosclerosis_ means inflammation of a tendon.

3. _achromatopnia_ refers to trauma to a joint, causing injury to the surrounding ligament.

4. _Meniere disease_ refers to muscular trauma that results from overuse or excessive, forcible stretch.

5. _strabismus_ means hunchback or humpback.

6. _anacusis_ is a malignant tumor that develops from bone marrow, usually in long bones or the pelvis, and occurs most commonly in adolescent boys.

7. _otitis media_ is also called *wryneck*.

8. _conjunctivitis_ is a disease characterized by excessive uric acid in the blood and around the joints.

9. _photophobia_ is a disease characterized by inflammatory changes in joints and related structures that result in crippling deformities.

10. _presbycusis_ refers to abnormal bone destruction that results in deformity; also called *osteitis deformans*.

11. _glaucoma_ is a fragment of necrosed bone that has become separated from surrounding tissue.

12. _vertigo_ means repair or replacement of a joint.

13. _retinal detachment_ is a grating sound made by the ends of bone rubbing together.

14. _hordeolum_ is a neuromuscular disorder characterized by muscular weakness and progressive fatigue.

15. _astigmatism_ means forward curvature of the lumbar spine; also called *swayback*.

16. _myringoplasty_ refers to a group of hereditary diseases characterized by gradual atrophy and weakness of muscle.

17. <u>tonometry</u> is connective tissue fibrosis that prevents normal mobility of the related tissue or joint.

18. <u>iridectomy</u> is abnormal sideward curvature of the spine to the left or right.

19. <u>Rinne</u> refers to rupture of the nucleus pulposus between two vertebrae.

20. <u>cataract</u> is pain or numbness resulting from compression of the median nerve within the carpal tunnel.

 Competency Verification: Check your answers in Appendix B, Answer Key, page 388. Review material that you did not answer correctly.

Correct Answers: _____ × 5 = _____ %

Pronunciation and Spelling

Use the following list to practice correct pronunciation and spelling of medical terms. First practice the pronunciation aloud. Then write the correct spelling of the term. The first word is completed for you.

Pronunciation	Spelling
1. ăb-DŬK-shŭn	*abduction*
2. ăr-thrō-KLĀ-zē-ă	arthro clasio
3. DOR-sĭ-flĕk-shŭn	dorsiflexion
4. făl-ăn-JĪ-tĭs	phalangitis
5. FĂSH-ē-ō-plăs-tē	fascioplasty
6. GOWT	gout
7. krĕp-ĭ-TĀ-shŭn	crepitation
8. lī-ō-mī-Ō-mă	leiomyoma
9. mī-ō-săr-KŌ-mă	myosarcoma
10. mī-ăs-THĒ-nē-ă GRĂV-ĭs	myasthenia gravis
11. or-thō-PĒ-dĭks	orthopedics
12. ŏs-te-o-ăr-THRŎP-ă-thē	osteoarthropathy
13. ŎS-tē-ō-klăst	osteoclast
14. PĂJ-ĕt dĭ-ZĒZ	paget disease
15. pĕl-VĬM-ĕ-trē	pelvimetry

(Continued)

Pronunciation	Spelling
16. ROO-mă-toyd ăr-THRĪ-tĭs	rheumatoid arthritis
17. sē-kwĕs-TRĔK-tō-mē	sequestrectomy
18. spŏn-dĭl-ō-mă-LĀ-shē-ă	spondylomalacia
19. stĕr-nō-KŎS-tăl	sternocostal
20. tōr-tĭ-KŎL-ĭs	torticollis

Competency Verification: Check your answers in Appendix B, Answer Key, on page 388. Review material that you did not answer correctly.

Correct Answers: _____ × 5 = _____ %

ABBREVIATIONS

The table that follows introduces abbreviations associated with the musculoskeletal system.

Abbreviation	Meaning	Abbreviation	Meaning
CTS	carpal tunnel syndrome	MG	myasthenia gravis
Fx	fracture	NSAIDs	nonsteroidal anti-inflammatory drugs
HNP	herniated nucleus pulposus (herniated disk)	RA	rheumatoid arthritis
L1, L2, to L5	first lumbar vertebra, second lumbar vertebra, and so on	S1, S2, to S5	first sacral vertebra, second sacral vertebra, and so on
MD	muscular dystrophy	THR	total hip replacement

CHART NOTES

Chart notes make up part of the medical record and are used in various types of health care facilities. The chart notes that follow were dictated by the patient's physician and reflect common clinical events using medical terminology to document the patient's care. Studying and completing the terminology and chart notes sections below will help you learn and understand terms associated with the medical specialty of orthopedics.

Terminology

The following terms are linked to chart notes in the medical specialty of orthopedics. Practice pronouncing each term aloud and then use a medical dictionary such as *Taber's Cyclopedic Medical Dictionary; Appendix A: Glossary of Medical Word Elements*, or other resources to define each term.

Term	Meaning
anteroposterior ăn-tĕr-ō-pŏs-TĒ-rē-ŏr	
bilateral bī-LĂT-ĕr-ăl	
degenerative dĕ-JĔN-ĕr-ă-tĭv	
hypertrophic hī-pĕr-TRŌF-ĭk	
intervertebral ĭn-tĕr-VĔRT-ĕ-brăl	
L5	
laminectomies lăm-ĭ-NĔK-tŏ-mēz	
lateral views LĂT-ĕr-ăl	
lipping LĬP-ĭng	
lumbar LŬM-băr	
lumbosacral lŭm-bō-SĀ-krăl	
S1	
sacroiliac sā-krō-ĬL-ē-ăk	
sacrum SĀ-krŭm	

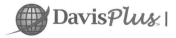 **DavisPlus** | Visit *Medical Terminology Express* at *DavisPlus* Online Resource Center. Use it to practice pronunciations and reinforce the meanings of the terms in this chart note.

Degenerative Intervertebral Disk Disease

Read the chart notes that follow aloud. Underline any term you have trouble pronouncing and any terms that you cannot define. If needed, refer to the Terminology section on page 313 for correct pronunciations and meanings of terms.

> Anteroposterior and lateral views of the lumbar spine and an AP view of the sacrum show a placement of L5 on S1. The L5-S1 intervertebral disk space contains a slight shadow of decreased density. There is now slight narrowing of the L3-4 and L4-5 spaces. Bilateral laminectomies appear to have been done at L5-S1. There is slight hypertrophic lipping of the upper margin of the body of L4. The sacroiliac joint spaces are well preserved. Lateral view of the lumbosacral spine taken with the spine in flexion and extension demonstrates slight motion at all of the lumbar and lumbosacral levels.
>
> Impression:
> 1. Degenerative, intervertebral disk disease at L5-S1, now also accompanied by slight narrowing of the L3-4 and L5-4 disk spaces.
> 2. Slight motion at all of the lumbar and lumbosacral levels.

Chart Note Analysis

From the preceding chart note, select the medical word that means

1. pertaining to the sacrum and ilium: _Sacroiliac_
2. designates the third and fourth lumbar vertebrae: _L3 L4_
3. bending motion of a limb: _flexion_
4. directional term indicating *from the front to the back*: _anteroposterior_
5. pertaining to two sides: _bilateral_
6. pertaining to an increase in the size of an organ or structure: _hypertropic_
7. pertaining to the lumbar vertebra and the sacrum: _lumbosacral_
8. pertaining to one side: _lateral_
9. extending motion of a limb: _extension_
10. pertaining to between vertebrae: _intervertebral_

> ✓ **Competency Verification:** Check your answers in Appendix B, Answer Key, on page 388. Review material that you did not answer correctly.
>
> **Correct Answers:** _____ × 10 = _____ %

Demonstrate What You Know!

To evaluate your understanding of how medical terms you have studied in this and previous chapters are used in a clinical environment, complete the numbered sentences by selecting an appropriate term from the list that follows.

ankylosis	calcaneodynia	gouty	muscles	rickets
arthrocentesis	carpoptosis	greenstick	NSAIDs	subluxation
articulate	degenerative	laminectomy	rheumatologist	talipes

1. _talipes_ is a congenital deformity of the foot.
2. The surgical puncture of a joint is known as _arthrocentesis_.
3. Partial or incomplete dislocation of a bone is known as a _subluxation_.
4. Immobility of joints is known as _ankylosis_.
5. A 52-year-old woman has arthritis and ankylosis. Her primary physician referred her to a specialist called a(n) _rheumatologist_.
6. A patient fell on her hand, resulting in a downward displacement of her wrist, a condition known as _carpoptosis_.
7. A joint is a place where two or more bones connect, or _articulate_, to allow motion between the parts.
8. _rickets_ is a form of osteomalacia in children caused by vitamin D deficiency.
9. _muscles_ are responsible for movement, maintaining posture, and the propulsion of substances through the body.
10. _degenerative_ refers to an impairment of a body structure.
11. A laboratory result with findings of excessive uric acid probably indicates _gouty_ arthritis.
12. The surgical procedure to excise part of the vertebrae is known as _laminectomy_.
13. _greenstick_ fractures usually occur in children because their growing bones are soft and tend to splinter rather than break completely.
14. _NSAIDs_ relieve pain and reduce inflammation in the treatment of musculoskeletal disorders.
15. A person with a symptom of heel pain has _calcaneodynia_.

Competency Verification: Check your answers in Appendix B, Answer Key, on page 388. Review material that you did not answer correctly.

Correct Answers: _____ × 6.67 = _____ %

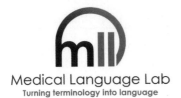

Medical Language Lab
Turning terminology into language

If you are not satisfied with your retention level of the musculoskeletal chapter, visit *DavisPlus* Student Online Resource Center and the Medical Language Lab to complete the website activities linked to this chapter.

Special Senses: Eyes and Ears

OBJECTIVES

Upon completion of this chapter, you will be able to:

- Describe types of medical treatment provided by ophthalmologists and otolaryngologists.
- Name the primary structures of the eyes and ears and discuss their functions.
- Identify combining forms, suffixes, and prefixes associated with the eyes and the ears.
- Recognize, pronounce, build, and spell pathological, diagnostic, and therapeutic terms and abbreviations associated with the eyes and ears.
- Demonstrate your knowledge of this chapter by successfully completing the activities in this chapter.

VOCABULARY PREVIEW

Term	Meaning
cataract KĂT-ă-răkt	Opacity of the lens of the eye, usually occurring as a result of aging, trauma, metabolic disease, or the adverse effect of certain medications or chemicals
cornea transplantation KOR-nē-ă	Procedure in which a damaged cornea is replaced by the cornea from the eye of a human cadaver; also known as *keratoplasty*
glaucoma glaw-KŌ-mă *glauc:* gray *–oma:* tumor	Eye disease in which increased eyeball pressure causes gradual loss of sight
ocular ŎK-ū-lăr *ocul:* eye *-ar:* pertaining to	Pertaining to the eye or sense of sight
radial keratotomy kĕr-ă-TŎT-ō-mē *kerat/o:* horny tissue; hard; cornea *-tomy:* incision	Surgery to correct myopia, or nearsightedness, by changing the shape of the cornea (transparent part of the eye that covers the iris and pupil)
sleep apnea ăp-NĔ-ă *a-:* without, not *-pnea:* breathing	Condition in which breathing stops for more than 10 seconds during sleep

Pronunciation Help	Long Sound	ā in rāte	ē in rēbirth	ī in īsle	ō in ōver	ū in ūnite
	Short Sound	ă in ălone	ĕ in ĕver	ĭ in ĭt	ŏ in nŏt	ŭ in cŭt

MEDICAL SPECIALTIES OF OPHTHALMOLOGY AND OTOLARYNGOLOGY

The medical specialty of **ophthalmology** is associated with the eyes, the organs of sight. The medical specialty of **otolaryngology** is associated with the ears, the organs of hearing.

Ophthalmology

Ophthalmology is the branch of medicine concerned with diagnosis and treatment of eye disorders. The medical specialist in ophthalmology is called an **ophthalmologist.** Although ophthalmologists specialize in treatment of the eyes only, it is important for them to be aware of other abnormalities that an eye examination may reveal. For example, the examination may reveal the first signs of a systemic illness, such as diabetes, even though it involves another part of the body. The ophthalmologist also prescribes corrective lenses and performs corrective eye surgeries. These surgeries include, but are not limited to,

cornea transplantation, **cataract** removal, repair of **ocular** muscle dysfunction, **glaucoma** treatment, lens removal, and **radial keratotomy**.

Two other health care practitioners, the **optometrist** and **optician,** specialize in providing corrective lenses for the eyes. These practitioners are not medical doctors, but they are licensed to examine and test the eyes and treat visual defects by prescribing corrective lenses. The optician also specializes in filling prescriptions for corrective lenses.

Otolaryngology

Otolaryngology is the oldest medical specialty in the United States. Fifty years ago, otolaryngology was practiced along with ophthalmology. During that time, the medical practice consisted mainly of removing tonsils and adenoids and irrigating (cleansing a canal by flushing it with water or other fluids) the sinuses and ear canals.

Today, otolaryngology is greatly expanded to include medical and surgical management of patients with disorders of the ear, nose, and throat (ENT) and related structures of the head and neck. Specialists in this practice are commonly called **ENT physicians**, or **otolaryngologists.** ENT physicians commonly treat disorders related to the sinuses, including allergies and disorders of the sense of smell. Their diagnostic techniques are used to detect the causes of symptoms such as hoarseness, hearing and breathing difficulty, and swelling around the head or neck. ENT physicians also treat sleep disorders, most commonly **sleep apnea**. Various types of procedures, including, but not limited to, surgery, may be performed to treat sleep apnea or snoring disorders.

EYES AND EARS QUICK STUDY

The major senses of the body are sight, hearing, smell, taste, and touch. These sensations are identified by specific body organs. Senses of smell and taste have been discussed in previous chapters. This chapter focuses on the eyes and ears, which include the senses of sight and hearing.

Eyes

The eyes and their accessory structures are receptor organs that provide vision. The eye is one of the most important sense organs of the body. The eyes provide most of the information about what we see as well as what we learn from printed material. Similar to other sensory organs, the eyes are constructed to detect stimuli in the environment and to transmit those observations to the brain for visual interpretation. (See *Eye Structures*, page 320.)

Ears

The ears and their accessory structures are receptor organs that enable us to hear and maintain balance. Each ear consists of three divisions: the external, middle, and inner ear. The external and middle ears conduct sound waves through the ear. The inner ear contains auditory structures that receive sound waves and transmit them to the brain for interpretation. The inner ear also contains specialized receptors that maintain balance and equilibrium in response to fluctuations in body position and motion. (See *Ear Structures,* page 321.)

ALERT: An extensive self-paced anatomy and physiology multimedia review is included in *TermPlus,* a powerful, interactive CD-ROM program that can be purchased separately from F.A. Davis Company.

MEDICAL WORD BUILDING

Constructing medical words using word elements related to the special senses of sight and hearing will enhance your understanding of those terms and reinforce your ability to use terms correctly.

Combining Forms

Begin your study of terminology related to the special senses by reviewing the organs of the eyes and ears and their associated combining forms (CFs), which are illustrated in the figures *Eye Structures* and *Ear Structures* that follow.

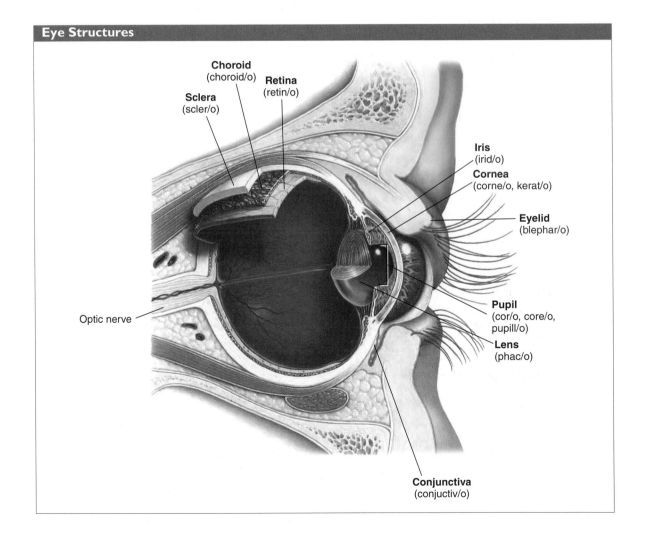

Eye Structures

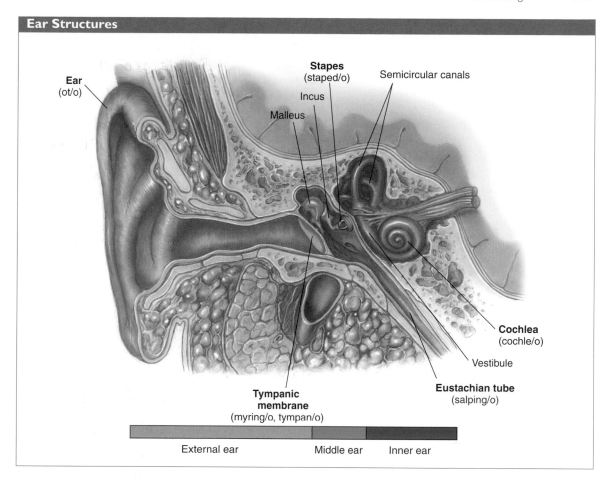

Ear Structures

Stapes
(staped/o)

Incus

Malleus

Semicircular canals

Ear
(ot/o)

Cochlea
(cochle/o)

Vestibule

Eustachian tube
(salping/o)

Tympanic
membrane
(myring/o, tympan/o)

External ear   Middle ear   Inner ear

In the table that follows, CFs are listed alphabetically, and other word parts are defined as needed. Review the medical word and study the elements that make up the term. Then complete the meaning of the medical words in the right-hand column. The first one is completed for you. You may also refer to *Appendix A: Glossary of Medical Word Elements* to complete this exercise.

Combining Form	Meaning	Medical Word	Meaning
Eye			
blephar/o	eyelid	**blephar/o**/spasm (BLĔF-ă-rō-spăzm) *-spasm:* involuntary contraction, twitching	*Involuntary contraction of the eyelid*

(Continued)

Combining Form	Meaning	Medical Word	Meaning
Eye			
choroid/o	choroid	**choroid**/o/pathy (kō-roy-DŎP-ă-thē) *-pathy:* disease	*choroid disease*
conjunctiv/o	conjunctiva	**conjunctiv**/itis (kŏn-jŭnk-tĭ-VĪ-tĭs) *-itis:* inflammation	*inflammation of conjunctiva*
corne/o	cornea	**corne**/itis (kor-nē-Ī-tĭs) *-itis:* inflammation	*inflammation of cornea*
cor/o	pupil	aniso/**cor**/ia (ăn-ī-sō-KŌ-rē-ă) *aniso:* unequal, dissimilar *-ia:* condition	*unequal pupil condition*
core/o		**core**/o/meter (kō-rē-ŎM-ě-těr) *-meter:* instrument for measuring the pupil	*instrument for measuring pupil*
pupill/o		**pupill**/ary (PŪ-pĭ-lěr-ē) *-ary:* pertaining to	*pertaining to pupil*
dacry/o	tear; lacrimal apparatus (duct, sac, or gland)	**dacry**/o/rrhea (dăk-rē-ō-RĒ-ă) *-rrhea:* discharge, flow	*lacrimal discharge*
lacrim/o		**lacrim**/ation (lăk-rĭ-MĀ-shŭn) *-ation:* process (of)	*process of tear*
dipl/o	double	**dipl**/opia (dĭp-LŌ-pē-ă) *-opia:* vision	*double vision*
irid/o	iris	**irid**/o/plegia (ĭr-ĭd-ō-PLĒ-jē-ă) *-plegia:* paralysis	*iris paralysis*
kerat/o	horny tissue; hard; cornea	**kerat**/o/plasty (KĚR-ă-tō-plăs-tē) *-plasty:* surgical repair	*surgical cornea repair*

Combining Form	Meaning	Medical Word	Meaning
Eye			
ocul/o	eye	intra/**ocul**/ar (ĭn-tră-ŎK-ū-lăr) *intra-:* in, within -*ar:* pertaining to	pertaining to within the eye
ophthalm/o		**ophthalm**/o/scope (ŏf-THĂL-mō-skōp) -*scope:* instrument for examining	instrument for examining eye
opt/o	eye, vision	**opt**/ic (ŎP-tĭk) -*ic:* pertaining to	pertaining to eye
retin/o	retina	**retin**/o/pathy (rĕt-ĭn-ŎP-ă-thē) -*pathy:* disease	retina disease
Ear			
acous/o	hearing	**acous**/tic (ă-KOOS-tik) -*tic:* pertaining to	pertaining to hearing
audi/o		**audi**/o/meter (aw-dē-ŎM-ĕ-tĕr) -*meter:* instrument for measuring	instrument for measuring hearing
audit/o		**audit**/ory (AW-dĭ-tō-rē) -*ory:* pertaining to	pertaining to hearing
myring/o	tympanic membrane (eardrum)	**myring**/o/tomy (mĭr-ĭn-GŎT-ō-mē) -*tomy:* incision	tympanic incision
tympan/o		**tympan**/o/plasty (tĭm-păn-ō-PLĂS-tē) -*plasty:* surgical repair	surgical repair of eardrum
ot/o	ear	**ot**/o/rrhea (ō-tō-RĒ-ă) -*rrhea:* discharge, flow	ear discharge
salping/o	tube (usually fallopian or eustachian [auditory] tubes)	**salping**/o/pharyng/eal (săl-pĭng-gō-fă-RĬN-jē-ăl) *pharyng:* pharynx (throat) -*eal:* pertaining to	pertaining to pharynx

Suffixes and Prefixes

In the table that follows, suffixes and prefixes are listed alphabetically, and other word parts are defined as needed. Review the medical word and study the elements that make up the term. Then complete the meaning of the medical words in the right-hand column. You may also refer to *Appendix A: Glossary of Medical Word Elements* to complete this exercise.

Word Element	Meaning	Medical Words	Meaning
Suffixes			
-acusis	hearing	an/**acusis** (ăn-ă-KŪ-sĭs) *an-:* without, not	*without hearing*
-cusis		presby/**cusis** (prĕz-bĭ-KŪ-sĭs) *presby:* old age	*old age hearing*
-opia	vision	ambly/**opia** (ăm-blē-Ō-pē-ă) *ambly:* dull, dim	*dull vision*
-opsia		heter/**opsia** (hĕt-ĕr-ŎP-sē-ă) *heter-:* different	*different vision*
-ptosis	prolapse, downward displacement	blephar/o/**ptosis** (blĕf-ă-rō-TŌ-sĭs) *blephar/o:* eyelid	*prolapsed eyelid*
Prefixes			
exo-	outside, outward	**exo**/tropia (ĕks-ō-TRŌ-pē-ă) *-tropia:* turning	*turning outward*
hyper-	excessive, above normal	**hyper**/opia (hī-pĕr-Ō-pē-ă) *-opia:* vision	*excessive vision*

 Competency Verification: Check your answers in Appendix B, Answer Key, pages 388–390. If you are not satisfied with your level of comprehension, review the terms in the table and retake the review.

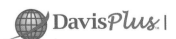 Visit the *Medical Terminology Express* online resource center at *DavisPlus* for an audio exercise of the terms in this table. Other activities are also available to reinforce content.

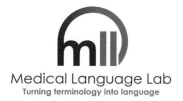

Medical Language Lab
Turning terminology into language

Visit the Medical Language Lab at *medicallanguagelab.com* to enhance your study and reinforce this chapter's word elements with the flash-card activity. We recommend you complete the flash-card activity before continuing with the next section.

Medical Terminology Word Building

In this section, combine the word parts you have learned to construct medical terms related to the eyes and the ears.

Use *ophthalm/o* (eye) to build words that mean:

1. paralysis of the eye ___ophthalmoplegia___

2. study of the eye ___ophthalmology___

Use *pupill/o* (pupil) to build a word that means:

3. examination of the pupil ___pupilloscopy___

Use *kerat/o* (cornea) to build words that mean:

4. softening of the cornea ___keratomalacia___

5. instrument for measuring the cornea ___keratometer___

Use *scler/o* (sclera) to build words that mean:

6. inflammation of the sclera ___scleritis___

7. softening of the sclera ___scleromalacia___

Use *irid/o* (iris) to build words that mean:

8. paralysis of the iris ___iridoplegia___

9. herniation of the iris ___iridocele___

Use *retin/o* (retina) to build words that mean:

10. disease of the retina ___retinopathy___

11. inflammation of the retina ___retinitis___

Use *blephar/o* (eyelid) to build words that mean:

12. paralysis of the eyelid ___blepharoplegia___

13. prolapse of the eyelid ___blepharoptosis___

14. surgical repair of the eyelid ___blepharoplasty___

Use *ot/o* (ear) to build a word that means:

15. flow of pus from the ear ___otopyorrhea___

Use *audi/o* (hearing) to build a word that means:

16. instrument for measuring hearing <u>audiometer</u>

Use *myring/o* (tympanic membrane [eardrum]) to build words that mean:

17. instrument for cutting the eardrum <u>Myringotome</u>

18. surgical repair of the tympanic membrane <u>myringoplasty</u>

Use *salping/o* (tube, usually fallopian or eustachian [auditory] tubes) to build words that means:

19. inflammation of the eustachian tube <u>Salpingitis</u>

20. pertaining to the eustachian tube and throat <u>Salpingopharyngeal</u>

 Competency Verification: Check your answers in Appendix B, Answer Key, page 390. Review material that you did not answer correctly.

Correct Answers: _____ × 5 = _____ %

MEDICAL VOCABULARY

The following tables consist of selected terms that pertain to diseases and conditions of the eyes and ears. Terms related to diagnostic, medical, and surgical procedures are included as well as pharmacological agents used to treat diseases. Recognizing and learning these terms will help you understand the connection between diseases and their treatments. Word analyses for selected terms are also provided.

Diseases and Conditions

Eye

achromatopsia
 ă-krō-mă-TŎP-sē-ă
    a-: without, not
 chromat: color
  -opsia: vision
	Congenital deficiency in color perception that is more common in men; also called *color blindness*

astigmatism
 ă-STĬG-mă-tĭzm
    a-: without, no
 stigmat: point, mark
  -ism: condition
	Refractive disorder in which excessive curvature of the cornea or lens causes light to be scattered over the retina, rather than focused on a single point, resulting in a distorted image (See Figure 13-1.)

cataract KĂT-ă-răkt	Degenerative disease that is due mainly to the aging process in which the lens of the eye becomes progressively cloudy, causing decreased vision, and that is treated with cataract surgery (phacoemulsification) (See Figure 13-2.)

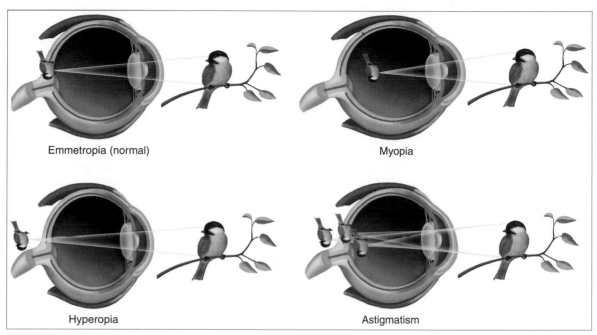

Figure 13-1 Refraction of the eye.

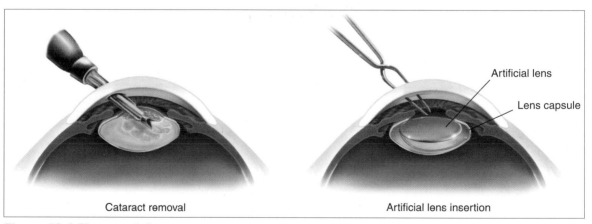

Figure 13-2 Phacoemulsification.

conjunctivitis kŏn-jŭnk-tĭ-VĪ-tĭs *conjunctiv:* conjunctiva *-itis:* inflammation	Inflammation of the conjunctiva that can be caused by bacteria, allergy, irritation, or a foreign body; also called *pinkeye*

diabetic retinopathy dī-ă-BĔT-ĭk rĕt-ĭn-ŎP-ă-thē *retin/o:* retina *-pathy:* disease	Retinal damage in diabetic patients marked by aneurysmal dilation and bleeding of blood vessels or the formation of new blood vessels causing visual changes
hordeolum hor-DĒ-ō-lŭm	Small, purulent, inflammatory infection of a sebaceous gland of the eyelid; also called *sty* (See Figure 13-3.)
macular degeneration MĂK-ū-lăr	Deterioration of the macula, resulting in loss of central vision; most common cause of visual impairment in persons older than age 50 (See Figure 13-4.)
photophobia fō-tō-FŌ-bē-ă *phot/o:* light *-phobia:* fear	Unusual intolerance and sensitivity to light that occurs in disorders such as meningitis, eye inflammation, measles, and rubella
retinal detachment RĔT-ĭ-năl *retin:* retina *-al:* pertaining to	Separation of the retina from the choroid, which disrupts vision and results in blindness if not repaired
strabismus stră-BĬZ-mŭs	Muscular eye disorder in which the eyes turn from the normal position so that they deviate in different directions (See Figure 13-5.)
esotropia ĕs-ō-TRŌ-pē-ă *eso-:* inward *-tropia:* turning	Strabismus in which there is deviation of the visual axis of one eye toward that of the other eye, resulting in diplopia; also called *cross-eye* or *convergent strabismus* (See Figure 13-5A.)
exotropia ĕks-ō-TRŌ-pē-ă *exo-:* outside, outward *-tropia:* turning	Strabismus in which there is deviation of the visual axis of one eye away from that of the other, resulting in diplopia; also called *wall-eye* or *divergent strabismus* (See Figure 13-5B.)

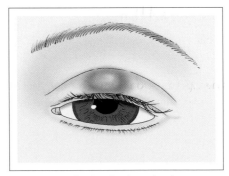

Figure 13-3 Hordeolum (sty).

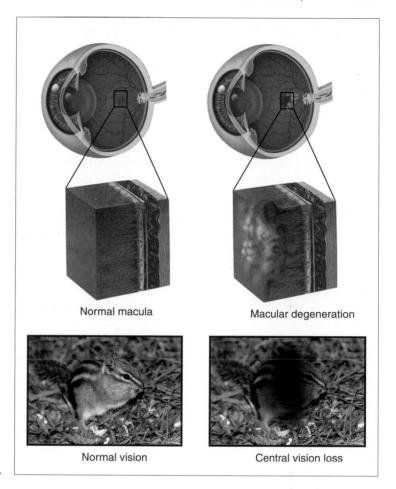

Normal macula

Macular degeneration

Normal vision

Central vision loss

Figure 13-4 Macular degeneration.

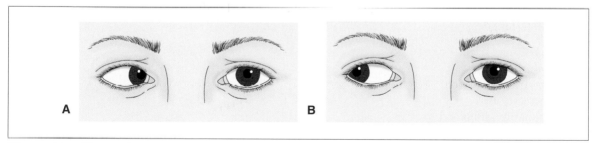

Figure 13-5 Types of strabismus. (A) Esotropia (affected eye turns inward). (B) Exotropia (affected eye turns outward).

Ear

hearing loss	Loss of sense or perception of sound
anacusis ăn-ă-KŪ-sĭs *an-:* without, not *-acusis:* hearing	Total deafness (complete hearing loss)
conductive	Results from any condition that prevents sound waves from being transmitted to the auditory receptors
presbycusis prĕz-bĭ-KŪ-sĭs *presby:* old age *cusis:* hearing	Hearing loss that gradually occurs in most individuals as they grow older
sensorineural sĕn-sō-rē-NŪ-răl	Inability of nerve stimuli to be delivered to the brain from the inner ear as a result of damage to the auditory (acoustic) nerve or cochlea; also called *nerve deafness*
Ménière disease mĕn-ē-ĀR	Rare disorder characterized by progressive deafness, vertigo, and tinnitus, possibly secondary to swelling of membranous structures within the labyrinth

otitis media (OM)
ō-TĪ-tĭs MĒ-dē-ă
  ot: ear
-itis: inflammation
med: middle
  -ia: condition
	Inflammation of the middle ear, which is commonly the result of an upper respiratory infection (URI) and may be treated with tympanostomy tube insertion
	
	Get a closer look at tympanostomy tube insertion on page 336.

otosclerosis ō-tō-sklĕ-RŌ-sĭs *ot/o:* ear *scler:* hardening; sclera (white of eye) *-osis:* abnormal condition; increase (used primarily with blood cells)	Progressive deafness secondary to ossification in the bony labyrinth of the inner ear
tinnitus tĭn-Ī-tĭs	Ringing or tinkling noise heard constantly or intermittently in one or both ears, even in a quiet environment, that usually results from damage to inner ear structures associated with hearing
vertigo VĔR-tĭ-gō	Sensation of moving around in space or a feeling of spinning or dizziness that usually results from inner ear structure damage associated with balance and equilibrium

Diagnostic Procedures

Eye

tonometry tōn-ŎM-ĕ-trē 　*ton/o:* tension *-metry:* act of measuring	Test to measure the pressure inside the eyes (intraocular pressure); used to screen for glaucoma (See Figure 13-6.)
visual acuity test ă-KŪ-ĭ-tē	Standard eye examination to determine the smallest letters a person can read on a Snellen chart, or E chart, at a distance of 20 feet (See Figure 13-7.)

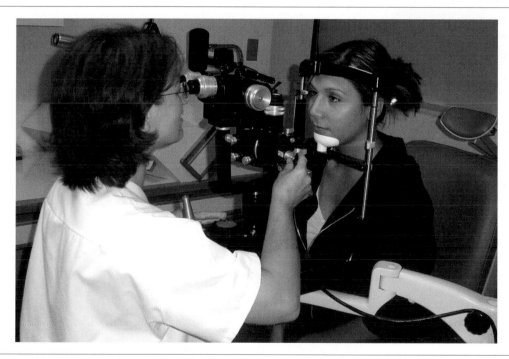

Figure 13-6 Tonometry.

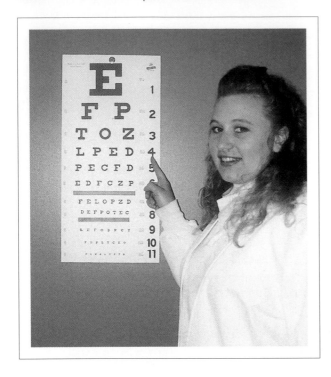

Figure 13-7 Snellen chart is used to assess visual acuity.

Ear

audiometry ăw-dē-ŎM-ĕ-trē *audi/o:* hearing *-metry:* act of measuring	Test that measures hearing acuity at various sound frequencies
otoscopy ō-TŎS-kŏ-pē *ot/o:* ear *-scopy:* visual examination	Visual examination of the external auditory canal and the tympanic membrane using an otoscope
tuning fork test	Hearing tests that use a tuning fork (instrument that produces a constant pitch when struck) that is struck and then placed against or near the bones on the side of the head to assess nerve and bone conduction of sound
Rinne RĬN-nē	Evaluates bone conduction of sound in one ear at a time
Weber WĔB-ĕr	Evaluates bone conduction of sound in both ears at the same time

Medical and Surgical Procedures

Eye

cataract surgery KĂT-ă-răkt	Excision of a lens affected by a cataract
phacoemulsification FĂK-ō-ē-mŭl-sĭ-fĭ-kā-shŭn	Excision of the lens by ultrasonic vibrations that break the lens into tiny particles, which are suctioned out of the eye; also called *small incision cataract surgery (SICS)* (See Figure 13-2.)
iridectomy ĭr-ĭ-DĔK-tŏ-mē *irid:* iris *-ectomy:* excision, removal	Excision of a portion of the iris used to relieve intraocular pressure in patients with glaucoma
laser iridotomy ĭr-ĭ-DŎT-ō-mē *irid/o:* iris *-tomy:* incision	Laser surgery that creates an opening on the rim of the iris to allow aqueous humor to flow between the anterior and posterior chambers to relieve intraocular pressure that occurs as a result of glaucoma; is replacing iridectomy because it is a safer procedure
laser photocoagulation fō-tō-kō-ăg-ū-LĀ-shŭn	Use of a laser beam to seal leaking or hemorrhaging retinal blood vessels to treat diabetic retinopathy

Ear

cochlear implant KŎK-lē-ăr *cochle:* cochlea *-ar:* pertaining to	Electronic transmitter surgically implanted into the cochlea of a deaf person to restore hearing
ear irrigation ĭr ĭr-ĭ-gā-shŭn	Process of flushing the external ear canal with sterile water or sterile saline solution to treat blockages of a foreign body or cerumen (ear wax) impaction (See Figure 13-8.)
myringoplasty mĭr-ĬN-gō-plăst-ē *myring/o:* tympanic membrane (eardrum) *-plasty:* surgical repair	Surgical repair of a perforated eardrum with a tissue graft to correct hearing loss; also called *tympanoplasty*
myringotomy mĭr-ĭn-GŎT-ō-mē *myring/o:* tympanic membrane (eardrum) *-tomy:* incision	Incision of the tympanic membrane (eardrum) to relieve pressure and drain fluid from the middle ear or to insert tympanostomy tubes in the eardrum via surgery Get a closer look at tympanostomy tube insertion on page 336.

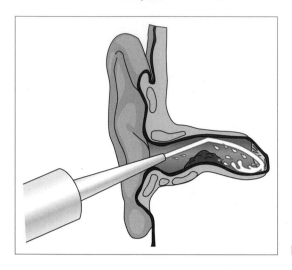

Figure 13-8 Ear irrigation.

Pharmacology

antiglaucoma agents ăn-tĭ-glaw-KŌ-mă	Reduce intraocular pressure by decreasing the amount of aqueous humor in the eyeball either by reducing its production or by increasing its outflow
miotics mī-ŎT-ĭks	Cause the pupil to constrict
mydriatics mĭd-rē-ĂT-ĭks	Cause the pupil to dilate and prepare the eye for an internal examination
vertigo and motion sickness agents VĔR-tĭ-gō	Decrease sensitivity of the inner ear to motion and prevent nerve impulses from the inner ear from reaching the vomiting center of the brain
wax emulsifiers ē-MŬL-sĭ-fī-ĕrs	Loosen and help remove impacted cerumen (ear wax)

Pronunciation Help	Long Sound	ā in rāte	ē in rēbirth	ī in īsle	ō in ōver	ū in ūnite
	Short Sound	ă in ălone	ĕ in ĕver	ĭ in ĭt	ŏ in nŏt	ŭ in cŭt

A Closer Look

Take a closer look at the following eye disorders and ear procedures to enhance your understanding of the medical terminology associated with them.

Glaucoma

Glaucoma is a condition in which the aqueous humor fails to drain properly and accumulates in the anterior chamber of the eye, causing elevated **intraocular pressure (IOP)**. The increased IOP leads to degeneration and atrophy of the retina and optic nerve. There are two forms of glaucoma: open-angle

A Closer Look—cont'd

and closed-angle. **Open-angle glaucoma** is the most common form. It results from degenerative changes that cause congestion and reduce flow of aqueous humor through the canal of Schlemm. This type of glaucoma is painless but destroys peripheral vision, causing tunnel vision. Closed-angle glaucoma is a medical emergency. This type of glaucoma is caused by an anatomically narrow angle between the iris and the cornea, which prevents outflow of aqueous humor from the eye into the lymphatic system, causing a sudden increase in IOP. Symptoms include severe pain, blurred vision, and photophobia. Glaucoma eventually leads to vision loss and, commonly, blindness. Treatment for glaucoma includes eyedrops **(miotics)** that cause the pupils to constrict, permitting aqueous humor to escape from the eye, relieving pressure. If miotics are ineffective, surgery may be necessary. The illustration that follows shows the normal flow of aqueous humor (*yellow arrows*) and an abnormal flow of aqueous humor (*red arrow*), causing destruction of the optic nerve.

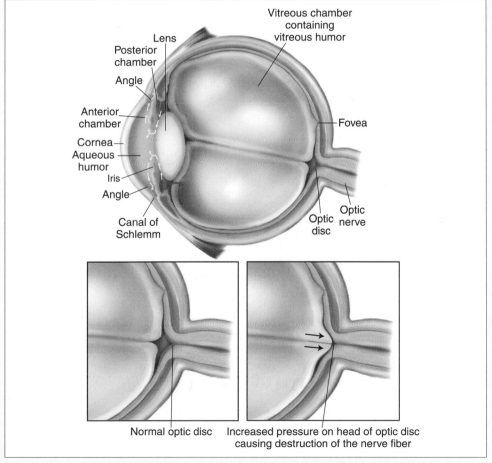

Glaucoma, with the eye showing a normal flow of aqueous humor (*yellow arrow*), causing destruction of the optic nerve.

(Continued)

A Closer Look—cont'd

Tympanostomy Tube Insertion

Tympanostomy tubes, also known as **ear tubes** or **pressure-equalizing (PE) tubes,** are plastic cylinders surgically inserted into the eardrum to drain fluid and equalize pressure between the middle and outer ear. PE tubes are most commonly used in children who have recurrent ear infections that do not respond to antibiotics, or when fluid remains behind the eardrum. Tympanostomy tube insertion is an outpatient surgery performed by an otolaryngologist while the child is under general anesthesia. As seen in the illustration that follows, a small opening is made in the eardrum (**tympanostomy,** or **myringotomy**) followed by tube insertion. The tube decreases the feeling of pressure in the ears, reduces pain, and allows air to enter the middle ear and fluid to flow out of the middle ear and into the ear canal. Postsurgical recovery is usually rapid with little pain or other symptoms. Tubes normally remain in the ears for 6 to 12 months. They commonly fall out on their own, or they may require surgical removal.

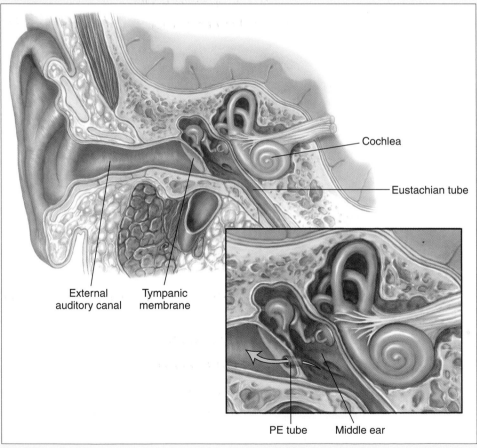

Placement of a pressure-equalizing (PE) tube.

Medical Vocabulary Recall

Match the medical terms below with the definitions in the numbered list.

achromatopsia	conjunctivitis	Ménière disease	photophobia	strabismus
anacusis	glaucoma	myringoplasty	presbycusis	tinnitus
astigmatism	hordeolum	otitis media	retinal detachment	tonometry
cataract	iridectomy	otosclerosis	Rinne	vertigo

1. **tinnitus** _____ means ringing in the ears.

2. **ostosclerosis** _____ is progressive deafness resulting from ossification in the bony labyrinth of the inner ear.

3. **achromatopsia** _____ means color blindness.

4. **Meniere disease** _____ is characterized by progressive deafness, vertigo, and tinnitus.

5. **Strabismus** _____ is a muscular eye disorder in which the eyes deviate in different directions.

6. **anacusis** _____ means total deafness.

7. **otitis media** _____ refers to middle ear infection, commonly seen in young children.

8. **conjunctivitis** _____ refers to pinkeye.

9. **photophobia** _____ means intolerance or unusual sensitivity to light.

10. **presbycusis** _____ is hearing loss that commonly occurs as people age.

11. **glaucoma** _____ refers to increased intraocular pressure caused by failure of the aqueous humor to drain.

12. **vertigo** _____ refers to a feeling of spinning or dizziness.

13. **retinal detachment** _____ refers to separation of the retina from the choroid.

14. **hordeolum** _____ is another term for sty.

15. **astigmatism** _____ is a refractive disorder in which light scatters over the retina resulting in a distorted image.

16. **myringoplasty** _____ is a surgical repair of the eardrum.

17. **tonometry** _____ measures intraocular pressure; used to diagnose glaucoma.

18. **iridectomy** _____ refers to excision of a portion of the iris.

19. **Rinne** _____ is a hearing test performed with a vibrating tuning fork.

20. **cataract** _____ refers to opacity (cloudiness) of the lens.

Competency Verification: Check your answers in Appendix B, Answer Key, on page 390. Review material that you did not answer correctly.

Correct Answers: _____ × **5** = _____ %

Pronunciation and Spelling

Use the following list to practice correct pronunciation and spelling of medical terms. Practice the pronunciation aloud and then write the correct spelling of the term. The first word is completed for you.

Pronunciation	Spelling
1. a-KOOS-tĭk nū-RŌ-mă	*acoustic neuroma*
2. ă-krō-mă-TŎP-sē-ă	achromatopsia
3. ă-STĬG-mă-tĭzm	astigmatism
4. AW-dĭ-tō-rē	auditory
5. blĕf-ă-rō-TŌ-sĭs	blepharoptosis
6. dăk-rē-ō-RĒ-ă	dacryorrhea
7. ĕks-ō-TRŌ-pē-ă	exotropia
8. FĂK-ō-ē-mŭl-sĭ-fĭ-kā-shŭn	phaccemulsification
9. glaw-KŌ-mă	glaucoma
10. hor-DĒ-ō-lŭm	hordeolum
11. ĭr-ĭd-ō-PLĒ-jē-ă	iridopleqia
12. kŏn-jŭnk-tĭ-VĪ-tĭs	conjunctivitis
13. mĕn-ē-ĀR	Meniere
14. ŏf-THĂL-mō-skōp	opthalmuscope
15. prĕz-bĭ-KŪ-sĭs	preshycusis
16. săl-pĭng-gō-fă-RĬN-jē-ăl	Salpingophorungeal
17. stră-BĬZ-mŭs	Strabismus
18. tĭm-păn-ō-PLĂS-tē	tumpanoplasty
19. tĭn-Ī-tĭs	tinnitus
20. VĔR-tĭ-gō	vertigo

 Competency Verification: Check your answers in Appendix B, Answer Key, on page 390. Review material that you did not answer correctly.

Correct Answers: _____ × 5 = _____ %

ABBREVIATIONS

The table that follows introduces abbreviations associated with the eyes and the ears.

Abbreviation	Meaning	Abbreviation	Meaning
ARMD	age-related macular degeneration	Myop	myopia
Ast	astigmatism	OM	otitis media
ENT	ear, nose, and throat	SICS	small incision cataract surgery
IOP	intraocular pressure	ST	esotropia

CHART NOTES

Chart notes make up part of the medical record and are used in various types of health care facilities. The chart notes that follow were dictated by the patient's physician and reflect common clinical events using medical terminology to document the patient's care. Studying and completing the terminology and chart notes sections below will help you learn and understand terms associated with the medical specialty of otolaryngology.

Terminology

The following terms are linked to chart notes in the specialty of otolaryngology. First, practice pronouncing each term aloud. Then use a medical dictionary such as *Taber's Cyclopedic Medical Dictionary; Appendix A: Glossary of Medical Word Elements,* or other resources to define each term.

Term	Meaning
cholesteatoma kō-lē-stē-ă-TŌ-mă	
ENT	
general anesthesia ăn-ĕs-THĒ-zē-ă	
mucoserous mū-kō-SĒR-ŭs	
otitis media ō-TĪ-tĭs MĒ-dē-ă	
postoperatively pōst-ŎP-ĕr-ă-tĭv-lē	
tympanoplasty tĭm-păn-ō-PLĂS-tē	

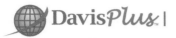 | Visit *Medical Terminology Express* at *DavisPlus* Online Resource Center. Use it to practice pronunciations and reinforce the meanings of the terms in this chart note.

Cholesteatoma

Read the chart note that follows aloud. Underline any term you have trouble pronouncing and any terms that you cannot define. If needed, refer to the Terminology section on page 339 for correct pronunciations and meanings of terms.

This 30-year-old white woman was seen by the ENT specialist for a diagnosis of mucoserous otitis media on the right. Patient was admitted to City Hospital and developed cholesteatoma. A tube was inserted for chronic adhesive otitis media with secondary cholesteatoma. Patient progressed favorably postoperatively, but the cholesteatoma continues to enlarge in size. Presently she is in the hospital for a right tympanoplasty under general anesthetic.

Chart Note Analysis

From the preceding chart note, select the medical word that means
1. of long duration: _Chronic_
2. composed of mucus and serum: _mucoserous_
3. surgical repair of the eardrum: _tympanoplasty_
4. inflammation of the inner ear: _otitis media_
5. abbreviation that refers to *ear, nose, and throat*: _ENT_
6. cystlike sac filled with cholesterol and epithelial cells: _Cholesteatoma_
7. agent that causes loss of sensation to the entire body and results in a loss of consciousness: _general anesthetic_
8. term denoting the name of a disease a person has or is believed to have: _diagnosis_
9. causing two surfaces to unite: _adhesive_
10. following a surgical procedure: _postoperatively_

✓ **Competency Verification:** Check your answers in Appendix B, Answer Key, on page 390. Review material that you did not answer correctly.

Correct Answers: _____ × 10 = _____ %

Demonstrate What You Know!

To evaluate your understanding of how medical terms you have studied in this and previous chapters are used in a clinical environment, complete the numbered sentences by selecting an appropriate term from the words below.

anacusis	cholesteatoma	exotropia	myringotomy	presbycusis
blepharoplasty	diagnosis	heteropsia	ophthalmoplegia	tympanitis
blepharoptosis	esotropia	mydriatics	otitis media	vertigo

1. When a person experiences a stroke and is unable to move his or her eyes, the condition is called _ophthalmoplegia_.

2. A deviation of one eye toward the other eye is a type of strabismus called _esotropia_.

3. An eye tuck, also called _blepharoplasty_ a cosmetic procedure to remove wrinkles from the eyelid.

4. Agents that dilate the pupil to prepare the eye for an internal examination are called _mydriatics_

5. A patient is diagnosed with an inequality of vision. The diagnosis is charted as _heteropsia_.

6. A deviation of one eye away from the other eye is a type of strabismus called _exotropia_.

7. If a stroke results in facial paralysis, the patient may experience drooping eyelids. This condition is charted as _blepharoptosis_.

8. _diagnosis_ is a term denoting the disease a person has or is believed to have.

9. The medical term for a cystlike sac filled with cholesterol is _cholesteatoma_.

10. The diagnosis for a patient with inflammation of an eardrum is _tympanitis_.

11. _vertigo_ refers to a feeling of spinning or dizziness.

12. _presbycusis_ is a gradual hearing loss that occurs as people age.

13. _otitis media_ is a middle ear infection commonly seen in young children.

14. _anacusis_ refers to a state of complete deafness.

15. _myringotomy_ is an incision of the eardrum to relieve pressure and release fluid in the middle ear.

 Competency Verification: Check your answers in Appendix B, Answer Key, on page 390. Review material that you did not answer correctly.

Correct Answers: _____ × 6.67 = _____ %

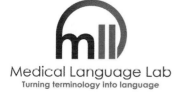
Medical Language Lab
Turning terminology into language

If you are not satisfied with your retention level of the special senses chapter, visit *DavisPlus* Student Online Resource Center and the Medical Language Lab to complete the website activities linked to this chapter.

Glossary of Medical Word Elements

Medical Word Element	Meaning	Medical Word Element	Meaning
A		-al	pertaining to
a-	without, not	albin/o	white
ab-	from, away from	albumin/o	albumin (protein)
abdomin/o	abdomen	-algesia	pain
-ac	pertaining to	-algia	pain
acous/o	hearing	allo-	other
acr/o	extremity	alveol/o	alveolus; air sac
acromi/o	acromion (projection of scapula)	ambly/o	dull, dim
		amni/o	amnion (amniotic sac)
-acusis	hearing	an-	without, not
-ad	toward	an/o	anus
ad-	toward	ana-	against; up; back
aden/o	gland	andr/o	male
adenoid/o	adenoids	aneurysm/o	widened blood vessel
adip/o	fat	angi/o	vessel (usually blood or lymph)
adren/o	adrenal glands	aniso-	unequal, dissimilar
adrenal/o	adrenal glands	ankyl/o	stiffness; bent, crooked
aer/o	air	ante-	before, in front of
agglutin/o	clumping, gluing		

(Continued)

Medical Word Element	Meaning	Medical Word Element	Meaning
anter/o	anterior, front	**B**	
anthrac/o	coal, coal dust	bacteri/o	bacteria (singular, *bacterium*)
anti-	against	balan/o	glans penis
aort/o	aorta	bas/o	base (alkaline, opposite of acid)
append/o	appendix	bi-	two
appendic/o	appendix	bi/o	life
aque/o	water	bil/i	bile, gall
-ar	pertaining to	-blast	embryonic cell
-arche	beginning	blast/o	embryonic cell
arter/o	artery	blephar/o	eyelid
arteri/o	artery	brachi/o	arm
arteriol/o	arteriole (small artery)	brachy-	short
arthr/o	joint	brady-	slow
-ary	pertaining to	bronch/o	bronchus (plural, *bronchi*)
-asthenia	weakness, debility	bronchi/o	bronchus (plural, *bronchi*)
astr/o	star	bronchiol/o	bronchiole
-ate	having the form of, possessing	bucc/o	cheek
atel/o	incomplete; imperfect	**C**	
ather/o	fatty plaque	calc/o	calcium
-ation	process (of)	calcane/o	calcaneum (heel bone)
atri/o	atrium	-capnia	carbon dioxide (CO_2)
audi/o	hearing	carcin/o	cancer
audit/o	hearing	cardi/o	heart
aur/o	ear	-cardia	heart condition
auricul/o	ear	carp/o	carpus (wrist bones)
auto-	self, own	caud/o	tail
azot/o	nitrogenous compounds		

Medical Word Element	Meaning	Medical Word Element	Meaning
cauter/o	heat, burn	-clast	to break
-cele	hernia, swelling	clavicul/o	clavicle (collar bone)
-centesis	surgical puncture	-cleisis	closure
cephal/o	head	-clysis	irrigation, washing
-ceps	head	coccyg/o	coccyx (tail bone)
-ception	conceiving	cochle/o	cochlea
cerebell/o	cerebellum	col/o	colon
cerebr/o	cerebrum	colon/o	colon
cervic/o	neck; cervix uteri (neck of uterus)	colp/o	vagina
		condyl/o	condyle
cheil/o	lip	coni/o	dust
chem/o	chemical; drug	conjunctiv/o	conjunctiva
chlor/o	green	-continence	to hold back
chol/e	bile, gall	contra-	against, opposite
cholangi/o	bile vessel	cor/o	pupil
cholecyst/o	gallbladder	core/o	pupil
choledoch/o	bile duct	corne/o	cornea
chondr/o	cartilage	coron/o	heart
chori/o	chorion	corp/o	body
choroid/o	choroid	corpor/o	body
chrom/o	color	cortic/o	cortex
chromat/o	color	cost/o	ribs
-cide	killing	crani/o	cranium (skull)
cine-	movement	crin/o	secrete
circum-	around	-crine	secrete
cirrh/o	yellow	cruci/o	cross
-cision	a cutting	cry/o	cold
-clasia	to break; surgical fracture	crypt/o	hidden
-clasis	to break; surgical fracture		

(Continued)

Medical Word Element	Meaning	Medical Word Element	Meaning
-cusia	hearing	dist/o	far, farthest
-cusis	hearing	dors/o	back (of body)
cutane/o	skin	duct/o	to lead; carry
cyan/o	blue	-duction	act of leading, bringing, conducting
cycl/o	ciliary body of eye; circular; cycle	duoden/o	duodenum (first part of small intestine)
-cyesis	pregnancy	-dynia	pain
cyst/o	bladder	dys-	bad; painful; difficult
cyt/o	cell		
-cyte	cell	**E**	
		-eal	pertaining to
D		ec-	out, out from
dacry/o	tear; lacrimal apparatus (duct, sac, or gland)	echo-	a repeated sound
dacryocyst/o	lacrimal sac	-ectasis	dilation, expansion
dactyl/o	fingers; toes	ecto-	outside, outward
de-	cessation	-ectomy	excision, removal
dent/o	teeth	-edema	swelling
derm/o	skin	electr/o	electricity
-derma	skin	-ema	state of; condition
dermat/o	skin	embol/o	embolus (plug)
-desis	binding, fixation (of a bone or joint)	-emesis	vomiting
di-	double	-emia	blood condition
dia-	through, across	emphys/o	to inflate
dipl-	double	en-	in, within
dipl/o	double	encephal/o	brain
diplo-	double	end-	in, within
dips/o	thirst	endo-	in, within
-dipsia	thirst	enter/o	intestine (usually small intestine)

Medical Word Element	Meaning	Medical Word Element	Meaning
epi-	above, upon	**G**	
epididym/o	epididymis	galact/o	milk
epiglott/o	epiglottis	gangli/o	ganglion (knot or knotlike mass)
episi/o	vulva	gastr/o	stomach
erot/o	sexual desire	-gen	forming, producing, origin
erythem/o	red	gen/o	forming, producing, origin
erythemat/o	red	-genesis	forming, producing, origin
erythr/o	red	genit/o	genitalia
eschar/o	scab	gest/o	pregnancy
-esis	condition	gingiv/o	gum(s)
eso-	inward	glauc/o	gray
esophag/o	esophagus	gli/o	glue; neuroglial tissue
esthes/o	feeling	-glia	glue; neuroglial tissue
-esthesia	feeling	-globin	protein
eti/o	cause	glomerul/o	glomerulus
eu-	good, normal	gloss/o	tongue
ex-	out, out from	gluc/o	sugar, sweetness
exo-	outside, outward	glucos/o	sugar, sweetness
extra-	outside	glyc/o	sugar, sweetness
F		glycos/o	sugar, sweetness
faci/o	face	gnos/o	knowing
fasci/o	band, fascia (fibrous membrane supporting and separating muscles)	-gnosis	knowing
		gon/o	seed (ovum or spermatozoon)
femor/o	femur (thigh bone)	gonad/o	gonads, sex glands
-ferent	to carry	-grade	to go
fibr/o	fiber, fibrous tissue	-graft	transplantation
fibul/o	fibula (smaller bone of lower leg)	-gram	record, writing
fluor/o	luminous, fluorescence	granul/o	granule

(Continued)

Medical Word Element	Meaning	Medical Word Element	Meaning
-graph	instrument for recording	**I**	
-graphy	process of recording	-ia	condition
-gravida	pregnant woman	-iac	pertaining to
gyn/o	woman, female	-iasis	abnormal condition (produced by something specified)
gynec/o	woman, female	iatr/o	physician; medicine; treatment
H		-iatry	medicine; treatment
hem/o	blood	-ic	pertaining to
hemangi/o	blood vessel	-ical	pertaining to
hemat/o	blood	-ice	noun ending
hemi-	one half	ichthy/o	dry, scaly
hepat/o	liver	-ician	specialist
hetero-	different	-icle	small, minute
hidr/o	sweat	-icterus	jaundice
hirsut/o	hairy	idi/o	unknown, peculiar
hist/o	tissue	-ile	pertaining to
histi/o	tissue	ile/o	ileum (third part of small intestine)
home/o	same, alike	ili/o	ilium (lateral, flaring portion of hip bone)
homeo-	same, alike		
homo-	same	im-	not
humer/o	humerus (upper arm bone)	immun/o	immune, immunity, safe
hydr/o	water	in-	in; not
hyp-	under, below, deficient	-ine	pertaining to
hyp/o	under, below, deficient	infer/o	lower, below
hyper-	excessive, above normal	infra-	below, under
hypn/o	sleep	inguin/o	groin
hypo-	under, below, deficient	insulin/o	insulin
hyster/o	uterus (womb)		

Medical Word Element	Meaning	Medical Word Element	Meaning
inter-	between	kinesi/o	movement
intra-	in, within	-kinesia	movement
-ion	the act of	kinet/o	movement
-ior	pertaining to	klept/o	to steal
irid/o	iris	kyph/o	humpback
-is	noun ending	**L**	
isch/o	to hold back, block	labi/o	lip
ischi/o	ischium (lower portion of hip bone)	labyrinth/o	labyrinth (inner ear)
-ism	condition	lacrim/o	tear; lacrimal apparatus (duct, sac, or gland)
iso-	same, equal	lact/o	milk
-ist	specialist	-lalia	speech, babble
-isy	state of; condition	lamin/o	lamina (part of vertebral arch)
-itic	pertaining to	lapar/o	abdomen
-itis	inflammation	laryng/o	larynx (voice box)
-ive	pertaining to	later/o	side, to one side
-ization	process (of)	lei/o	smooth
J		leiomy/o	smooth muscle (visceral)
jaund/o	yellow	-lepsy	seizure
jejun/o	jejunum (second part of small intestine)	lept/o	thin, slender
		leuk/o	white
K		lingu/o	tongue
kal/i	potassium (an electrolyte)	lip/o	fat
kary/o	nucleus	lipid/o	fat
kerat/o	horny tissue; hard; cornea	-listhesis	slipping
ket/o	ketone bodies (acids and acetones)	-lith	stone, calculus
		lith/o	stone, calculus
keton/o	ketone bodies (acids and acetones)	lob/o	lobe

(Continued)

Medical Word Element	Meaning	Medical Word Element	Meaning
log/o	study of	melan/o	black
-logist	specialist in the study of	men/o	menses, menstruation
-logy	study of	mening/o	meninges (membranes covering brain and spinal cord)
lord/o	curve, swayback		
-lucent	to shine; clear	meningi/o	meninges (membranes covering brain and spinal cord)
lumb/o	loins (lower back)		
lymph/o	lymph	ment/o	mind
lymphaden/o	lymph gland (node)	meso-	middle
lymphangi/o	lymph vessel	meta-	change, beyond
-lysis	separation; destruction; loosening	metacarp/o	metacarpus (hand bones)
		metatars/o	metatarsus (foot bones)
M		-meter	instrument for measuring
macro-	large	metr/o	uterus (womb); measure
mal-	bad	metri/o	uterus (womb)
-malacia	softening	-metry	act of measuring
mamm/o	breast	mi/o	smaller, less
-mania	state of mental disorder, frenzy	micr/o	small
mast/o	breast	micro-	small
mastoid/o	mastoid process	mono-	one
maxill/o	maxilla (upper jaw bone)	morph/o	form, shape, structure
meat/o	opening, meatus	muc/o	mucus
medi-	middle	multi-	many, much
medi/o	middle	muscul/o	muscle
mediastin/o	mediastinum	mut/a	genetic change
medull/o	medulla	my/o	muscle
mega-	enlargement	myc/o	fungus (plural, *fungi*)
megal/o	enlargement	mydr/o	widen, enlarge
-megaly	enlargement	myel/o	bone marrow; spinal cord

Medical Word Element	Meaning	Medical Word Element	Meaning
myos/o	muscle	onc/o	tumor
myring/o	tympanic membrane (eardrum)	onych/o	nail
myx/o	mucus	oophor/o	ovary
N		-opaque	obscure
narc/o	stupor; numbness; sleep	ophthalm/o	eye
nas/o	nose	-opia	vision
nat/o	birth	-opsia	vision
natr/o	sodium (an electrolyte)	-opsy	view of
necr/o	death, necrosis	opt/o	eye, vision
neo-	new	optic/o	eye, vision
nephr/o	kidney	or/o	mouth
neur/o	nerve	orch/o	testis (plural, *testes*)
neutr/o	neutral; neither	orchi/o	testis (plural, *testes*)
nid/o	nest	orchid/o	testis (plural, *testes*)
noct/o	night	-orexia	appetite
nucle/o	nucleus	orth/o	straight
nulli-	none	-ory	pertaining to
nyctal/o	night	-ose	pertaining to; sugar
O		-osis	abnormal condition; increase (used primarily with blood cells)
obstetr/o	midwife	-osmia	smell
ocul/o	eye	oste/o	bone
odont/o	teeth	ot/o	ear
-oid	resembling	-ous	pertaining to
-ole	small, minute	ovari/o	ovary
olig/o	scanty	ox/i	oxygen
-oma	tumor	ox/o	oxygen
omphal/o	navel (umbilicus)	-oxia	oxygen

(Continued)

Medical Word Element	Meaning	Medical Word Element	Meaning
P		-phagia	swallowing, eating
pan-	all	phalang/o	phalanges (bones of fingers and toes)
pancreat/o	pancreas		
para-	near, beside; beyond	pharmaceu-tic/o	drug, medicine
-para	to bear (offspring)	pharyng/o	pharynx (throat)
parathyroid/o	parathyroid glands	-phasia	speech
-paresis	partial paralysis	-phil	attraction for
patell/o	patella (kneecap)	phil/o	attraction for
path/o	disease	-philia	attraction for
-pathy	disease	phleb/o	vein
pector/o	chest	-phobia	fear
ped/i	foot; child	-phonia	voice
ped/o	foot; child	-phoresis	carrying, transmission
pedicul/o	lice	-phoria	feeling (mental state)
pelv/i	pelvis	phot/o	light
pelv/o	pelvis	phren/o	diaphragm; mind
pen/o	penis	-phylaxis	protection
-penia	decrease, deficiency	-physis	growth
-pepsia	digestion	pil/o	hair
per-	through	pituitar/o	pituitary gland
peri-	around	-plakia	plaque
perine/o	perineum (area between scrotum [or vulva in the female] and anus)	plas/o	formation, growth
		-plasia	formation, growth
peritone/o	peritoneum	-plasm	formation, growth
-pexy	fixation (of an organ)	-plasty	surgical repair
phac/o	lens	-plegia	paralysis
phag/o	swallowing, eating	pleur/o	pleura
-phage	swallowing, eating		

Medical Word Element	Meaning	Medical Word Element	Meaning
-plexy	stroke	pub/o	pelvis bone (anterior part of pelvic bone)
-pnea	breathing	pulmon/o	lung
pneum/o	air; lung	pupill/o	pupil
pneumon/o	air; lung	py/o	pus
pod/o	foot	pyel/o	renal pelvis
-poiesis	formation, production	pylor/o	pylorus
poli/o	gray; gray matter (of brain or spinal cord)	pyr/o	fire
poly-	many, much	**Q, R**	
polyp/o	small growth	quadri-	four
-porosis	porous	rachi/o	spine
post-	after, behind	radi/o	radiation, x-ray; radius (lower arm bone on thumb side)
poster/o	back (of body), behind, posterior	radicul/o	nerve root
-potence	power	rect/o	rectum
-prandial	meal	ren/o	kidney
pre-	before, in front of	reticul/o	net, mesh
presby/o	old age	retin/o	retina
primi-	first	retro-	backward, behind
pro-	before, in front of	rhabd/o	rod-shaped (striated)
proct/o	anus, rectum	rhabdomy/o	rod-shaped (striated) muscle
prostat/o	prostate gland	rhin/o	nose
proxim/o	near, nearest	rhytid/o	wrinkle
pseudo-	false	roentgen/o	x-rays
psych/o	mind	-rrhage	bursting forth (of)
-ptosis	prolapse, downward displacement	-rrhagia	bursting forth (of)
ptyal/o	saliva	-rrhaphy	suture
-ptysis	spitting	-rrhea	discharge, flow

(Continued)

Medical Word Element	Meaning	Medical Word Element	Meaning
-rrhexis	rupture	sigmoid/o	sigmoid colon
-rrhythm/o	rhythm	sin/o	sinus, cavity
rube/o	red	sinus/o	sinus, cavity
S		-sis	state of; condition
sacr/o	sacrum	somat/o	body
salping/o	tube (usually fallopian or eustachian [auditory] tubes)	somn/o	sleep
		son/o	sound
-salpinx	tube (usually fallopian or eustachian [auditory] tubes)	-spadias	slit, fissure
		-spasm	involuntary contraction, twitching
sarc/o	flesh (connective tissue)		
-sarcoma	malignant tumor of connective tissue	sperm/i	spermatozoa, sperm cells
		sperm/o	spermatozoa, sperm cells
scapul/o	scapula (shoulder blade)	spermat/o	spermatozoa, sperm cells
-schisis	a splitting	sphygm/o	pulse
schiz/o	split	-sphyxia	pulse
scler/o	hardening; sclera (white of eye)	spin/o	spine
scoli/o	crooked, bent	spir/o	breathe
-scope	instrument for examining	splen/o	spleen
-scopy	visual examination	spondyl/o	vertebra (backbone)
scot/o	darkness	squam/o	scale
seb/o	sebum, sebaceous	staped/o	stapes
semi-	one half	-stasis	standing still
semin/i	semen; seed	steat/o	fat
semin/o	semen; seed	sten/o	narrowing, stricture
sept/o	septum	-stenosis	narrowing, stricture
sequestr/o	separation	stern/o	sternum (breast bone)
ser/o	serum	steth/o	chest
sial/o	saliva, salivary gland	sthen/o	strength
sider/o	iron		

Medical Word Element	Meaning	Medical Word Element	Meaning
stomat/o	mouth	thromb/o	blood clot
-stomy	forming an opening (mouth)	thym/o	thymus gland
sub-	under, below	thyr/o	thyroid gland
sudor/o	sweat	thyroid/o	thyroid gland
super-	upper, above	tibi/o	tibia (larger bone of lower leg)
super/o	upper, above	-tic	pertaining to
supra-	above; excessive; superior	-tocia	childbirth, labor
sym-	union, together, joined	-tome	instrument to cut
syn-	union, together, joined	tom/o	to cut, slice
synapt/o	synapsis, point of contact	-tomy	incision
synov/o	synovial membrane; synovial fluid	ton/o	tension
		tonsill/o	tonsils
T		tox/o	poison
tachy-	rapid	-toxic	poison
tars/o	tarsals	toxic/o	poison
ten/o	tendon	trache/o	trachea (windpipe)
tend/o	tendon	trans-	across, through
tendin/o	tendon	tri-	three
-tension	to stretch	trich/o	hair
test/o	testis (plural, *testes*)	-tripsy	crushing
thalam/o	thalamus	-trophy	development, nourishment
thec/o	sheath (usually refers to meninges)	-tropia	turning
		-tropin	stimulate
thel/o	nipple	tubercul/o	a little swelling
therapeut/o	treatment	tympan/o	tympanic membrane (eardrum)
-therapy	treatment	**U**	
therm/o	heat	-ula	small, minute
thorac/o	chest	-ule	small, minute
-thorax	chest		

(Continued)

Medical Word Element	Meaning	Medical Word Element	Meaning
uln/o	ulna (lower arm bone on opposite side of thumb)	ven/o	vein
		ventr/o	belly, belly side
ultra-	excess, beyond	ventricul/o	ventricle (of heart or brain)
-um	structure, thing	venul/o	venule (small vein)
umbilic/o	umbilicus, navel	-verse	to turn
ungu/o	nail	-version	turning
uni-	one	vertebr/o	vertebra (backbone)
ur/o	urine, urinary tract	vesic/o	bladder
ureter/o	ureter	vesicul/o	seminal vesicle
urethr/o	urethra	viscer/o	internal organs
-uria	urine	vitr/o	vitreous body (of eye)
urin/o	urine, urinary tract	vitre/o	glassy
-us	condition; structure	vulv/o	vulva
uter/o	uterus (womb)		
uvul/o	uvula	**W, X, Y, Z**	
		xanth/o	yellow
V		xen/o	foreign, strange
vagin/o	vagina	xer/o	dry
valv/o	valve	xiph/o	sword
varic/o	dilated vein	-y	condition; process
vas/o	vessel; vas deferens; duct		
vascul/o	vessel (usually blood or lymph)		

Answer Key

CHAPTER 1

Introduction to Medical Terminology

Review Activity 1-1: Matching Word Elements

1. J	**3.** G	**5.** I	**7.** E	**9.** B
2. D	**4.** H	**6.** F	**8.** C	**10.** A

Review Activity 1-2: Understanding Medical Word Elements

1. root, combining form, suffix, and prefix
2. arthr

Identify the following statements as either true or false. If false, rewrite the statement correctly in the space provided.

3. False—A combining vowel is usually an "o."
4. False—A word root links a suffix that begins with a vowel.
5. True
6. True
7. False—Whenever a prefix stands alone, it will be followed by a hyphen.
8. True

Underline the word root in each of following combining forms.

9. <u>splen</u>/o	**12.** <u>neur</u>/o	**15.** <u>hydr</u>/o
10. <u>hyster</u>/o	**13.** <u>ot</u>/o	
11. <u>enter</u>/o	**14.** <u>dermat</u>/o	

Review Activity 1-3: Identifying Word Roots and Combining Forms

1. <u>nephr</u>itis
2. <u>arthr</u>odesis
3. <u>dermat</u>itis
4. <u>arthr</u>ocentesis
5. <u>gastr</u>ectomy
6. nephr (word root)
7. <u>hepat</u>/o
8. arthr (word root)
9. <u>oste</u>/o/arthr
10. <u>cholangi</u>/o

Review Activity 1-4: Defining Medical Words

1. *breast*
2. inflammation
3. colon
4. bone
5. after
6. joint
7. disease
8. pre-
9. gastr/o
10. -pathy
11. mast/o
12. -scope
13. appendix
14. intestine (usually small intestine)
15. -centesis

Review Activity 1-5: Defining and Building Medical Words

Term	Definition
1. col/itis	*inflammation (of) colon*
2. gastr/o/scope	instrument for examining the stomach
3. hepat/itis	inflammation of the liver
4. pre/nat/al	pertaining to (the period) before birth
5. tonsill/ectomy	excision of the tonsils
6. tonsill/itis	inflammation of the tonsils

Write the number for the rule that applies to each listed term and a short summary of the rule.

Term	Rule	Summary of Rule
7. append/ectomy	*1*	*A WR links a suffix that begins with a vowel.*
8. arthr/o/centesis	2	A CF links a suffix that begins with a consonant.
9. col/ectomy	1	A WR links a suffix that begins with a vowel.
10. colon/o/scope	2	A CF links a suffix that begins with a consonant.
11. gastr/itis	1	A WR links a suffix that begins with a vowel.
12. gastr/o/enter/o/ col/itis	3, 1	A CF links multiple roots to each other. This rule holds true even if the next word root begins with a vowel. A WR links a suffix that begins with a vowel.
13. arthr/o/pathy	2	A CF links a suffix that begins with a consonant.
14. oste/o/arthr/itis	3, 1	A CF links multiple roots to each other. This rule holds true even if the next word root begins with a vowel. A WR links a suffix that begins with a vowel.
15. oste/o/chondr/itis	3, 1	A CF links multiple roots to each other. This rule holds true even if the next word root begins with a vowel. A WR links a suffix that begins with a vowel.

Review Activity 1-6: Understanding Pronunciations

1. macron	**3.** long	**5.** k	**7.** is	**9.** second
2. breve	**4.** short	**6.** n	**8.** eye	**10.** separate

Review Activity 1-7: Plural Suffixes

Singular	Plural	Rule
1. sarcoma	*sarcomata*	*Retain the* ma *and add* ta.
2. thrombus	thrombi	Drop *us* and add *i*.
3. appendix	appendices	Drop *ix* and add *ices*.
4. diverticulum	diverticula	Drop *um* and add *a*.
5. ovary	ovaries	Drop *y* and add *ies*.
6. diagnosis	diagnoses	Drop *is* and add *es*.
7. lumen	lumina	Drop *en* and add *ina*.
8. vertebra	vertebrae	Retain the *a* and add *e*.
9. thorax	thoraces	Drop the *x* and add *ces*.
10. spermatozoon	spermatozoa	Drop *on* and add *a*.

Review Activity 1-8: Common Suffixes

Surgical Suffixes

Term	Meaning
arthr/o/**centesis**	*surgical puncture of a joint*
oste/o/**clasis**	surgical breaking or fracture of a bone to correct a deformity; also called *osteoclasia*
arthr/o/**desis**	binding or fixation of a joint
append/**ectomy**	excision or removal of the appendix
thromb/o/**lysis**	separation, destruction, or loosening of a blood clot
mast/o/**pexy**	surgical fixation of the breast(s)
rhin/o/**plasty**	surgical repair of the nose (to change shape or size)
my/o/**rrhaphy**	suture of a muscle

(Continued)

Term	Meaning
trache/o/**stomy**	forming an opening (mouth) into the trachea
oste/o/**tome**	instrument to cut bone
trache/o/**tomy**	incision of the trachea
lith/o/**tripsy**	crushing a stone or calculus

Diagnostic Suffixes

Term	Meaning
electr/o/cardi/o/**gram**	*record of electrical activity of the heart*
cardi/o/**graph**	instrument to record electrical activity of the heart
angi/o/**graphy**	process of recording images of blood vessels (recording images of blood vessels after injection of a contrast medium)
pelv/i/**meter**	instrument for measuring the pelvis
pelv/i/**metry**	act of measuring the pelvis
endo/**scope**	instrument for examining within (instrument for examining inside a hollow organ or cavity)
endo/**scopy**	visual examination within; visual examination of a cavity or canal using a specialized lighted instrument called an *endoscope*

Pathological Suffixes

Term	Meaning
neur/**algia** ot/o/**dynia**	*pain in a nerve; pain along the path of a nerve* pain in the ear (earache)
hepat/o/**cele**	hernia or swelling of the liver
bronchi/**ectasis**	dilation or expansion of a bronchus or bronchi
lymph/**edema**	swelling of lymph tissue (swelling and accumulation of tissue fluid)
hyper/**emesis**	excessive or above normal vomiting
an/**emia**	without blood (blood condition caused by iron deficiency or decrease in red blood cells)

Term	Meaning
chol/e/lith/**iasis**	presence or formation of gallstones (in the gallbladder or common bile duct)
gastr/**itis**	inflammation of the stomach
chol/e/**lith**	gallstone
chondr/o/**malacia**	softening of cartilage
cardi/o/**megaly**	enlargement of the heart
neur/**oma**	tumor composed of nerve cells
cyan/**osis**	abnormal condition of blueness (bluish discoloration of the skin and mucous membrane)
my/o/**pathy**	disease of muscle
erythr/o/**penia**	abnormal decrease or deficiency in red (blood cells)
hem/o/**phobia**	fear of blood
hemi/**plegia**	paralysis of one half (paralysis of one side of the body)
hem/o/**rrhage**	bursting forth of blood (loss of large amounts of blood within a short period, either externally or internally)
men/o/**rrhagia**	bursting forth of menses (profuse discharge of blood during menstruation)
dia/**rrhea**	discharge or flow through (frequent discharge or flow of fluid fecal matter from the bowel)
arteri/o/**rrhexis**	rupture of an artery
arteri/o/**stenosis**	narrowing or stricture of an artery
hepat/o/**toxic**	poisonous or toxic to the liver
dys/**trophy**	bad development or nourishment (abnormal condition caused by defective nutrition or metabolism)

Review Activity 1-9: Common Prefixes

Term	Meaning
a/mast/ia	*without a breast*
an/esthesia	without feeling (partial or complete loss of sensation with or without loss of consciousness)

(Continued)

Term	Meaning
circum/duction	act of leading around (movement of a part, such as an extremity, in a circular direction)
peri/odont/al	pertaining to around a tooth
dia/thermy	process of generating heat through (some part of the body)
trans/vagin/al	pertaining to through or across the vagina
dipl/opia	double vision
diplo/bacteri/al	pertaining to a paired bacteria
dys/phonia	difficulty in speaking
endo/crine	secrete within (gland that secretes hormones directly into the bloodstream)
intra/muscul/ar	pertaining to within the muscle
homo/graft	transplantation of same (transplantation of tissue between the same species)
homeo/plasia	formation or growth of new tissue similar to tissue already existing in a part
hypo/derm/ic	pertaining to under the skin (under or inserted under the skin, as in a hypodermic injection)
macro/cyte	abnormally large erythrocyte, such as those found in pernicious anemia
micro/scope	instrument for examining small (minute) objects
mono/therapy	one treatment
uni/nucle/ar	pertaining to one nucleus
post/nat/al	pertaining to (the period) after birth
pre/nat/al	pertaining to (the period) before birth
pro/gnosis	before knowing (prediction of the course and end of a disease and the estimated chance of recovery)
primi/gravida	woman pregnant for the first time
retro/version	turning backward (tipping backward of an organ, such as the uterus, from its normal position)
super/ior	pertaining to upper or above (toward the head or upper portion of a structure)

Medical Vocabulary Recall

1. rhinoplasty	**5.** appendectomy	**9.** myopathy	**13.** neuroma
2. primigravida	**6.** hyperemesis	**10.** postnatal	**14.** chondromalacia
3. pelvimetry	**7.** mastopexy	**11.** dysphonia	**15.** hemophobia
4. hepatocele	**8.** gastritis	**12.** tracheotomy	

CHAPTER 2

Body Structure

Figure 2-2: Anatomical Position, Directional Terms, and Body Planes.

1. Median plane
2. Frontal plane
3. Horizontal plane

Figure 2-4: Regions and Quadrants. (A) Four Quadrants of the Abdomen.

1. Right upper quadrant
2. Right lower quadrant
3. Left upper quadrant
4. Left lower quadrant

Combining Forms

Medical Word	Meaning
Body Regions	
abdomin/al	*pertaining to the abdomen*
caud/ad	toward the tail; in a posterior direction
cephal/ad	toward the head
cervic/al	pertaining to the neck of the body or the neck of the uterus
crani/al	pertaining to the cranium or skull
gastr/ic	pertaining to the stomach
ili/ac	pertaining to the ilium
inguin/al	pertaining to the groin
lumb/ar	pertaining to the loins or lower back
pelv/i/meter pelv/ic	instrument for measuring the pelvis pertaining to the pelvis
spin/al	pertaining to the spine or spinal column
thorac/ic	pertaining to the chest
umbilic/al	pertaining to the umbilicus or navel

(Continued)

Medical Word	Meaning
Directional Terms	
anter/ior	pertaining to the front of the body, an organ, or a structure
dist/al	pertaining to a point farthest from the center, a medial line, or the trunk; opposite of proximal
dors/al	pertaining to the back or posterior (of the body)
infer/ior	pertaining to below or lower; toward the tail
later/al	pertaining to the side
medi/al	pertaining to the middle
poster/ior	pertaining to back or posterior side (of the body)
proxim/al	nearest the point of attachment, center of the body, or point of reference
super/ior	pertaining to above or higher; toward the head
ventr/al	pertaining to the belly side or front (of the body)
Other CFs Related to Body Structure	
cyt/o/meter	instrument for counting and measuring cells
hist/o/lysis	separation, destruction, or disintegration of tissue
nucle/ar	pertaining to a nucleus
radi/o/graphy	process of recording an x-ray

Suffixes and Prefixes

Medical Words	Meaning
Suffixes	
medi/**ad**	toward the middle or center
coron/**al**	pertaining to the heart
cost/**algia** thorac/o/**dynia**	pain in the ribs pain in the chest
path/o/**gen** carcin/o/**genesis**	forming, producing, or origin of a disease forming, producing, or origin of cancer
hist/o/**logist**	specialist in study of tissues
eti/o/**logy**	study of the causes (of disease)

Medical Words	Meaning
Suffixes	
cyt/o/**lysis**	destruction, dissolution, or separation of a cell
therm/o/**meter**	instrument for measuring heat
hyper/**plasia**	excessive growth of tissue
hepat/o/**toxic**	pertaining to poison in the liver
Prefixes	
bi/later/al	pertaining to or affecting two sides
epi/gastr/ic	pertaining to above or on the stomach
infra/cost/al	pertaining to below or under the ribs
trans/vagin/al	pertaining to or across the vagina

Medical Terminology Word Building

1. caudad
2. caudal
3. thoracocentesis
4. thoracic
5. thoracoplasty
6. gastric
7. gastroplasty
8. pelvic
9. pelvimeter
10. abdominal
11. abdominoplasty
12. cranial
13. cranioplasty
14. medial
15. mediad
16. cytology
17. cytologist
18. cytolysis
19. histology
20. histologist

Medical Vocabulary Recall

1. CT scan
2. fluoroscopy
3. US
4. MRI
5. PET
6. endoscope
7. inflammation
8. SPECT
9. tomography
10. radiopharmaceutical
11. endoscopy
12. nuclear scan
13. adhesion
14. radiography
15. sepsis

Pronunciation and Spelling

1. *bilateral*
2. adhesion
3. cervical
4. cranial
5. distal
6. endoscope
7. fluoroscopy
8. inflammation
9. lumbar
10. radiopharmaceutical
11. radiography
12. sepsis
13. sigmoidoscope
14. speculum
15. tomography

Demonstrate What You Know!

1. i	4. h	7. c	10. e	13. l
2. n	5. a	8. b	11. k	14. f
3. j	6. m	9. d	12. o	15. g

CHAPTER 3

Integumentary System

Combining Forms

Medical Word	Meaning
adip/o/cele **lip/o**/cyte **steat**/oma	*hernia containing fat or fatty tissue* cell containing fat or fatty tissue tumor composed of fat
sub/**cutane**/ous **dermat/o**/logist hypo/**derm**/ic	pertaining to beneath the skin specialist or physician who studies or treats skin disorders pertaining to under or inserted under the skin, as in a hypodermic injection
cyan/osis	abnormal condition of blue (skin)
erythem/a **erythemat**/ous **erythr/o**/cyte	redness of skin caused by capillary dilation pertaining to redness (of the skin) red blood cell
hidr/osis **sudor**/esis	abnormal condition of sweat condition of profuse sweating
ichthy/**osis**	abnormal condition of dry, scaly (skin)
kerat/osis	abnormal condition of a horny growth, or abnormal condition of the skin characterized by overgrowth and thickening of skin
melan/oma	black tumor (malignant tumor of melanocytes)
dermat/o/**myc**/osis	abnormal condition of a fungal infection of the skin
onych/o/malacia	abnormal softening of nails
pil/o/nid/al **trich/o**/pathy	pertaining to growth of hair in a cyst or other internal structure disease of the hair
scler/o/derma	hardening of the skin or chronic disease with abnormal hardening of the skin
seb/o/rrhea	discharge or flow of sebum (secreted by sebaceous glands)
squam/ous	pertaining to scales (scalelike)
therm/al	pertaining to heat, such as thermal burn caused by heat
xer/o/derma	dry skin or skin condition characterized by excessive roughness and dryness

Suffixes and Prefixes

Medical Words	Meaning
Suffixes	
leuk/o/**cyte**	white blood cell
py/o/**derma**	pyogenic infection of the skin
carcin/**oma**	cancerous tumor
dia/**phoresis**	carrying or transmitting across or condition of profuse sweating; also called *sudoresis* or *hyperhidrosis*
dermat/o/**plasty**	surgical repair of the skin
cry/o/**therapy**	treatment using cold as a destructive medium
Prefixes	
an/hidr/osis	abnormal condition of absence of sweat
epi/derm/oid	resembling or pertaining to the epidermis
homo/graft	transplantation of tissue from an individual of one species to an individual of the same species; also called *allograft*
hyper/hidr/osis	abnormal condition of excessive or profuse sweating; also called *diaphoresis* or *sudoresis*

Medical Terminology Word Building

1. adipoma, lipoma
2. adipocyte, lipocyte
3. ichthyosis
4. onychoma
5. onychopathy
6. onychomalacia
7. trichopathy
8. trichosis
9. xeroderma
10. xerosis
11. erythrocyte
12. leukocyte
13. melanocyte
14. anhidrosis
15. hyperhidrosis

Medical Vocabulary Recall

1. verruca
2. vitiligo
3. tinea
4. pressure ulcer
5. eczema
6. autograft
7. biopsy
8. dermabrasion
9. hirsutism
10. cryosurgery
11. débridement
12. scabies
13. alopecia
14. comedo
15. metastasize

Pronunciation and Spelling

1. *abrasion*
2. abscess
3. acne
4. alopecia
5. biopsy
6. cryotherapy
7. diaphoresis
8. epidermoid
9. erythematous
10. furuncle
11. keloid
12. hematoma
13. hirsutism
14. lesions
15. onychomalacia
16. petechia
17. scabies
18. psoriasis
19. seborrhea
20. vitiligo

Chart Note Analysis

1. macule
2. intermittent
3. syncope
4. vulgaris
5. colitis
6. chronic
7. sclerosed
8. enteritis
9. pruritus
10. Bartholin glands
11. psoriasis
12. erythematous
13. sinusitis
14. papule
15. diaphoresis

Demonstrate What You Know!

1. dermis
2. sudoriferous
3. onychopathy
4. mycosis
5. xenograft
6. epidermis
7. dermatologist
8. sebaceous
9. carcinoma
10. ichthyosis
11. onychomalacia
12. antibiotic
13. lipocyte
14. psoriasis
15. pyoderma

CHAPTER 4

Respiratory System

Combining Forms

Medical Word	Meaning
Upper Respiratory Tract	
adenoid/ectomy	*excision of the adenoids*
laryng/o/scope	instrument for examining the larynx
nas/al **rhin**/o/rrhea	pertaining to the nose discharge from the nose (runny nose), often the result of a cold or allergy
pharyng/o/spasm	twitching or involuntary contractions of the pharynx (throat)
tonsill/ectomy	excision of the tonsils
trache/o/tomy	incision of the trachea
Lower Respiratory Tract	
alveol/ar	pertaining to an alveolus (or alveoli)
bronch/o/scopy **bronchi**/ectasis	visual examination of the bronchus (or bronchi) through a bronchoscope expansion or dilation of a bronchus (or bronchi)
bronchiol/itis	inflammation of the bronchiole(s)
phren/algia	pain in the diaphragm
pleur/o/dynia	pain in the pleura
pneum/o/melan/osis **pneumon**/ia	abnormal condition of blackening of the lung tissue (caused by inhalation of coal dust or other black particles) abnormal condition of the lungs
pulmon/o/logist	physician or medical specialist who treats pulmonary diseases
thorac/o/pathy	disease of the thorax

Medical Word	Meaning
Other Related Combining Forms	
aer/o/phagia	swallowing air
cyan/osis	abnormal condition of blue (skin)
mastoid/itis	inflammation of one of the mastoid bones, usually an extension of a middle ear infection
muc/oid	resembling mucus
myc/osis	any disease induced by a fungus
orth/o/**pnea**	(labored) breathing that improves when standing or sitting up
py/o/thorax	pus in the chest

Suffixes and Prefixes

Medical Words	Meaning
Suffixes	
chondr/**oma**	tumor composed of cartilage
rhin/o/**plasty**	surgical repair of the nose
laryng/o/**plegia**	paralysis of the larynx (voice box)
Prefixes	
a/pnea	not breathing
brady/pnea	slow breathing
dys/pnea	bad, painful, or difficult breathing
eu/pnea	normal, unlabored breathing
tachy/pnea	rapid breathing

Medical Terminology Word Building

1. rhinoplasty
2. rhinorrhea
3. laryngoplegia
4. laryngitis
5. bronchiectasis
6. bronchoscopy
7. pleurodynia *or* pleuralgia
8. pleuritis
9. cyanosis
10. dyspnea
11. bradypnea
12. tachypnea
13. eupnea
14. pyothorax
15. aerophagia

Medical Vocabulary Recall

1. pleurisy
2. croup
3. hypoxemia
4. corticosteroids
5. CF
6. stridor
7. asthma
8. bronchodilators
9. pneumothorax
10. ABGs
11. epistaxis
12. anosmia
13. PFT
14. Mantoux
15. atelectasis

Pronunciation and Spelling

1. *acidosis*
2. aerophagia
3. anosmia
4. asphyxia
5. asthma
6. atelectasis
7. bradypnea
8. bronchiectasis
9. bronchodilators
10. bronchoscopy
11. emphysema
12. corticosteroids
13. coryza
14. crackle
15. dyspnea
16. hypoxemia
17. hypoxia
18. pertussis
19. pleurisy
20. rhonchi

Demonstrate What You Know!

1. tracheotomy
2. alveoli
3. laryngectomy
4. emphysema
5. laryngoscope
6. pharyngitis
7. bronchioles
8. apnea
9. rhonchi
10. O_2
11. pneumonia
12. phrenalgia
13. hypoxia
14. diaphragm
15. tachypnea

Chart Note Analysis

1. polypoid
2. meatus
3. biopsy
4. metastatic
5. polypectomy
6. snare
7. hemorrhage
8. anesthesia
9. cm
10. carcinoma

CHAPTER 5

Cardiovascular System

Combining Forms

Medical Word	Meaning
aneurysm/ectomy	*excision of an aneurysm (to repair a weak area in the aorta that is likely to rupture if left in place)*
aort/o/stenosis	narrowing or stricture of the aorta
arter/itis	inflammation of the arteries
arteri/o/scler/osis	hardening of an artery; disorder characterized by thickening, loss of elasticity, and calcification of arterial walls
ather/oma	tumor of fatty plaque; fatty degeneration or thickening of the larger arterial walls, as in atherosclerosis
atri/um	structure of the atrium (a cavity, such as the atrium of the heart)
cardi/o/megaly **coron**/ary	enlargement of the heart pertaining to the heart
phleb/itis **ven**/ous	inflammation of a vein pertaining to the veins or blood passing through them
thromb/o/lysis	destruction or breaking up of a thrombus (blood clot)

Medical Word	Meaning
varic/ose	pertaining to a dilated vein
vas/o/spasm	involuntary contraction or spasm of a blood vessel
vascul/ar	pertaining to or composed of blood vessels
intra/**ventricul**/ar	within a ventricle (of the heart)

Suffixes and Prefixes

Medical Word	Meaning
Suffixes	
tachy/**cardia**	rapid heart rate
electr/o/cardi/o/**gram**	record of electrical activity of the heart
electr/o/cardi/o/**graph**	instrument for recording electrical activity of the heart
angi/o/**graphy**	process of recording (radiography) the heart and blood vessels
aort/o/**stenosis**	narrowing of the aorta
Prefixes	
brady/cardi/ac	pertaining to a slow heart (rate)
endo/cardi/um	structure (serous membrane that lines the interior of the heart) within the heart
epi/cardi/um	structure (outermost layer of the heart) above the heart
peri/cardi/um	structure (fibrous sac) around the heart

Medical Terminology Word Building

1. atheroma
2. atherosclerosis
3. phlebitis
4. phlebothrombosis
5. venous
6. venospasm
7. cardiologist
8. electrocardiograph
9. cardiomegaly
10. angiopathy
11. angioma
12. aortostenosis
13. arteriostenosis
14. tachycardia
15. bradycardia

Medical Vocabulary Recall

1. varicose veins
2. fibrillation
3. thrombolytics
4. embolus
5. HF
6. DVT
7. HTN
8. arrhythmia
9. statin
10. bruit
11. stroke
12. rheumatic heart disease
13. Holter monitor
14. Raynaud disease
15. endarterectomy

Pronunciation and Spelling

1. *aneurysm*
2. arrhythmia
3. atherosclerosis
4. bruit
5. cardiomegaly
6. diastole
7. electrocardiography
8. fibrillation
9. infarction
10. hypertension
11. ischemia
12. myocardial
13. tachycardia
14. thrombus
15. varicose

Demonstrate What You Know!

1. cardiologist
2. arteriole
3. angioplasty
4. statin
5. tricuspid
6. oxygen
7. arteriosclerosis
8. cardiomegaly
9. phlebitis
10. nitrate
11. ischemia
12. arteriostenosis
13. aneurysm
14. tachycardia
15. MI

Chart Note Analysis

1. apnea
2. postoperative
3. anxiety
4. thyroiditis
5. syncope
6. desiccated
7. fibrillation
8. malaise
9. sinus tachycardia
10. EKG
11. dyspnea
12. mg

CHAPTER 6

Blood, Lymphatic, and Immune Systems

Combining Forms

Medical Word	Meaning
Blood System	
agglutin/ation	*process by which particles are caused to adhere and form into clumps*
embol/ectomy	excision of an embolus, may be done surgically or by use of enzymes that dissolve the clot
erythr/o/cyte	red blood cell
hem/o/phobia **hemat**/oma	fear of blood tumor composed of blood (usually clotted)
leuk/o/cyte	white blood cell
myel/o/gen/ic	pertaining to, producing, or originating in bone marrow
thromb/o/lysis	dissolution of a blood clot
ven/ous	pertaining to a vein

Medical Word	Meaning
Lymphatic and Immune Systems	
aden/o/pathy	disease of a gland
immun/o/gen	substance that produces immunity or an immune response
lymph/o/poiesis	formation of lymphocytes or lymphoid tissue
lymphaden/itis	inflammation of a lymph gland
lymphangi/oma	tumor of a lymph vessel
phag/o/cyte	cell that ingests (and destroys microorganisms and other cell debris)
splen/o/megaly	enlargement of the spleen
thym/oma	tumor of the thymus gland

Suffixes and Prefixes

Medical Words	Meaning
Suffixes	
leuk/**emia**	white blood; hematological malignancies of bone marrow cells
macr/o/**phage**	eating or swallowing large (pathogens); monocyte that transforms into a phagocyte capable of ingesting pathogens
ana/**phylaxis**	against protection; exaggerated, life-threatening hypersensitivity (allergic) reaction to a previously encountered antigen
hem/o/**poiesis**	formation or production of blood also called *hematopoiesis*
hem/o/**stasis**	standing still of blood
Prefixes	
macro/cyte	large (red) cell
micro/cyte	small (red) cell
mono/nucle/osis	abnormal increase of mononuclear (leukocytes in the blood)

Medical Terminology Word Building

1. hematoma
2. hematopoiesis
3. hematologist
4. thrombectomy
5. thromboid
6. thrombolysis
7. erythrocytes
8. leukocytes *or* leucocytes
9. phagocytes
10. lymphopoiesis
11. lymphocytes
12. lymphadenopathy
13. immunology
14. immunogen
15. agglutination
16. agglutinogen
17. splenomegaly
18. hepatosplenomegaly
19. myelogenic
20. anaphylaxis

Medical Vocabulary Recall

1. anemia
2. mononucleosis
3. thrombolytics
4. SLE
5. lymphadenitis
6. HIV
7. lymphangiography
8. tissue typing
9. Hodgkin disease
10. AIDS
11. leukemia
12. ELISA
13. lymphedema
14. hemophilia
15. anticoagulants

Pronunciation and Spelling

1. *adenopathy*
2. agglutination
3. anaphylaxis
4. anticoagulant
5. erythrocyte
6. hematoma
7. hemostasis
8. immunogen
9. leukemia
10. lymphangiography
11. macrocyte
12. mononucleosis
13. phagocyte
14. splenomegaly
15. vaccination

Chart Note Analysis

1. dyspnea
2. antiretroviral therapy
3. chills, night sweats
4. Tylenol
5. hemoglobin
6. persistent
7. *Pneumocystis*
8. WNL
9. CD4
10. sputum

Demonstrate What You Know!

1. hematology
2. hemopoiesis
3. oncology
4. lymphocytes
5. phagocytes
6. aplastic
7. immunosuppressants
8. HIV
9. pernicious
10. antigen
11. splenomegaly
12. lymphadenitis
13. immunodeficiency
14. pathogen
15. agglutination

CHAPTER 7

Digestive System

Combining Forms

Medical Word	Meaning
Oral Cavity	
dent/ist orth/**odont**/ist	*specialist in treatment of the teeth* dental specialist who prevents and corrects abnormally positioned or misaligned teeth
gingiv/itis	inflammation of gums
hypo/**gloss**/al sub/**lingu**/al	pertaining to under the tongue pertaining to under the tongue

Medical Word	Meaning
Oral Cavity	
or/al **stomat**/o/pathy	pertaining to the mouth disease of the mouth
ptyal/ism	condition of excessive salivation
sial/o/rrhea	excessive flow of saliva; also called *hypersalivation* or *ptyalism*
Esophagus, Pharynx, and Stomach	
esophag/o/scope	instrument for examining the esophagus
gastr/o/scopy	visual examination of the stomach
pharyng/o/tonsill/itis	inflammation of the pharynx (throat) and tonsils
pylor/o/tomy	incision of the pylorus (lower portion of the stomach)
Small Intestine	
duoden/o/scopy	visual examination of the duodenum (a type of endoscopic procedure)
enter/o/pathy	disease of the intestine (usually small); any intestinal disease
jejun/o/rrhaphy	suture of the jejunum
ile/o/stomy	surgical creation of an opening in the ileum (to drain urine or feces into an exterior pouch)
Large Intestine	
peri/**an**/al	pertaining to around the anus
append/ectomy	removal of the appendix
appendic/itis	inflammation of the appendix
col/o/stomy **colon/o**/scopy	creation of an opening between the colon and the abdominal wall visual examination of the colon using a long, flexible endoscope (a type of endoscopic procedure)
proct/o/logist	physician who specializes in treating disorders of the colon, rectum, and anus
rect/o/cele	herniation or protrusion of the rectum; also called *proctocele*
sigmoid/o/tomy	incision of sigmoid colon
Accessory Organs of Digestion	
cholangi/ole	small terminal portion of the bile duct
chol/e/lith	gallstone

(Continued)

Medical Word	Meaning
Accessory Organs of Digestion	
cholecyst/itis	inflammation of the gallbladder
choledoch/o/tomy	incision of the common bile duct
hepat/itis	inflammation of the liver
pancreat/o/lysis	destruction of the pancreas by pancreatic enzymes

Suffixes and Prefixes

Medical Words	Meaning
Suffixes	
gastr/**algia** gastr/o/**dynia**	pain in the stomach pain in the stomach
hyper/**emesis**	excessive vomiting
chol/e/lith/**iasis**	presence or formation of gallstones
hepat/o/**megaly**	enlargement of the liver
an/**orexia**	without appetite; loss of appetite
cirrh/**osis**	abnormal condition of yellowness
dys/**pepsia**	difficult or painful digestion; also called *indigestion*
dys/**phagia**	difficulty swallowing or eating
post/**prandial**	following a meal
dia/**rrhea**	frequent, watery bowel movements
Prefixes	
endo/scopy	visual examination within (an organ or cavity using an endoscope)
hemat/emesis	vomiting blood
hypo/gastr/ic	pertaining to below the stomach

Medical Terminology Word Building

1. esophagospasm
2. esophagostenosis
3. gastritis
4. gastrodynia *or* gastralgia
5. gastropathy
6. jejunectomy
7. ileitis
8. jejunoileal
9. enteritis
10. enteropathy
11. colorectal
12. coloptosis
13. proctostenosis *or* rectostenosis
14. proctocele *or* rectocele
15. proctoplegia *or* proctoparalysis
16. cholecystitis
17. cholelithiasis
18. hepatoma
19. hepatomegaly
20. pancreatitis

Medical Vocabulary Recall

1. stool guaiac
2. nasogastric intubation
3. polyp
4. ascites
5. Crohn disease
6. lithotripsy
7. fistula
8. jaundice
9. barium enema
10. IBD
11. hematochezia
12. volvulus
13. cirrhosis
14. barium swallow
15. IBS

Pronunciation and Spelling

1. *appendicitis*
2. ascites
3. bilirubin
4. borborygmus
5. cholangiopancre-atography
6. cholecystectomy
7. choledochoplasty
8. cholelithiasis
9. cirrhosis
10. colostomy
11. Crohn disease
12. duodenitis
13. enteropathy
14. esophagogastro-duodenoscopy
15. gastroesophageal
16. glossectomy
17. hepatitis
18. ileorectal
19. jaundice
20. sigmoidotomy

Chart Note Analysis

1. postprandial
2. anorectal
3. angulation
4. polyp
5. diverticulum
6. dysphagia
7. enteritis
8. ileostomy
9. hematemesis
10. carcinoma

Demonstrate What You Know!

1. sublingually
2. orthodontist
3. gastroesophagitis
4. bariatric
5. sigmoidoscopy
6. hemorrhoids
7. pylorotomy
8. constipation
9. hematemesis
10. bile ducts
11. nausea
12. stool
13. stones
14. stomach
15. GERD

CHAPTER 8

Urinary System

Combining Forms

Medical Word	Meaning
cyst/o/scopy vesic/o/cele	*visual examination of the bladder* hernial protrusion of the urinary bladder; also called *cystocele*
glomerul/o/pathy	disease of the glomerulus
meat/us	opening or tunnel through any part of the body, such as the external opening of the urethra

(Continued)

Medical Word	Meaning
hydr/o/**nephr**/osis **ren**/al	abnormal condition of water in the kidney(s) pertaining to the kidney
pyel/o/plasty	surgical repair of the renal pelvis
ur/emia	excessive levels of urea and other nitrogenous waste products in the blood; also called *azotemia*
urin/ary	pertaining to urine or the urinary tract
ureter/o/stenosis	narrowing or stricture of a ureter
urethr/o/cele	hernia or swelling of the urethra

Suffixes and Prefixes

Medical Words	Meaning
Suffixes	
azot/**emia**	nitrogenous compounds in the blood
lith/**iasis**	abnormal condition of a stone or calculus
dia/**lysis**	process of removing toxic wastes from blood when kidneys are unable to do so
nephr/o/**pathy**	disease of the kidney(s)
nephr/o/**pexy**	surgical fixation of a kidney
nephr/o/**ptosis**	downward displacement or dropping of a kidney
lith/o/**tripsy**	crushing of a stone
olig/**uria**	diminished or scanty capacity to form and pass urine
Prefixes	
an/uria	without urine
poly/uria	excessive urination
supra/ren/al	pertaining to the area above the kidney

Medical Terminology Word Building

1. nephrolith
2. nephropathy
3. nephrohydrosis *or* hydronephrosis
4. pyelectasis *or* pyelectasia
5. pyelopathy
6. ureterocele
7. ureteroplasty
8. cystitis
9. cystoscope
10. azoturia
11. azotemia
12. urethrostenosis
13. urethrotome
14. urography
15. uropathy

Medical Vocabulary Recall

1. UA
2. Wilms tumor
3. azoturia
4. dysuria
5. diuresis
6. retrograde pyelography
7. hydronephrosis
8. interstitial nephritis
9. BUN
10. enuresis
11. catheterization
12. VCUG
13. uremia
14. renal hypertension
15. dialysis

Pronunciation and Spelling

1. *azotemia*
2. catheterization
3. cystoscopy
4. cystourethroscope
5. glomerulonephritis
6. incontinence
7. lithotripsy
8. nephrolithotomy
9. nephroptosis
10. nephrosclerosis
11. oliguria
12. polyuria
13. proteinuria
14. pyeloplasty
15. pyonephrosis
16. retrograde pyelography
17. ureterectasis
18. ureterostenosis
19. urethrocele
20. urologist

Chart Note Analysis

1. cystitis
2. nocturia
3. hematuria
4. cystoscopy
5. epigastric
6. urgency
7. appendectomy
8. cholelithiasis
9. cholecystitis
10. choledocholithiasis
11. polyuria
12. incontinence
13. choledocholithotomy
14. cholecystectomy
15. gallbladder

Demonstrate What You Know!

1. edema
2. diuretic
3. urinary
4. pyelopathy
5. intravenous
6. hematuria
7. pyuria
8. anuria
9. urologist
10. continence
11. nephromegaly
12. hernia
13. pus
14. lithotomy
15. nephrologist

CHAPTER 9

Reproductive System

Combining Forms

Medical Word	Meaning
Female Reproductive System	
amni/o/centesis	*surgical puncture of the amniotic sac (to remove fluid for laboratory analysis)*
cervic/itis	inflammation of cervix uteri
colp/o/scopy	examination of the vagina and cervix with an optical magnifying instrument
vagin/o/cele	herniation into the vagina; also called *colpocele*
galact/o/rrhea	discharge or flow of milk
lact/o/gen	(substance that stimulates) formation or production of milk
gynec/o/logist	physician specializing in treating disorders of the female reproductive system
hyster/ectomy	excision of the uterus
uter/o/vagin/al	pertaining to the uterus and vagina
mamm/o/gram	radiography of the breast
mast/o/pexy	surgical fixation of the breast(s)
men/o/rrhagia	bursting forth of menses; heavy menstrual bleeding
endo/**metr**/itis	inflammation of the endometrium
pre/**nat**/al	pertaining to (the period) before birth
oophor/oma	ovarian tumor
ovari/o/tomy	incision of an ovary
perine/o/rrhaphy	suture of the perineum, which is performed to repair a laceration that occurs spontaneously or is made surgically during the delivery of the fetus
salping/ectomy	excision of a fallopian tube
vulv/o/pathy	disease of the vulva
episi/o/tomy	incision of the perineum, which is performed to enlarge the vaginal opening for delivery of a fetus

Medical Word	Meaning
Male Reproductive System	
andr/o/gen	substance producing or stimulating the development of male characteristics
balan/itis	inflammation of the glans penis
gonad/o/tropin	gonad-stimulating hormone that stimulates the function of the testes and ovaries
olig/o/sperm/ia	condition of scanty sperm cells
crypt/**orch**/ism	condition of a hidden testicle; failure of the testicles to descend into the scrotum
orchi/o/pexy	surgical fixation of one or both testes
orchid/ectomy	excision of one or both testes
test/algia	pain in one or both testes
prostat/itis	inflammation of the prostate gland
spermat/o/cide	agent that kills spermatozoa; also called *spermicide*
sperm/i/cide	agent that kills spermatozoa; also called *spermatocide*
a/**sperm**/ia	failure to form semen or ejaculate
varic/o/cele	dilated or enlarged vein of the spermatic cord
vas/ectomy	removal of all or part of the vas deferens
vesicul/itis	inflammation of the seminal vesicle

Suffixes and Prefixes

Medical Words	Meaning
Suffixes	
men/**arche**	initial menstrual period
pseudo/**cyesis**	false pregnancy; condition in which a woman believes she is pregnant when she is not
primi/**gravida**	woman during her first pregnancy
multi/**para**	woman who has delivered more than one viable infant
hemat/o/**salpinx**	blood in the fallopian tube
dys/**tocia**	painful, difficult childbirth
Prefix	
retro/version	tipping back of an organ

Medical Terminology Word Building

1. gynecopathy
2. gynecologist
3. cervicovaginitis
4. cervicectomy
5. colposcope
6. colposcopy
7. hysterrhexis
8. hysteropathy
9. metrorrhagia
10. metritis
11. salpingocele
12. salpingitis
13. salpingopexy
14. prostatomegaly
15. prostatodynia, prostatalgia
16. orchidopathy, orchiopathy
17. orchialgia, orchiodynia, orchidalgia
18. balanorrhea
19. balanitis
20. balanoplasty

Medical Vocabulary Recall

1. cryptorchidism
2. PSA
3. sterility
4. anorchism
5. candidiasis
6. chlamydia
7. circumcision
8. cerclage
9. lumpectomy
10. endometriosis
11. mammography
12. gonorrhea
13. syphilis
14. TSS
15. trichomoniasis
16. D&C
17. phimosis
18. impotence
19. preeclampsia
20. fistula

Pronunciation and Spelling

1. *cerclage*
2. cervicitis
3. chlamydia
4. circumcision
5. epispadias
6. gonadotropin
7. gynecologist
8. hysterosalpingo-oophorectomy
9. mammography
10. oophoroma
11. orchiopexy
12. Papanicolaou
13. perineorrhaphy
14. phimosis
15. prostatitis
16. pseudocyesis
17. spermicide
18. syphilis
19. trichomoniasis
20. varicocele

Chart Note Analysis

1. metastases (singular, *metastasis*)
2. postmenopausal
3. lesion
4. neoplastic
5. Premarin
6. mastectomy
7. menstrual
8. laparoscopy
9. gravida 4
10. para 4

Demonstrate What You Know!

1. ovaries
2. galactorrhea
3. hysterectomy
4. obstetrics
5. colpocystocele
6. infertility
7. fallopian tube
8. dystocia
9. fertilization
10. cryptorchidism
11. spermicide
12. urologists
13. prostatitis
14. aspermia
15. sperm

CHAPTER 10

Endocrine System

Combining Forms

Medical Word	Meaning
aden/oma	*tumor composed of glandular tissue*
adrenal/ectomy **adren**/al	excision or removal of one or both adrenal glands pertaining to the adrenal glands
hypo/**calc**/emia	deficiency of calcium in the blood

Medical Word	Meaning
gluc/o/genesis hyper/**glyc**/emia	forming or producing glucose (sugar) greater than normal amount of glucose in the blood
pancreat/itis	inflammation of the pancreas
parathyroid/ectomy	excision or removal of one or both parathyroid glands
hypo/**pituitar**/ism	condition of inadequate levels of pituitary hormone in the body
thym/oma	tumor of the thymus gland
thyr/o/megaly **thyroid**/ectomy	enlargement of the thyroid gland excision of the thyroid gland
toxic/o/logist	specialist in the study of poisons or toxins

Suffixes and Prefixes

Medical Words	Meaning
Suffixes	
endo/**crine**	to secrete internally or within
hirsut/**ism**	condition of excessive hair growth in unusual places, especially in women
thyr/o/**toxic**	pertaining to toxic activity of the thyroid gland
Prefixes	
hyper/thyroid/ism	excessive secretion of the thyroid gland
poly/dipsia	excessive thirst

Medical Terminology Word Building

1. hyperglycemia
2. hypoglycemia
3. glycogenesis
4. pancreatitis
5. pancreatolysis
6. pancreatopathy
7. thyroiditis
8. thyromegaly
9. parathyroidectomy
10. adrenalectomy

Medical Vocabulary Recall

1. total calcium
2. type 1 diabetes
3. cretinism
4. exophthalmos
5. insulinoma
6. myxedema
7. TFT
8. Cushing syndrome
9. panhypopituitarism
10. HRT
11. Addison disease
12. FBG
13. pheochromocytoma
14. pancreatitis
15. type 2 diabetes

Pronunciation and Spelling

1. *adenoma*
2. adrenalectomy
3. diabetes
4. exophthalmos
5. glucose
6. hypocalcemia
7. hyperglycemia
8. insulinoma
9. mellitus
10. myxedema
11. pancreatitis
12. peripheral
13. pituitarism
14. polydipsia
15. toxicologist

Demonstrate What You Know!

1. hypocalcemia
2. hypersecretion
3. insulin
4. aerobic
5. ulceration
6. hormones
7. RAIU
8. Graves
9. GTT
10. homeostasis
11. toxicologist
12. pancreas
13. hyperglycemia
14. FBG
15. thymoma

Chart Note Analysis

1. erythema
2. antibiotic
3. vascular
4. calcaneal
5. ulceration
6. peripheral diabetic neuropathy
7. malleolus
8. trophic
9. type 1 diabetes mellitus
10. anaerobic

CHAPTER 11

Nervous System

Combining Forms

Medical Word	Meaning
cerebr/o/spin/al	*pertaining to the brain and spine or spinal cord*
encephal/itis	inflammation of the brain
gli/oma	tumor composed of neuroglial tissue (supportive tissue of the nervous system)
mening/o/cele	herniation or saclike protrusion of the meninges through the skull or vertebral column
meningi/oma	tumor composed of meninges
myel/algia	pain of the spinal cord or its membranes
neur/o/lysis	destruction of a nerve

Suffixes and Prefixes

Medical Words	Meaning
Suffixes	
epi/**lepsy**	seizure disorder
a/**phasia**	absence of speech
Prefixes	
dys/phagia	difficulty speaking or impairment in the production of speech
hemi/paresis	paralysis of one half of the body (right half or left half)
para/plegia	paralysis of both legs and the lower part of the body
quadri/plegia	paralysis of all four extremities

Medical Terminology Word Building

1. neuroma
2. neurolysis
3. encephalitis
4. encephaloma
5. encephalocele
6. myelalgia, myelodynia
7. myelocele
8. cerebrospinal
9. aphasia
10. dysphasia

Medical Vocabulary Recall

1. Bell palsy
2. stroke
3. epilepsy
4. thalamotomy
5. LP
6. TIA
7. Parkinson disease
8. poliomyelitis
9. sciatica
10. spina bifida
11. hydrocephalus
12. neuroblastoma
13. Alzheimer disease
14. anticonvulsants
15. dementia
16. shingles
17. anesthetics
18. antiparkinsonian
19. craniotomy
20. paralysis

Pronunciation and Spelling

1. *Alzheimer*
2. cerebrovascular
3. craniotomy
4. epilepsy
5. lumbar
6. palsy
7. poliomyelitis
8. paralysis
9. paraplegia
10. neuroblastoma
11. quadriplegia
12. spina bifida occulta
13. sciatica
14. seizure
15. shingles

Chart Note Analysis

1. anorexia
2. deglutition
3. diplopia
4. jaundice
5. vertigo
6. paralysis
7. adenocarcinoma
8. cholecystoje-junostomy
9. biliary
10. metastasis
11. aphasia
12. pruritus

Demonstrate What You Know!

1. meningomyelocele
2. quadriplegia
3. meningitis
4. paresis
5. cognition
6. CNS
7. vertigo
8. PNS
9. myelalgia
10. homeostasis
11. flaccid
12. neurosurgeon
13. TIAs
14. aphasia
15. diplopia

CHAPTER 12

Musculoskeletal System

Combining Forms

Medical Word	Meaning
Muscles and Related Structures	
fasci/o/plasty	*surgical repair of fascia*
fibr/oma	tumor of fibrous tissue
leiomy/oma	tumor of smooth muscle
lumb/o/cost/al	pertaining to the lumbar region and the ribs
muscul/ar **my/o**/rrhexis	pertaining to muscles rupture of a muscle
ten/o/tomy **tend/o**/plasty **tendin**/itis	incision of a tendon surgical repair of a tendon inflammation of a tendon, usually resulting from strain; also called *tendonitis*
Bones of the Upper Extremities	
carp/o/ptosis	downward displacement of the wrist; also called *dropped wrist*
cervic/al	pertaining to the neck
sub/**cost**/al	beneath the ribs
crani/o/tomy	incision through the cranium, usually to gain access to the brain during neurosurgical procedures
humer/al	pertaining to the humerus
metacarp/ectomy	excision or resection of one or more metacarpal bones
phalang/itis	inflammation of one or more phalanges
spondyl/itis	inflammation of any of the vertebrae, usually characterized by stiffness and pain
vertebr/al	pertaining to a vertebra or the vertebral column
stern/o/cost/al	pertaining to the sternum and ribs
Bones of the Lower Extremities	
calcane/o/dynia	painful condition of the heel
femor/al	pertaining to the femur
fibul/ar	pertaining to the fibula

Medical Word	Meaning
Bones of the Lower Extremities	
patell/ectomy	excision of the patella
pelv/i/metry **pelv**/is	measurement of the pelvic dimensions or proportions refers to the hip bone
radi/o/graph	x-ray image
tibi/al	pertaining to the tibia (shin bone)
Other Related Structures	
ankyl/osis	immobility of a joint
arthr/o/desis	surgical fixation of a joint
cost/o/chondr/itis	inflammation of cartilage of the anterior chest wall (ribs)
lamin/ectomy	excision of the lamina (bony arches of one or more vertebrae)
myel/o/cele	herniation of the spinal cord
orth/o/ped/ics	branch of medicine concerned with prevention and correction of musculoskeletal system disorders
oste/o/porosis	porous bone

Suffixes and Prefixes

Medical Words	Meaning
Suffixes	
arthr/o/**clasia**	surgical breaking of adhesions to improve mobility of a joint
oste/o/**clast**	cell that breaks down bone
hemi/**plegia**	paralysis of one side of the body
my/o/**sarcoma**	malignant tumor of muscle tissue
Prefixes	
dia/physis	shaft or middle region of a long bone
peri/oste/um	layer that covers the surface of a bone

Medical Terminology Word Building

1. osteocytes
2. ostealgia, osteodynia
3. osteoarthropathy
4. osteogenesis
5. cervical
6. cervicobrachial
7. cervicofacial
8. myeloma
9. myelosarcoma
10. myelography
11. myelomalacia
12. suprasternal
13. sternoid
14. chondroblast
15. arthritis
16. osteoarthritis
17. pelvimeter
18. myospasm
19. myopathy
20. myorrhexis

Medical Vocabulary Recall

1. osteoporosis
2. tendinitis
3. sprain
4. strain
5. kyphosis
6. Ewing sarcoma
7. torticollis
8. gout
9. RA
10. Paget disease
11. sequestrum
12. arthroplasty
13. crepitation
14. myasthenia gravis
15. lordosis
16. muscular dystrophy
17. contracture
18. scoliosis
19. herniated disk
20. CTS

Pronunciation and Spelling

1. *abduction*
2. arthroclasia
3. dorsiflexion
4. phalangitis
5. fascioplasty
6. gout
7. crepitation
8. leiomyoma
9. myosarcoma
10. myasthenia gravis
11. orthopedics
12. osteoarthropathy
13. osteoclast
14. Paget disease
15. pelvimetry
16. rheumatoid arthritis
17. sequestrectomy
18. spondylomalacia
19. sternocostal
20. torticollis

Chart Note Analysis

1. sacroiliac
2. L3-L4
3. flexion
4. anteroposterior
5. bilateral
6. hypertrophic
7. lumbosacral
8. lateral
9. extension
10. intervertebral

Demonstrate What You Know!

1. talipes
2. arthrocentesis
3. subluxation
4. ankylosis
5. rheumatologist
6. carpoptosis
7. articulate
8. rickets
9. muscles
10. degenerative
11. gouty
12. laminectomy
13. greenstick
14. NSAIDs
15. calcaneodynia

CHAPTER 13

Special Senses: Eyes and Ears

Combining Forms

Medical Word	Meaning
Eye	
blephar/o/spasm	*involuntary contraction of the eyelid*
choroid/o/pathy	disease of the choroid (layer between the retina and the sclera)

Medical Word	Meaning
Eye	
conjunctiv/itis	inflammation of the conjunctiva; also called *pinkeye*
corne/itis	inflammation of the cornea; also called *keratitis*
aniso/**cor**/ia **core**/o/meter **pupill**/ary	inequality of pupil size instrument for measuring the pupil pertaining to the pupil
dacry/o/rrhea	excessive secretion of tears
lacrim/ation	secretion and discharge of tears
dipl/opia	two images of an object seen at the same time; also called *double vision*
irid/o/plegia	paralysis of the sphincter of the iris
kerat/o/plasty	surgical repair of the cornea; also called *corneal transplant*
intra/**ocul**/ar **ophthalm**/o/scope	pertaining to within the eyeball instrument for examining the eye
opt/ic	pertaining to the eye or vision
retin/o/pathy	disease of the retina
Ear	
acous/tic **audi**/o/meter **audit**/ory	pertaining to hearing instrument for measuring levels of hearing pertaining to sense of hearing
myring/o/tomy **tympan**/o/plasty	incision of the tympanic membrane surgical repair of the tympanic membrane
ot/o/rrhea	discharge from the ear
salping/o/pharyng/eal	pertaining to the eustachian tube and pharynx

Suffixes and Prefixes

Medical Words	Meaning
Suffixes	
an/**acusis** presby/**cusis**	without hearing; total deafness hearing loss associated with old age

(Continued)

Medical Words	Meaning
Suffixes	
ambly/**opia**	reduction or dimness of vision usually in one eye with no apparent pathological condition; also called *lazy eye*
heter/**opsia**	inequality of vision in the two eyes
blephar/o/**ptosis**	downward displacement or drooping of the upper eyelid
Prefixes	
exo/tropia	abnormal turning outward of one or both eyes; also called *divergent strabismus*
hyper/opia	excess (farsighted) vision

Medical Terminology Word Building

1. ophthalmoplegia, ophthalmoparalysis
2. ophthalmology
3. pupilloscopy
4. keratomalacia
5. keratometer
6. scleritis
7. scleromalacia
8. iridoplegia, iridoparalysis
9. iridocele
10. retinopathy
11. retinitis
12. blepharoplegia
13. blepharoptosis
14. blepharoplasty
15. otopyorrhea
16. audiometer
17. myringotome
18. myringoplasty
19. salpingitis
20. salpingopharyngeal

Medical Vocabulary Recall

1. tinnitus
2. otosclerosis
3. achromatopsia
4. Ménière disease
5. strabismus
6. anacusis
7. otitis media
8. conjunctivitis
9. photophobia
10. presbycusis
11. glaucoma
12. vertigo
13. retinal detachment
14. hordeolum
15. astigmatism
16. myringoplasty
17. tonometry
18. iridectomy
19. Rinne
20. cataract

Pronunciation and Spelling

1. *acoustic neuroma*
2. achromatopsia
3. astigmatism
4. auditory
5. blepharoptosis
6. dacryorrhea
7. exotropia
8. phacoemulsification
9. glaucoma
10. hordeolum
11. iridoplegia
12. conjunctivitis
13. Ménière
14. ophthalmoscope
15. presbycusis
16. salpingopharyngeal
17. strabismus
18. tympanoplasty
19. tinnitus
20. vertigo

Chart Note Analysis

1. chronic
2. mucoserous
3. tympanoplasty
4. otitis media
5. ENT
6. cholesteatoma
7. general anesthetic
8. diagnosis
9. adhesive
10. postoperatively

Demonstrate What You Know!

1. ophthalmoplegia
2. esotropia
3. blepharoplasty
4. mydriatics
5. heteropsia
6. exotropia
7. blepharoptosis
8. diagnosis
9. cholesteatoma
10. tympanitis
11. vertigo
12. presbycusis
13. otitis media
14. anacusis
15. myringotomy

Abbreviations and Symbols

ABBREVIATIONS

The following table lists common abbreviations used in health care and related fields along with their meanings.

Abbreviation	Meaning	Abbreviation	Meaning
A		AED	automatic external defibrillator
A&P	anatomy and physiology; auscultation and percussion	AF	atrial fibrillation
		AGN	acute glomerulonephritis
A, B, AB, O	blood types in ABO blood group	AI	artificial insemination
AAA	abdominal aortic aneurysm	AICD	automatic implantable cardioverter defibrillator
AB, Ab, ab	antibody; abortion	AIDS	acquired immune deficiency syndrome
ABG	arterial blood gas(es)		
a.c.*	before meals	AK	above the knee
ACL	anterior cruciate ligament	ALL	acute lymphocytic leukemia
ACTH	adrenocorticotropic hormone	ALS	amyotrophic lateral sclerosis (also called *Lou Gehrig disease*)
ad lib.	as desired		
AD*	right ear	ALT	alanine aminotransferase
ADH	antidiuretic hormone (vasopressin)	AM, a.m.	in the morning (before noon)
		AML	acute myelogenous leukemia
ADHD	attention-deficit hyperactivity disorder	ANS	autonomic nervous system
		AOM	acute otitis media
AE	above the elbow		

(Continued)

Abbreviation	Meaning	Abbreviation	Meaning
AP	anteroposterior	BPH	benign prostatic hyperplasia; benign prostatic hypertrophy
ARDS	acute respiratory distress syndrome	BS	blood sugar
ARF	acute renal failure	BSE	breast self-examination
ARMD, AMD	age-related macular degeneration	BSO	bilateral salpingo-oophorectomy
AS	aortic stenosis	BUN	blood urea nitrogen
AS*	left ear	Bx, bx	biopsy
ASD	atrial septal defect	**C**	
ASHD	arteriosclerotic heart disease	C1, C2 (and so on)	first cervical vertebra, second cervical vertebra (and so on)
AST	angiotensin sensitivity test	CA	cancer; chronological age; cardiac arrest
Ast	astigmatism		
AU*	both ears	Ca	calcium; cancer
AV	atrioventricular; arteriovenous	CABG	coronary artery bypass graft
B		CAD	coronary artery disease
Ba	barium	CAH	chronic active hepatitis; congenital adrenal hyperplasia
BBB	bundle-branch block		
BC	bone conduction	CAT	computed axial tomography
BCC	basal cell carcinoma	Cath	catheterization; catheter
BE	barium enema; below the elbow	CBC	complete blood count
BG	blood glucose	CC	cardiac catheterization; chief complaint
b.i.d.*	twice a day	cc*	cubic centimeters (same as milliliters; 1/1,000 of a liter)
BK	below the knee		
BKA	below-knee amputation	CCU	coronary care unit
BM	bowel movement	CDH	congenital dislocation of the hip
BMI	body mass index	CF	cystic fibrosis
BMR	basal metabolic rate	CHD	coronary heart disease
BNO	bladder neck obstruction	chemo	chemotherapy
BP, B/P	blood pressure	CHF	congestive heart failure

Abbreviation	Meaning	Abbreviation	Meaning
Chol	cholesterol	CVS	chorionic villus sampling
CK	creatine kinase (cardiac enzyme); conductive keratoplasty	CXR	chest x-ray; chest radiograph
		cysto	cystoscopy
CKD	chronic kidney disease	**D**	
CLL	chronic lymphocytic leukemia	dc, DC, D/C*	discharge; discontinue
cm	centimeter (1/100 of a meter)	D&C	dilation and curettage
CML	chronic myelogenous leukemia	Decub.	decubitus (lying down)
CNS	central nervous system	derm	dermatology
c/o	complains of, complaints	DES	diffuse esophageal spasm; drug-eluting stent
CO	cardiac output	DEXA, DXA	dual-energy x-ray absorptiometry
CO_2	carbon dioxide	DI	diabetes insipidus; diagnostic imaging
COPD	chronic obstructive pulmonary disease	diff	differential count (white blood cells)
CP	cerebral palsy	DJD	degenerative joint disease
CPAP	continuous positive airway pressure	DKA	diabetic ketoacidosis
CPD	cephalopelvic disproportion	DM	diabetes mellitus
CPK	creatine phosphokinase (enzyme released into the bloodstream after a heart attack)	DMARDs	disease-modifying antirheumatic drugs
CPR	cardiopulmonary resuscitation	DNA	deoxyribonucleic acid
CRF	chronic renal failure	D.O., DO	Doctor of Osteopathy
C&S	culture and sensitivity	DOE	dyspnea on exertion
CS, C-section	cesarean section	DPI	dry powder inhaler
CSF	cerebrospinal fluid	D.P.M.	Doctor of Podiatric Medicine
CT	computed tomography	DPT	diphtheria, pertussis, tetanus
CTS	carpal tunnel syndrome	DRE	digital rectal examination
CV	cardiovascular	DVT	deep vein thrombosis; deep venous thrombosis
CVA	cerebrovascular accident; costovertebral angle	Dx	diagnosis
CVD	cardiovascular disease		

(Continued)

Abbreviation	Meaning	Abbreviation	Meaning
E		FTND	full-term normal delivery
EBV	Epstein-Barr virus	FVC	forced vital capacity
ECCE	extracapsular cataract extraction	Fx	fracture
ECG, EKG	electrocardiogram; electrocardiography	**G**	
ECHO	echocardiogram; echocardiography; echoencephalogram; echoencephalography	G	gravida (pregnant)
		g, gm	gram
		GB	gallbladder
		GBS	gallbladder series (x-ray studies)
ED	erectile dysfunction; emergency department	GC	gonococcus (*Neisseria gonorrhoeae*)
EEG	electroencephalogram; electroencephalography	GER	gastroesophageal reflux
		GERD	gastroesophageal reflux disease
EENT	eyes, ears, nose, and throat	GH	growth hormone
EF	ejection fraction	GI	gastrointestinal
EGD	esophagogastroduodenoscopy	GTT	glucose tolerance test
ELT	endovenous laser ablation; endoluminal laser ablation	GU	genitourinary
		GVHD	graft-versus-host disease
EMG	electromyography	GVHR	graft-versus-host reaction
ENT	ears, nose, and throat	GYN	gynecology
EOM	extraocular movement	**H**	
ERCP	endoscopic retrograde cholangiopancreatography	H_2O	water
		HAV	hepatitis A virus
ESRD	end-stage renal disease	Hb, Hgb, hgb	hemoglobin
ESWL	extracorporeal shock-wave lithotripsy	HBV	hepatitis B virus
		HCG	human chorionic gonadotropin
F		HCl	hydrochloric acid
FBS	fasting blood sugar	HCT, Hct	hematocrit
FECG, FEKG	fetal electrocardiogram	HCV	hepatitis C virus
FH	family history	HD	hemodialysis; hip disarticulation; hearing distance
FS	frozen section		
FSH	follicle-stimulating hormone		

Abbreviation	Meaning	Abbreviation	Meaning
HDL	high-density lipoprotein	Ig	immunoglobulin
HDN	hemolytic disease of the newborn	IM	intramuscular; infectious mononucleosis
HDV	hepatitis D virus	IMP	impression (synonymous with diagnosis)
HEV	hepatitis E virus		
HF	heart failure	IOL	intraocular lens
HIV	human immunodeficiency virus	IOP	intraocular pressure
HMD	hyaline membrane disease	IPPB	intermittent positive-pressure breathing
HNP	herniated nucleus pulposus (herniated disk)	IRDS	infant respiratory distress syndrome
HPV	human papillomavirus		
HRT	hormone replacement therapy	IT	inhalation therapy; intensive therapy
hs*	half-strength		
h.s.*	at bedtime	IUD	intrauterine device
HSG	hysterosalpingography	IV	intravenous
HSV	herpes simplex virus	IVC	intravenous cholangiogram; intravenous cholangiography
HTN	hypertension	IVF	in vitro fertilization
Hx	history	IVF-ET	in vitro fertilization and embryo transfer
I, J		IVP	intravenous pyelogram; intravenous pyelography
IAS	interatrial septum		
IBD	inflammatory bowel disease	IVU	intravenous urography
IBS	irritable bowel syndrome	**K**	
ICD	implantable cardioverter-defibrillator	K	potassium (an electrolyte)
ICP	intracranial pressure	KD	knee disarticulation
ICU	intensive care unit	KUB	kidneys, ureters, bladder
I&D	incision and drainage; irrigation and débridement	**L**	
ID	intradermal	L	liter
IDDM	insulin-dependent diabetes mellitus	L1, L2 (and so on)	first lumbar vertebra, second lumbar vertebra (and so on)

(Continued)

Abbreviation	Meaning	Abbreviation	Meaning
LA	left atrium	MI	myocardial infarction
LASIK	laser-assisted in situ keratomileusis	ml, mL	milliliter (1/1,000 of a liter)
LAT, lat	lateral	mm	millimeter (1/1,000 of a meter)
LBBB	left bundle-branch block	mm Hg	millimeters of mercury
LD	lactate dehydrogenase; lactic acid dehydrogenase (cardiac enzyme)	MR	mitral regurgitation
		MRA	magnetic resonance angiogram; magnetic resonance angiography
LDL	low-density lipoprotein	MRI	magnetic resonance imaging
LES	lower esophageal sphincter	MSH	melanocyte-stimulating hormone
LFT	liver function test	MUGA	multiple-gated acquisition (scan)
LH	luteinizing hormone	MVP	mitral valve prolapse
LLQ	left lower quadrant	MVR	mitral valve replacement; massive vitreous retraction (blade); microvitreoretinal
LMP	last menstrual period		
LOC	loss of consciousness	Myop	myopia (nearsightedness)
LP	lumbar puncture	**N**	
LPR	laryngopharyngeal reflux	Na	sodium (an electrolyte)
LS	lumbosacral spine	NB	newborn
LSO	left salpingo-oophorectomy	NCV	nerve conduction velocity
lt	left	NG	nasogastric
LUQ	left upper quadrant	NIDDM	non–insulin-dependent diabetes mellitus
LV	left ventricle		
lymphos	lymphocytes	NIHL	noise-induced hearing loss
M		NK	natural killer cell
MDI	metered-dose inhaler	NMT	nebulized mist treatment
MEG	magnetoencephalography	NPO, n.p.o.*	nothing by mouth
MG	myasthenia gravis	NSAID	nonsteroidal anti-inflammatory drug
mg	milligram (1/1,000 of a gram)		
mg/dl, mg/dL	milligram per deciliter	NSR	normal sinus rhythm

Abbreviation	Meaning	Abbreviation	Meaning
O		PCNL	percutaneous nephrolithotomy
O₂	oxygen	Pco₂	partial pressure of carbon dioxide
OB	obstetrics	PCP	*Pneumocystis* pneumonia; primary care physician; phencyclidine (hallucinogen)
OCP	oral contraceptive pill		
OD	overdose	PE	physical examination; pulmonary embolism; pressure-equalizing (tube)
OD*	right eye		
O.D.	Doctor of Optometry		
OM	otitis media	PERRLA	pupils equal, round, and reactive to light and accommodation
OP	outpatient; operative procedure		
OR	operating room	PET	positron emission tomography
ORTH, ortho	orthopedics	PFT	pulmonary function test
OS*	left eye	PGH	pituitary growth hormone
os	opening; mouth	pH	symbol for degree of acidity or alkalinity
OSA	obstructive sleep apnea		
OU*	both eyes	PID	pelvic inflammatory disease
		PIH	pregnancy-induced hypertension
P		PKD	polycystic kidney disease
P	phosphorus; pulse	PMH	past medical history
PA	posteroanterior; pernicious anemia; pulmonary artery; physician assistant	PMI	point of maximum impulse
		PMN, PMNL	polymorphonuclear leukocyte
PAC	premature atrial contraction	PMP	previous menstrual period
PAD	peripheral artery disease	PMS	premenstrual syndrome
Pap	Papanicolaou (test)	PND	paroxysmal nocturnal dyspnea
para 1, 2, 3 (and so on)	unipara, bipara, tripara (and so on) (number of viable births)	PNS	peripheral nervous system
		p.o.*	by mouth
PBI	protein-bound iodine	Po₂	partial pressure of oxygen
pc, p.c.*	after meals	poly	polymorphonuclear leukocyte
PCL	posterior cruciate ligament	post	posterior

(Continued)

Abbreviation	Meaning	Abbreviation	Meaning
p.r.n.*	as required	RF	rheumatoid factor
PSA	prostate-specific antigen	RGB	Roux-en-Y gastric bypass
PT	prothrombin time; physical therapy	RIA	radioimmunoassay
		RK	radial keratotomy
pt	patient	RLQ	right lower quadrant
PTCA	percutaneous transluminal coronary angioplasty	R/O	rule out
		ROM	range of motion
PTH	parathyroid hormone (also called *parathormone*)	RP	retrograde pyelogram; retrograde pyelography
PTHC	percutaneous transhepatic cholangiography	RSO	right salpingo-oophorectomy
PTT	partial thromboplastin time	rt	right
PUD	peptic ulcer disease	RUQ	right upper quadrant
PVC	premature ventricular contraction	RV	residual volume; right ventricle
PVD	peripheral vascular disease	**S**	
Q		S1, S2 (and so on)	first sacral vertebra, second sacral vertebra (and so on)
q.2h.*	every 2 hours	SA, S-A	sinoatrial
qAM*	every morning	SaO$_2$	arterial oxygen saturation
q.d.*	every day	SCC	squamous cell carcinoma
q.h.*	every hour	SD	shoulder disarticulation
q.i.d.*	four times a day	SIADH	syndrome of inappropriate antidiuretic hormone
q.o.d.*	every other day		
qPM*	every evening	SICS	small incision cataract surgery
R		SIDS	sudden infant death syndrome
RA	right atrium; rheumatoid arthritis	SLE	systemic lupus erythematosus; slit-lamp examination
RAI	radioactive iodine		
RAIU	radioactive iodine uptake	SMAS	superficial musculoaponeurotic system (flap)
RBC, rbc	red blood cell	SNS	sympathetic nervous system
RD	respiratory distress	SOB	shortness of breath
RDS	respiratory distress syndrome		

Abbreviation	Meaning	Abbreviation	Meaning
sono	sonogram	TPR	temperature, pulse, and respiration
sp. gr.	specific gravity	TRAM	transverse rectus abdominis muscle
SPECT	single-photon emission computed tomography	TSE	testicular self-examination
ST	esotropia	TSH	thyroid-stimulating hormone
stat., STAT	immediately	TSS	toxic shock syndrome
STI	sexually transmitted infection	TURP	transurethral resection of the prostate
subcu*, Sub-Q*, subQ*	subcutaneous (injection)	TVH	total vaginal hysterectomy
Sx	symptom	TVH-BSO	total vaginal hysterectomy–bilateral salpingo-oophorectomy
T		Tx	treatment
T1, T2 (and so on)	first thoracic vertebra, second thoracic vertebra (and so on)	**U**	
T_3	triiodothyronine (thyroid hormone)	UA	urinalysis
		UC	uterine contractions
T_4	thyroxine (thyroid hormone)	UGI	upper gastrointestinal
T&A	tonsillectomy and adenoidectomy	UGIS	upper gastrointestinal series
TAH	total abdominal hysterectomy	U&L, U/L	upper and lower
TB	tuberculosis	ung	ointment
TFT	thyroid function test	UPP	uvulopalatopharyngoplasty
THA	total hip arthroplasty	URI	upper respiratory infection
ther	therapy	US	ultrasound; ultrasonography
THR	total hip replacement	UTI	urinary tract infection
TIA	transient ischemic attack	UV	ultraviolet
TIBC	total iron–binding capacity	**V**	
t.i.d.*	three times a day	VA	visual acuity
TKA	total knee arthroplasty	VC	vital capacity
TKR	total knee replacement	VCUG	voiding cystourethrography
TN	trigeminal neuralgia	VD	venereal disease

(Continued)

Abbreviation	Meaning	Abbreviation	Meaning
VF	visual field	WN	well-nourished
VSD	ventricular septal defect	WNL	within normal limits
VT	ventricular tachycardia	**X, Y, Z**	
VUR	vesicoureteral reflux	XP, XDP	xeroderma pigmentosum
W		XT	exotropia
WBC, wbc	white blood cell		
WD	well-developed		

*Although these abbreviations are currently found in medical records and clinical notes, they are easily misinterpreted. The Joint Commission (formerly JCAHO) requires their discontinuance. Instead, The Joint Commission recommends the full terms be written out. For a summary of these abbreviations, see the following table.

Summary of Discontinued Abbreviations

As noted above, The Joint Commission has recommended the discontinuance of certain abbreviations that are easily misinterpreted in medical records. The following table lists these abbreviations along with their meanings.

Abbreviation	Meaning
Medication and Therapy Time Schedule	
a.c.	before meals
b.i.d.	twice a day
hs	half-strength
h.s.	at bedtime
NPO, n.p.o.	nothing by mouth
p.c.	after meals
p.o.	by mouth (orally)
p.r.n.	as required
qAM	every morning
q.d.	every day
q.h.	every hour
q.2h.	every 2 hours
q.i.d.	four times a day
q.o.d.	every other day
qPM	every evening
t.i.d.	three times a day
Other Related Abbreviations	
AD	right ear
AS	left ear
AU	both ears
cc	cubic centimeters; same as mL (1/1,000 of a liter) *Use mL for milliliters or write out the meaning.*
dc, DC, D/C	discharge; discontinue
OD	right eye

(Continued)

Abbreviation	Meaning
Other Related Abbreviations	
OS	left eye
OU	both eyes
subcu, Sub-Q, subQ	subcutaneous (injection)
U	unit

Common Symbols

The following table lists some common symbols used in health care and related fields.

Symbol	Meaning	Symbol	Meaning
@	at	×	multiplied by; magnification
+	plus, positive	pH	degree of acidity or alkalinity
$\bar{a}\,\bar{a}$	of each	=	equals
−	minus, negative	℞	prescription, treatment, therapy
′	foot	≈	approximately equal
±	plus or minus; either positive or negative; indefinite	$\bar{s}$	without
″	inch	°	degree
Ø	no	→	to, in the direction of
$\bar{c}$	with	%	percent
#	number; following a number; pounds	↑	increase(d), up
Δ	change; heat	♀	female
÷, /	divided by	↓	decrease(d), down
$\bar{p}$	after	♂	male

Drug Classifications

The table that follows provides a quick reference of common drug categories. Prescription and over-the-counter drugs that are used to treat symptoms, signs, and diseases of the various body systems are included.

Drug Classification	Description
anesthetics ăn-ĕs-THĔT-ĭks	Produce partial or complete loss of sensation with or without loss of consciousness
general	Produce complete loss of feeling with loss of consciousness
local	Produce loss of feeling and affect a local area only
antacids ănt ĂS ĭds	Neutralize acids in the stomach
antibiotics ăn-tĭ-bī-ŎT-ĭks	Treat bacterial infections of the urinary tract by acting on the bacterial membrane or one of its metabolic processes
anticoagulants ăn-tĭ-kō-ĂG-ū-lănts	Prevent the clotting or coagulation of blood
anticonvulsants ăn-tĭ-kŏn-VŬL-sănts	Prevent or control seizures
antidiarrheals ăn-tĭ-dī-ă-RĒ-ălz	Control loose stools and relieve diarrhea by absorbing excess water in the bowel or slowing peristalsis in the intestinal tract
antiemetics ăn-tĭ-ē-MĔT-ĭks	Control nausea and vomiting by blocking nerve impulses to the vomiting center of the brain
antifungals ăn-tĭ-FŬN-gălz	Treat vaginal fungal infections, such as candidiasis
antiglaucoma agents ăn-tĭ-glaw-KŌ-mă	Reduce intraocular pressure by lowering the amount of aqueous humor in the eyeball—either decreasing production or increasing outflow

(Continued)

Drug Classification	Description
antiparkinsonian agents ăn-tĭ-păr-kĭn-SŌN-ē-ăn	Reduce signs and symptoms associated with Parkinson disease
antipruritics ăn-tĭ-proo-RĬT-ĭks	Reduce severe itching
antipsychotics ăn-tĭ-sī-KŎT-ĭks	Alter neurotransmitters in the brain to alleviate symptoms of delusions and hallucinations
antispasmodics ăn-tē-spăz-MŎD-ĭks	Decrease spasms in the urethra and bladder (caused by urinary tract infections and catheterization) by relaxing the smooth muscles lining their walls, allowing normal emptying of the bladder
beta blockers BĀ-tă	Slow the heart rate and reduce the force with which the heart muscle contracts, thereby lowering blood pressure
bone reabsorption inhibitors	Reduce the reabsorption of bones in treatment of weak and fragile bones as seen in osteoporosis and Paget disease
bronchodilators brŏng-kō-DĪ-lā-tŏrs	Dilate constricted airways by relaxing muscle spasms in the bronchial tubes through oral administration or inhalation via a metered-dose inhaler (MDI)
corticosteroids kor-tĭ-kō-STĒR-oydz	Suppress the inflammatory reaction that causes swelling and narrowing of the bronchi
diuretics dī-ū-RĔT-ĭks	Block reabsorption of sodium by the kidneys, increasing the amount of salt and water excreted in the urine (causes reduction of fluid retained in the body and prevents edema)
estrogens ĔS-trō-jĕnz	Treat symptoms of menopause (hot flashes, vaginal dryness) through hormone replacement therapy (HRT)
expectorants ĕk-SPĔK-tō-rănts	Improve the ability to cough up mucus from the respiratory tract
gold salts	Treat rheumatoid arthritis by inhibiting activity within the immune system, preventing further disease progression
gonadotropins gŏn-ă-dō-TRŌ-pĭns	Hormonal preparation used to increase sperm count in infertility cases
hormone replacement therapy (HRT)	Synthetic hormone used to correct a deficiency of estrogen, progesterone, testosterone, or testosterone hormone; relieve symptoms of menopause; and prevent osteoporosis in women
immunizations ĭm-ū-nĭ-ZĀ-shŭns	Vaccination or injection of immune globulins to induce immunity to a particular infectious disease
immunosuppressants ĭm-ū-nō-sū-PRĔS-ănts	Suppress the immune response to prevent organ rejection after transplantation or slow the progression of autoimmune disease

Drug Classification	Description
insulins ĬN-sŭ-lĭns	Replace insulin in patients with type 1 diabetes or severe type 2 diabetes
laxatives LĂK-să-tĭvz	Relieve constipation and facilitate passage of feces through the lower gastrointestinal tract
metered-dose inhaler (MDI)	Device that enables the patient to self-administer a specific amount of medication into the lungs through inhalation
miotics mī-ŎT-ĭks	Cause the pupil to constrict
muscle relaxants	Relieve muscle spasms, pain, and stiffness
mydriatics mĭd-rē-ĂT-ĭks	Cause the pupil to dilate and prepare the eye for an internal examination
nebulized mist treatment (NMT) NĔB-ū-līzd	Method of administering medication directly into the lungs using a device (nebulizer) that produces a fine spray; also called *aerosol therapy*
nitrates NĪ-trāts	Relieve chest pain associated with angina and ease symptoms of heart failure
nonsteroidal anti-inflammatory drugs (NSAIDs) nŏn-STĒR-oyd-ăl ăn-tē-ĭn-FLĂM-ă-tō-rē	Relieve mild to moderate pain and reduce inflammation in treatment of musculoskeletal conditions, such as sprains and strains, and inflammatory disorders, including rheumatoid arthritis, osteoarthritis, bursitis, gout, and tendinitis
oral contraceptives (OCPs) kŏn-tră-SĔP-tĭvz	Prevent ovulation in order to avoid pregnancy; also known as *birth control pills*
spermicides SPĔR-mĭ-sīdz	Destroy sperm by creating a highly acidic environment in the uterus; used as a method of birth control
statins STĂ-tĭnz	Reduce cholesterol levels in the blood and block production of an enzyme in the liver that produces cholesterol
thrombolytics thrŏm-bō-LĬT-ĭks	Dissolve blood clots in a process known as *thrombolysis*
vaccinations văk-sĭ-NĀ-shŭnz	Introduction of altered antigens (viruses or bacteria) into the body to produce an immune response and protect against disease
vertigo and motion sickness drugs VĔR-tĭ-gō	Decrease sensitivity of the inner ear to motion and prevent nerve impulses from the inner ear from reaching the vomiting center of the brain
wax emulsifiers ē-MŬL-sĭ-fī-ĕrs	Loosen and help remove impacted cerumen (ear wax)

Medical Specialties

Medical Specialty	Medical Specialist	Description of Medical Specialty
Allergy	Allergist	Diagnosis and treatment of allergic disorders caused by hypersensitivity to foods, pollens, dusts, and medicines
Anesthesiology	Anesthesiologist	Administration of agents capable of bringing about loss of sensation with or without loss of consciousness
Cardiology	Cardiologist	Diagnosis and treatment of heart and vascular disorders
General practice (GP)	General practitioner (GP)	Coordination of total health care delivery to all members of the family, regardless of sex, including counseling; also known as *family medicine* *The GP encompasses several branches of medicine, including internal medicine, preventive medicine, pediatrics, surgery, obstetrics, and gynecology.*
Geriatrics	Geriatrician	Understanding of the physiological characteristics of aging and the diagnosis and treatment of diseases affecting elderly patients; also known as *gerontology*
Gynecology	Gynecologist	Diagnosis and treatment of diseases of the female reproductive organs
Hematology	Hematologist	Diagnosis and treatment of diseases of the blood and blood-forming tissues
Immunology	Immunologist	Study of various elements of the immune system and their functions *Immunology includes treatment of immunodeficiency diseases such as acquired immune deficiency syndrome (AIDS) and autoimmune diseases such as systemic lupus erythematosus (SLE), allergies, and various cancer types related to the immune system.*

(Continued)

Medical Specialty	Medical Specialist	Description of Medical Specialty
Internal medicine	Internist	Study of the physiological and pathological characteristics of internal organs and the diagnosis and treatment of these organs
Neonatology	Neonatologist	Care and treatment of neonates
Nephrology	Nephrologist	Diagnosis and management of kidney disease, kidney transplantation, and dialysis therapies
Neurosurgery	Neurosurgeon	Surgery of the brain, spinal cord, and peripheral nerves
Obstetrics	Obstetrician	Care of women during pregnancy, childbirth, and postnatal care
Oncology	Oncologist	Diagnosis, treatment, and prevention of cancer *Oncologists are internal medicine physicians who specialize in the treatment of solid tumors (e.g., carcinomas and sarcomas) and liquid tumors (including hematological malignancies such as leukemias).*
Ophthalmology	Ophthalmologist	Diagnosis and treatment of eye diseases, including prescribing corrective lenses
Optometry	Optometrist	Primary eye care, including testing the eyes for visual acuity, diagnosing and managing eye health, prescribing corrective lenses, and recommending eye exercises *An optometrist, licensed by the state, is not a medical doctor but is known as a Doctor of Optometry (OD).*
Orthopedics	Orthopedist	Prevention, diagnosis, care, and treatment of musculoskeletal disorders *Musculoskeletal disorders include injury to or disease of bones, joints, ligaments, muscles, and tendons.*
Otolaryngology	Otolaryngologist	Medical and surgical management of disorders of the ear, nose, and throat (ENT) and related structures of the head and neck
Pathology	Pathologist	Study and cause of disease *A pathologist usually specializes in autopsy or in clinical or surgical pathology.*
Pediatrics	Pediatrician	Diagnosis and treatment of disease in infants, children, and adolescents

Medical Specialty	Medical Specialist	Description of Medical Specialty
Physiatry	Physiatrist	Prevention, diagnosis, and treatment of disease or injury and the rehabilitation from resultant impairment and disability; also called *physical medicine* *Physiatrists are physicians who use physical agents such as light, heat, cold water, therapeutic exercise, mechanical apparatus, and, sometimes, pharmaceutical agents.*
Plastic surgery	Plastic surgeon	Surgery to alter, replace, and restore a body structure because of a defect or for cosmetic reasons
Pulmonology	Pulmonologist	Diagnosis and treatment of diseases involving the lungs, its airways and blood vessels, and the chest wall (thoracic cage); also called *pulmonary medicine*
Psychiatry	Psychiatrist	Diagnosis, treatment, and prevention of disorders of the mind
Radiology	Radiologist	Diagnosis using x-ray and other diagnostic procedures, such as ultrasound (US), computed tomography (CT), and magnetic resonance imaging (MRI) *Radiology also employs various radiation techniques to treat disease through other subspecialties of radiology, such as interventional radiology and nuclear medicine.*
Rheumatology	Rheumatologist	Diagnosis and treatment of inflammatory and degenerative diseases of the joints
Surgery	Surgeon	Use of operative procedures to treat deformity, injury, and disease
Thoracic surgery	Thoracic surgeon	Use of operative procedures to treat disease or injury of the thoracic area
Urology	Urologist	Diagnosis and treatment of the male urinary and reproductive systems and the female urinary system

Index of Diagnostic, Medical, and Surgical Procedures

This index lists the diagnostic, medical, and surgical procedures covered in the textbook along with page numbers. Diagnostic procedures help the physician determine a patient's health status, evaluate the factors influencing that status, and determine a method of treatment. Medical and surgical procedures are performed to treat a specific disorder that is diagnosed by the physician.

DIAGNOSTIC PROCEDURES

MEDICAL AND SURGICAL PROCEDURES

Index of Oncological Terms

Following is a list of oncological disorders, diagnostic and surgical procedures and illustrations, and common abbreviations related to the medical specialty of oncology. For easy reference, page numbers for all oncological terms are included in the list.

Index

RULES FOR SINGULAR AND PLURAL SUFFIXES

This table presents common singular suffixes, the rules for forming plurals, and examples of each.

Rule		Example	
Singular	Plural	Singular	Plural
-a	Retain *a* and add *e*.	pleur*a*	pleur*ae*
-ax	Drop *x* and add *ces*.	thor*ax*	thor*aces*
-en	Drop *en* and add *ina*.	lum*en*	lum*ina*
-is	Drop *is* and add *es*.	diagnos*is*	diagnos*es*
-ix	Drop *ix* and add *ices*.	append*ix*	append*ices*
-ex	Drop *ex* and add *ices*.	ap*ex*	ap*ices*
-ma	Retain *ma* and add *ta*.	carcino*ma*	carcinoma*ta*
-on	Drop *on* and add *a*.	gangli*on*	gangli*a*
-um	Drop *um* and add *a*.	bacteri*um*	bacteri*a*
-us	Drop *us* and add *i*.	bronch*us*	bronch*i*
-y	Drop *y* and add *ies*.	deformit*y*	deformit*ies*